"This is the book for which Christian schools of Nursing have been waiting. This third edition of *Called to Care* has been updated to address changes in nursing and provides a sound theology of Christian worldview. The updated format—including examples, questions, objectives, and case studies—provides structure for ease in classroom applications. Because the writing is clear and the content is accessible, this book also has general interest to Christian nurses beyond a classroom setting. I found it a pleasure to read. I plan to give it to my faculty members and to use it in our senior nursing synthesis courses for both our prelicensure and RN students."

Amy Rex Smith, professor and dean of the School of Nursing, Belhaven University

"The authors of the third edition of *Called to Care* clearly describe the theological foundation of nursing from a Christian worldview. As in previous editions, the text fills a critical need for nurses seeking to develop and explain their nursing philosophy and integrate their Christian faith in nursing practice. The biblical foundation of nursing is threaded throughout the text, assisting readers in reflecting on God as the source of their worldview and calling to nursing, supporting their motivation to be nurses. The authors encourage nurses to carefully consider biblical and theological truth when evaluating nursing theories they incorporate into their practice. Implications for caring for the whole person regardless of culture are emphasized in the text. The authors define culture, describe the person as a cultural being, and support the Christian nurse's role in providing Christ-centered care for diverse populations from a biblical perspective, emphasizing that people from all cultures should be respected and treated with kindness. The case studies and discussion questions following each chapter are good teaching tools, making this an excellent textbook for schools of nursing to include as a resource for their curriculum."

Shirlene Newbanks, associate faculty, School of Nursing at Indiana Wesleyan University

"The third edition of *Called to Care* once again allows students and nurses to consider nursing and the concepts of the nursing metaparadigm (nursing, person, health, environment) from a Christian, biblical perspective. Shelly, Miller, and Fenstermacher contend that 'there is a relationship between what a person believes about God and how nursing care is delivered.' I couldn't agree more. Their assertion that spirituality, from the Christian worldview, 'is essentially relationship—a relationship of the whole person to a personal God and to other people (or spirits),' brings clarity to a complex concept. This third edition, like the first two, is an easy-to-read introductory text for anyone wanting to appreciate what is Christian nursing. I was again inspired that my calling as a nurse is from God."

Kathy Schoonover-Shoffner, PhD, RN, national director of Nurses Christian Fellowship USA and editor in chief of the *Journal of Christian Nursing*

"In this long-awaited third edition, authors Shelly, Miller, and Fenstermacher revive the beloved classic that presents a Christian worldview for nursing. This book has been a staple of faith-based nursing programs for decades. Readers will find chapters and content consistent with prior editions along with some new applications and stories. The vision set forth by this text remains true to the timeless Christian message that as nurses we embrace a worthy calling to bring compassion, comfort, and shalom to the persons we serve."

Kristen L. Mauk, professor of nursing and graduate program director at Colorado Christian University, coauthor of *Nursing as Ministry*

"This new edition of *Called to Care* carefully examines nursing's historical roots, theoretical tenets, and contemporary context through a Scripture-based lens while engaging readers with vignettes, case studies, and discussion points. This thoughtful and timely invitation for reflection on nursing as Christian caring is very relevant for Christian nurses, nursing students, and nurse educators."

Sue Kim, professor at the College of Nursing, Yonsei University, Seoul, Korea, and board member of Korea Nurses Christian Fellowship

Praise for the Second Edition

"In the increasingly complex and challenging world of health care, a nurse's faith can be a necessary point of reference to avoid being just swept along in the tide of change. This book can assist quicker development of a sufficiently mature and thought-through Christian faith to enable a nurse to cope explicitly with the challenges of life, suffering, death, and an unending succession of new ethical issues, and to support others in doing so. The original biblically well-referenced discussion of nursing and concepts relevant to it, illustrated by nursing stories, gives a coherent Christian perspective on nursing. . . . This book is a welcome resource."

Pat Ashworth, former senior lecturer in nursing, University of Ulster, Northern Ireland

"While the core Christian message has not changed since the first edition, the world within and beyond health care certainly has—and with it, the concrete implications of a Christian worldview. Even those familiar with the original edition will want to read the latest work of these champions of caring with heart and mind."

John F. Kilner, professor emeritus of bioethics and contemporary culture, Trinity International University

"Courageous nurses will find this new edition an essential companion that lights the way in practice and academic settings influenced by modern and postmodern worldviews."

Diane Elliott-Lee, RN, MSN, coauthor of *Courage: The Backbone of Leadership*

"To my mind, the first edition of *Called to Care* has become a classic for Christian nurses. . . . The book offers a valid challenge to those who propose to interpret notions like 'good nursing care' from the perspective of different worldviews. Shelly and Miller show a broad and deep knowledge of the literature and make a well-argued case for the strengths and weaknesses in many trends in nursing theory and practice. For those who want to interact with what the Christian tradition of nursing looks like today, *Called to Care* is as good a starting point as any."

Bart Cusveller, Viaa Christian University of Applied Sciences, Zwolle, Netherlands

JUDITH ALLEN SHELLY, ARLENE B. MILLER,
and KIMBERLY H. FENSTERMACHER

CALLED
TO CARE

THIRD EDITION

•••

A CHRISTIAN VISION
FOR NURSING

ivp
Academic
An imprint of InterVarsity Press
Downers Grove, Illinois

InterVarsity Press
P.O. Box 1400, Downers Grove, IL 60515-1426
ivpress.com
email@ivpress.com

InterVarsity Press® is the book-publishing division of InterVarsity Christian Fellowship/USA®, a movement of
students and faculty active on campus at hundreds of universities, colleges, and schools of nursing in the United States
of America, and a member movement of the International Fellowship of Evangelical Students. For information about
local and regional activities, visit intervarsity.org.

Scripture quotations, unless otherwise noted, are from the New Revised Standard Version Bible,
copyright © 1989 National Council of the Churches of Christ in the United States of America. Used by permission.
All rights reserved worldwide.

While any stories in this book are true, some names and identifying information may have been changed to protect
the privacy of individuals.

The publisher cannot verify the accuracy or functionality of website URLs used in this book beyond the date
of publication.

Cover design and image composite: David Fassett
Interior design: Daniel van Loon
Images: Florence Nightingale window: © SuperStock / Alamy Stock Photo
        gold background: © Katsumi Murouchi / Moment Collection / Getty Images
        blue background: © R. Tsubin / Moment Collection / Getty Images

ISBN 978-1-5140-0092-2 (print)
ISBN 978-1-5140-0093-9 (digital)

Printed in the United States of America ♾

InterVarsity Press is committed to ecological stewardship and to the conservation of natural resources in all our
operations. This book was printed using sustainably sourced paper.

Library of Congress Cataloging-in-Publication Data
A catalog record for this book is available from the Library of Congress.

P	27	26	25	24	23	22	21	20	19	18	17	16	15	14	13	12	11	10	9	8	7	6	5	4	3	2	1
Y	44	43	42	41	40	39	38	37	36	35	34	33	32	31	30	29	28	27	26	25	24	23	22	21			

WE DEDICATE THIS BOOK
to all the faithful nurses who put their lives on the
line by caring for patients with Covid-19
during the pandemic.

"This is my commandment, that you love one another as
I have loved you. No one has greater love than this,
to lay down one's life for one's friends."

JOHN 15:12-13

CONTENTS

PREFACE TO THE
THIRD EDITION

CALLED TO CARE CELEBRATED ITS TWENTIETH BIRTHDAY IN 2019. A third edition is long overdue. While the basic concepts in the previous editions still stand strong, nursing has changed radically in the last twenty years. The third edition addresses those changes—both in concepts and in practice. The text is revised and rewritten to reflect current nursing education and practice.

We welcome Kimberly Fenstermacher, PhD, CRNP, chief nursing administrator, assistant dean of nursing, and associate professor of nursing at Messiah University, to our writing team. Kim is on the cutting edge of those changes and maintains a strong voice for Christian nursing in the midst of this new nursing environment.

PREFACE

THIS BOOK BEGAN AS A CONVERSATION. It was the summer of 1984 at the Nurses Christian Fellowship conference in Burton, Ohio. We (Arlene and Judy) began to talk about our hopes and dreams for nursing—and our concerns. We concluded the conversation by agreeing that, if trends continued as they were, nursing as we knew it would cease to exist in ten years. Then we prayed for the profession we both loved.

We sensed a deep kindred spirit. Colleagues had quickly dismissed most of the concerns we shared when we expressed them in other settings. What a relief to find another person who shared the vision! The conversation grew into a friendship, and we kept talking. We observed and discussed nursing trends. We watched paradigms shift—both economic and philosophical. We studied changing values in nursing. To a great extent, nursing as we knew it did cease to exist.

In 1993 we coauthored *Values in Conflict: Christian Nursing in a Changing Profession*, but even before that manuscript was off the press, we sensed it was only the beginning. We immediately began thinking about another book on the theological foundations of nursing.

We believe that, as nurses, we cannot separate our professional roles from our profession of faith—regardless of what our culture tells us about keeping religion private. Furthermore, we are convinced that Christian faith is the very heart of nursing theory and practice. This book is addressed primarily to nurses who call themselves Christians and are trying to think through the implications of that commitment in their professional lives. We hope that others will also find it helpful.

The book is organized around the nursing metaparadigm.[1] We begin with a brief overview in chapters one through three; then we carefully examine and

---

[1]"A metaparadigm is the most general statement of a discipline and functions as a framework in which the more restricted structures of conceptual models develop." *Miller-Keane Encyclopedia and Dictionary of Medicine, Nursing, and Allied Health*, 7th ed., s.v. "metaparadigm." Retrieved September 23, 2020, from https://medical-dictionary.thefreedictionary.com/metaparadigm.

expand each concept in the metaparadigm—the person (chaps. 4–6), the environment (chaps. 7–9), health (chaps. 10–12), and nursing practice (chaps. 13–15)—identifying the implications of the Christian worldview as it relates to each area. We will also continually revisit the effects of modernism and postmodernism as they impinge on each concept. Since their influence is complex and pervasive, it may seem as if we are beating the same drum over and over. Our intent, however, is to demonstrate the subtle ways in which our Christian assumptions can shift to other paradigms as we move from one concept to another.

PART ONE

NURSING

THE CALL TO CARE

1

CARING AND
THE CHRISTIAN STORY

Purpose: To examine the relationship between Christian faith and nursing

Objectives: After reading this chapter and completing the exercises, you should be able to:
1. Describe the historical relationship between Christian faith and nursing
2. Define Christian nursing
3. Identify your motivation for being a nurse
4. Describe the relationship between personal faith and nursing care

Keywords: paradigm, story, narrative, history

JOHN, AN EMERGENCY-DEPARTMENT STAFF NURSE in an inner-city hospital, was on his way to work when the car in front of him suddenly swerved off the road into a tree. He called 911 and stopped to help. John found an unconscious man of about thirty lying face down on the road, bleeding heavily from a leg wound. He felt a weak pulse and checked his airway. The man's arms showed fresh track marks suggesting recent IV drug use. A syringe lay beside him. John suspected that the man had probably overdosed on heroin. He had no gloves with him and did not carry Narcan, but when help seemed long in coming, he began to care for the man's wounds, applying pressure on the leg wound. Afterward, John's colleagues said he had been irresponsible. But all John could think about was, *If Jesus encountered this accident, would he risk touching the wounds of a man, possibly Hepatitis C positive, and love him?*

In another situation, Rosene, a new nurse in an extended-care facility, felt repulsed at first by what she viewed as the "concentrated assemblage of helpless humanity" who surrounded her. But then she prayerfully determined that she would get to know her patients and see the image of God in each one. She gradually began to enjoy the people in her care.[1]

Rick, a nurse caring for Covid-19 patients, is also a deacon in his church, but he has chosen to isolate himself from his church and family to protect them from the virus. "My ministry right now is to my patients and colleagues," he explains.

Joy, an American nurse living in Turkey, saw starving babies in an orphanage and organized an ongoing project to provide them with nourishing formula.[2]

A common thread weaves throughout these stories, which are based on real nurses' accounts. Each of the nurses responded from a theological commitment. They saw those in their care as valuable human beings who reflected the image of God. They saw hope in the midst of hopeless situations. They viewed health as a holistic concept that radiates from a vital relationship with God and includes physical integrity, emotional stability, and participation in the life of the community. They were motivated by the desire to share the love of God, which each had personally experienced, and saw nursing as compassionate service to God and their neighbors. In sum, each of these nurses practiced nursing from a Christian worldview—the framework of ideas and beliefs through which a Christian interprets the world and interacts with it.

How does what we believe about God and the world affect the nursing care we provide? Is there a relationship between the way a society understands the nature of God and the type of health care that develops in that society? These are important questions for us to consider. We assert that there *is* a direct relationship between what a person believes about God and how nursing care is delivered. If the faith perspective changes, health care practices will follow in the same direction. In fact, we are living in the midst of such changes in North America right now.

From its earliest beginnings, the profession of nursing developed out of a Christian worldview. It is important to see that *the changes we are experiencing in health care stem from a growing paradigm shift in our culture.* By paradigm shift, we mean that the worldview, or the way a person or culture

---

[1]Rosene M. Dunkle, "Beyond Appearances: Caring in the Land of the Living Dead," *Journal of Christian Nursing* (1995): 4-6.
[2]Joy Sterling, "The American Milk Mama," *Journal of Christian Nursing* 13, no. 1 (1996): 28-30.

sees human beings, and the world around us, is changing. A paradigm is "a philosophical and theoretical framework of a scientific school or discipline within which theories, laws, and generalizations, and the experiments performed in support of them are formulated."[3] A paradigm shift is a fundamental change in the basic concepts and practices of a discipline.[4] To fully appreciate this shift, we must first look at who we are and how nursing developed in the first place.

How Did We Get Here?

With the rise of empiricism, in which all knowledge is derived from experimentation and sense experience, science blossomed and gave rise to high hopes for conquering drudgery and disease. Optimism ran high in mid–nineteenth century England. Progress toward better things in all areas of life was possible. And thus the positivist worldview that dominated the scientific community undoubtedly influenced Florence Nightingale as she went to Crimea in 1854.[5] By applying good principles of sanitation, she made a major difference in the death rate of British soldiers (from 42 percent to 2 percent). She also used statistics to successfully influence change in the care of wounded British soldiers.[6] But the spectacular success of science and high hopes of the philosophers had an unsettling effect on the common people—and that troubled Nightingale. She wrote to her friend John Stuart Mill, "Many years ago, I had a large and very curious acquaintance among the artisans of the North of England and of London. I learned that they were without any religion

---

[3]Merriam-Webster, s.v. "paradigm," accessed December 14, 2020, www.merriam-webster.com /dictionary/paradigm.

[4]Thomas Kuhn, *The Structure of Scientific Revolutions: 50th Anniversary Edition* (Chicago: University of Chicago Press, 2012).

[5]Positivism and empiricism are two related philosophical theories. Positivism describes the nature of knowledge, i.e., the verification of knowledge through scientific methods. Empiricism, on the other hand, describes the source and origin of knowledge. Positivism is built on the theory of empiricism.

[6]Edwin W. Kopf, "Florence Nightingale as Statistician," *Publications of the American Statistical Association* 15, no. 116 (1916): 388-404; Joshua Hammer, "Thou Shalt Not Underestimate Florence Nightingale," *Smithsonian* 50, no. 10 (March 2020): 24-33, 78-79. "Nightingale set about collecting statistics in Crimea. She treated this activity—counting the number of soldiers killed, injured or diseased—in the same way biologists collected specimens of butterflies and fossils on field trips. Like many collectors, she employed other people to collect statistics on her behalf, running a team of data-gatherers at the Crimea." "Florence Nightingale: The Pioneer Statistician," Science Museum, December 10, 2018, https://www.sciencemuseum.org.uk/objects-and-stories/florence -nightingale-pioneer-statistician.

whatever—though diligently seeking after one, principally in Comte and his school. Any return to what is called Christianity appeared impossible."[7]

Florence Nightingale seemed most concerned about the ethical implications of religious belief. In her book *Suggestions for Thought* she attempted to develop an alternative concept of God that would appeal to the disenchanted "artisans" (merchants and craftsmen) so they would have a basis for morality. Her theology was far from orthodox—she dismissed the incarnation, the Trinity, and the atonement as "abortions of a comprehension of God's plan."[8] However, she considered herself a Christian and her work a "call from God."[9]

The twentieth century brought another set of philosophical and theological influences into nursing. The progressive optimism prior to World War I gave way to the realities of violence, war, and human evil. New philosophers reacted against modern optimism built on the foundations laid by empiricism then began tearing them down. The results were nihilism, existentialism, and eventually postmodernism.[10] It became clear that all the knowledge that mattered in life could not be measured, counted, or weighed. This philosophical ferment laid the foundation for the tensions we face in nursing today.

Do the philosophical and theological underpinnings of nursing really matter? Absolutely! For just as Florence Nightingale observed that the common people in her day were becoming atheists and thereby losing their basis for ethical behavior, nurses today are affected by the philosophies and worldviews of our time. The spirit of service and compassion that once motivated nurses to enter the profession has evolved into a professionalism that demands power, status, and appropriate compensation.[11] We see the effects in

---

[7]Florence Nightingale, quoted in Michael D. Calabria and Janet A. Macrae, *Suggestions for Thought by Florence Nightingale* (Philadelphia: University of Pennsylvania Press, 1994), ix.

[8]Calabria and Macrae, *Suggestions for Thought*, 13.

[9]JoAnn G. Widerquist, "Florence Nightingale's Calling," *Second Opinion*, January 1992, 108-21.

[10]Nihilism is the rejection of all religious and moral principles; it is the belief that life is meaningless. Existentialism is a philosophical theory or approach that emphasizes the existence of the individual person as a free and responsible agent determining their own development through acts of the will. "Postmodernism is 'post' because it denies the existence of any ultimate principles, and it lacks the optimism of a scientific, philosophical, or religious truth which will explain everything for everybody—a characteristic of the so-called 'modern' mind." Center for Theology and the Natural Sciences and Richard P. Whaite, "Postmodernism," Counterbalance Foundation, accessed September 23, 2020, counterbalance.org/gengloss/postm-body.html.

[11]Suzanne Gordon and Sioban Nelson, "An End to Angels: Moving Away from the Virtue Script Toward a Knowledge-Based Identity for Nurses," *American Journal of Nursing* 105, no. 5 (2005): 62-69.

a health care system controlled by the bottom line, and many health care providers entering their professions for the paycheck rather than sensing a call to serve.

A Brief History of Nursing

Nursing has its roots in the early Christian church. Although some forms of health care were provided in ancient cultures,[12] nurse historian Patricia Donahue states, "The history of nursing first becomes continuous with the beginning of Christianity."[13] Nurse historians Dolan, Fitzpatrick, and Herrmann state, "The teachings and example of Jesus Christ had a profound influence on the emergence of gifted nurse leadership as well as on the expansion of the role of nurses. Christ stressed the need to love God and one's neighbor. The first organized group of nurses was established as a direct response to Jesus' example and challenge."[14]

The impetus for this movement came when the first-century Christians began to teach that all believers were to care for the poor, the sick, and the disenfranchised (e.g., Mt 25:31-46; Heb 13:1-3; Jas 1:27). As the churches grew, they appointed deacons to care for the needy within the church.[15] Eventually, more men and women were added to the roll of deacons, and their designated responsibilities grew to include caring for the sick.[16] Phoebe, the deacon mentioned in Romans 16:1-2, is often considered the first visiting nurse.[17]

By the third century, organized groups of deacons were caring for the sick, mentally ill, and lepers in the community.[18] In the fourth century the church began establishing hospitals. Most of these hospitals did not have a physician; they were staffed by nurses. There were several periods when the early church

---

[12]These health care providers included midwives, shamans, and wise women, but none of these roles meet the criteria for professional nursing as defined in this chapter.

[13]Patricia Donahue, *Nursing: The Finest Art—An Illustrated History* (St. Louis: Mosby, 1985), 93.

[14]Josephine Dolan, M. Louise Fitzpatrick, and Eleanor Krohn Herrmann, *Nursing in Society: A Historical Perspective*, 15th ed. (Philadelphia: W. B. Saunders, 1983), 43.

[15]James Monroe Barnett, *The Diaconate: A Full and Equal Order* (Valley Forge, PA: Trinity Press, 1995), 28-42.

[16]David Zersen, "Parish Nursing: 20th-Century Fad?," *Journal of Christian Nursing* (1994): 19-21, 45.

[17]Dolan et al., *Nursing in Society*, 45.

[18]Mary Haazig, "Historical Presence of the Nurse in the Church," in *Oneness in Purpose—Diversity in Practice* (Park Ridge, IL: National Parish Nurse Resource Center, 1989), 3.

did not condone the practice of medicine, which they viewed as a pagan art.[19] Nurse historians Lavinia Dock and Isabel Stewart state, "The age-old custom of hospitality . . . was practiced with religious fervor by the early Christians. . . . Their houses were opened wide to every afflicted applicant and, not satisfied with receiving needy ones, the deacons, men and women alike, went out to search and bring them in."[20]

Nursing in the Middle Ages centered in monasteries. Women and men who wanted to serve God and care for the sick joined together in monastic orders. In the late Middle Ages, the Knights Hospitallers of St. John, a military nursing order, built a hospital in Jerusalem, as well as others along the route of the Crusades. While the original intent was to care for pilgrims to Jerusalem, they also cared for Christian crusaders, Muslims, and Jews.[21]

The Renaissance through the eighteenth century brought a dark period in the history of nursing. As Catholic religious orders were disbanded or suppressed in Protestant countries, hospitals deteriorated. Nursing ceased to be a public role; it moved out of the church and into the home. However, some religious orders in southern Europe continued providing nursing care, including those established by Saint Francis de Sales (1567–1622) and Saint Vincent de Paul (1581–1660).[22] But, care deteriorated even among the religious orders as nuns were not allowed to touch any part of the human body except the head and extremities and were often forced to work twenty-four-hour shifts.[23]

By the nineteenth century, except for a few nursing orders of nuns, nursing was disorganized and corrupt. Dolan, Fitzpatrick and Herrmann describe hospitals in Philadelphia in 1884: "Hospital patients were penniless folk, usually homeless and friendless. In most of the city hospitals the nursing was done by inmates usually over 50 years old, many being 70 or 80. . . . There was practically no night nursing, except for the 'night watchers' provided for women in childbirth and the dying."[24]

---

[19]Bonnie Bullough and Vern L. Bullough, "Our Roots: What We Should Know About Nursing's Christian Pioneers," *Journal of Christian Nursing* (1987): 11-12.

[20]Lavinia L. Dock and Isabel Maitland Stewart, *A Short History of Nursing, From the Earliest Times to the Present Day* (New York: Putnam, 1931), 51.

[21]Verna Benner Carson, *Spiritual Dimensions of Nursing Practice* (Philadelphia: W. B. Saunders, 1989), 57.

[22]Carson, *Spiritual Dimensions*, 59-60.

[23]Dock and Stewart, *Short History of Nursing*, 99.

[24]Dolan et al., *Nursing in Society*, 137.

Charles Dickens portrayed nineteenth-century nursing in the character of Sairey Gamp in his novel *Martin Chuzzlewit*.[25] A self-seeking alcoholic, Gamp has become the symbol of nursing at its worst. Dickens focused public attention on the nursing care being provided by alcoholics, prostitutes, and other women who were uncaring and immoral.

Reform again came through the work of the Christian church. Elizabeth Seton (1774–1821) established the Widow's Society, a Protestant mission in New York, to care for poor women in their homes—to nurse and comfort them. She later joined the Catholic Church and eventually established the Sisters of Charity at Emmitsburg, Maryland. Mother Mary Catherine McAuley (1778–1841) founded the Sisters of Mercy, who ministered to the poor and sick in Dublin, Ireland, and the order eventually spread to other countries, including the United States. Elizabeth Fry (1780–1845), an American Quaker in London, began a campaign of prison reform that eventually developed into the Society of Protestant Sisters of Charity, whose primary objective was to supply nurses for the sick of all classes in their homes.[26]

Fry had a strong influence on a German Lutheran pastor, Theodor Fliedner (1800–1845), and his wife, Frederika. Seeing the pressing needs of the poor and the sick in their community, the Fliedners decided that the church must care for these people. They turned a little garden house into a home for outcast girls and eventually organized a community of deaconesses to visit and nurse the sick in their homes. That experiment quickly grew into the Kaiserswerth Institute for the Training of Deaconesses, with a huge complex of buildings, including a hospital, and educational programs for nurses and teachers.[27]

About the same time, Florence Nightingale (1820–1910), felt God calling her to future service. She responded to that call by becoming a nurse, studying first at the Kaiserswerth Institute, then at Catholic hospitals in Paris. Nightingale went on to single-handedly reform nursing, bringing it back to its Christian roots and setting high educational and practice standards.[28]

---

[25]Charles Dickens, *Martin Chuzzlewit* (New York: Books, Inc., 1868). Sairey Gamp is introduced in chapter 19 and continues as a key figure for the remainder of the book.

[26]Dolan et al., *Nursing in Society*, 137–39.

[27]Abdel Ross Wentz, *Fliedner the Faithful* (Philadelphia: Board of Publication of the United Lutheran Church in America, 1936), 55–83.

[28]Mary Lewis Coakley, "Florence Nightingale: A One-Woman Revolution," *Journal of Christian Nursing* (1989): 20–25.

However, her theological influence also set the stage for an ongoing struggle between those of her followers who wanted to be viewed as "professional" (secular) and those who understood nursing as a calling from God—a conflict Nightingale herself did not envision.

About this same period, churches in Europe and the United States began establishing hospitals with schools of nursing. William Passavant (1821–1894), a Lutheran pastor and pioneer in hospital development, visited Kaiserswerth. He brought deaconesses to Pittsburgh, Pennsylvania, to staff his first hospital and teach in the nursing school, rather than choosing secular nurses. Passavant described the tension that he observed between Christian service and professionalism in an address given in 1899:

> The deaconess has a Biblical office, the nurse a worldly vocation. The one serves through love; the other for her support. In the one case we have an exercise of charity as wide in extent as the sufferings and misery of mankind; in the other, a usefulness circumscribed by the narrow circle of obedient help given to the physicians and surgeons. Above all, the deaconess cares for the body in order to reach the soul. She works for eternity. The trained nurse, like the man whose vocation brings him to the sick-bed, is, as a rule, quite content to pass by unnoticed the possibilities of an eternal future in the demands of the present welfare of the patient.[29]

Influential nursing leaders at the turn of the nineteenth century railed against the idea of nursing as a religious calling for several reasons.[30] British empiricism left many thinking people of the time disillusioned with the church and placing their hopes in science. Also most nurses in the religious orders and deaconess communities worked under oppressive conditions, resulting in chronic fatigue and a high mortality rate among nurses.[31]

At the same time, the American social context included a strong sense of progress and an assumption that freedom and democracy would eventually create a pure, rational society. But rapid industrialization had left society with a loss of community and large populations of disenfranchised poor.

---

[29]William Passavant, quoted in C. Golder, *The History of the Deaconess Movement* (Cincinnati: Jennings and Pye, 1903), 585.

[30]See, for example, Diane Hamilton, "Constructing the Mind of Nursing," *Nursing History Review* 2 (1994): 3-28; and Dock and Stewart, *Short History of Nursing*, 241-83.

[31]Dock and Stewart, *Short History of Nursing*, 256-57.

Upper-middle-class women, as keepers of the culture's mores and unable to hold paying jobs, became social reformers. Out of these developments, public health nursing arose. Nurse historian Diane Hamilton comments about these nurse reformers ("inventors"):

> Thus, both nursing and religion, if pursued compassionately, healed wounded minds, bodies, and spirits. Although the nurse inventors intended an unyielding boundary between religion and nursing, the kindred missions of religion and nursing rendered the boundary translucent. The reformers envisioned that secular nursing would emulate the values of the religious sisters without accepting their rules, regulations, and cloistered life. Compassion, once associated with God's authority, would, according to the nurse inventors, be replaced with compassion based on commitment to the authority of humanity and its social progress.[32]

Other nursing leaders during the same period insisted that the intimacy inherent in nursing practice required religious goodness, credulity, discipline, and obedience. Charlotte Aikens, in a 1924 nursing ethics text, acknowledged "religion" (defined as "the relation which an individual fixes between his soul and his God") as the basis for nursing ethics.[33] Rebecca McNeill wrote in the *American Journal of Nursing* in 1910 that the "ideal nurse" must be a Christian.[34]

Adding to the tension between the secular and religious influences in nursing was the common practice of deaconess hospitals' establishing schools of nursing based on the Nightingale system, so that, until the establishment of baccalaureate nursing programs, the two philosophies—service and professionalism—developed side by side. As a baccalaureate nursing student in the early sixties, I (Judy) felt caught in the middle of this tension. When I wrote a class paper for a course in nursing leadership, I chose to defend the idea of *service*. In doing so, I raised the ire of my instructor.

At the end of the nineteenth century and beginning of the twentieth, the evangelical missionary movement developed. Early missionaries went to Asia and Africa, communicating the gospel primarily through education and health care. Florence Nightingale also sent out "missioners" to all

---

[32]Hamilton, "Constructing the Mind of Nursing," 21-22.
[33]Charlotte A. Aikens, *Studies in Ethics for Nurses* (Philadelphia: W. A. Saunders, 1924), 51-52.
[34]Rebecca H. McNeill, "The Ideal Nurse," *American Journal of Nursing* 10, no. 3 (1910): 393.

English-speaking countries.[35] Although they determined to be secular, most drew their motivation from Christian faith and often worked through religious orders or mission hospitals. As missionary activity spread around the world, nursing worldwide could trace its roots to both Florence Nightingale and a Christian paradigm.

Over time, revisionist approaches to nursing history have attempted to bypass the Christian roots of nursing. Some nursing histories look instead to animistic "medicine men and women" and shamans, Greek and Roman goddesses, Egyptian priestesses, Ayurvedic medicine, and healing traditions based on *chi* energy.[36]

What Is Nursing?

Nursing and medicine are two distinct professions with very different histories and foci. Western medicine developed out of a Greek, and later Cartesian, body-mind dualism that viewed the body as object.[37] The role of the nurse, however, grew out of a Christian understanding of the human person as created in the image of God and viewed the person as a living unity and the "temple of the Holy Spirit" (1 Cor 3:16).

Medicine has traditionally focused on the scientific dimension of the human body, relegating the spiritual and psychosocial dimensions to religion and psychology. The uniqueness of nursing has been its emphasis on caring for the whole person as embodied. It is defined as both an art and a science. Anne Bishop and John Scudder insist that nursing is neither an art nor a science but a *practice* that draws on both the arts and sciences.[38] Nursing, even in our most scientifically oriented periods, has always been concerned with the whole person. Nurse theorist Patricia Benner asserts, "Nurses deal with not only normality and pathophysiology but also with the lived social and skilled body in promoting health, growth, and development and in caring for the sick and dying."[39] In other words, nurses work from an understanding of

---

[35]Dock and Stewart, *Short History of Nursing*, 87-91.

[36]See, for example, Lynn Keegan, *The Nurse as Healer* (Albany, NY: Delmar, 1994), 182-88.

[37]Bullough and Bullough, "Our Roots," 12.

[38]Anne H. Bishop and John R. Scudder, "Nursing as a Practice Rather Than an Art or Science," *Nursing Outlook*, March–April 1997, 82-85.

[39]Patricia Benner, ed., *Interpretive Phenomenology: Embodiment, Caring, and Ethics in Health and Illness* (Thousand Oaks, CA: Sage, 1994), xvii.

the self as embodied and are concerned with how we relate to one another and function in the world through our bodies.

The classic definition of nursing, developed by theorist Virginia Henderson and adopted by the International Council of Nurses, states, "The unique function of the nurse is to assist the individual, sick or well, in the performance of those activities contributing to health or his recovery (or to peaceful death) that he would perform unaided if he had the necessary strength, will or knowledge. And to do this in such a way as to help him gain independence as rapidly as possible."[40]

Henderson further elaborates by listing fourteen activities that a nurse assists patients to perform.[41] Eight of these activities pertain directly to bodily functions. The remaining six relate to safety and finding meaning and purpose in life—enabling the embodied person to function in relation to other people and the environment in a healthy way.

While not completely denying the need for physical care, several more recent nurse theorists, influenced by Eastern philosophy and existentialism, define nursing by focusing more on a person's relationship to the environment and to the world, and less on the physical care. In the theoretical assertions of some nurse theorists, we see a worldview that is in contrast to a Christian view of nursing. For example, Martha Rogers, credited for developing the science of unitary human beings theory, states, "Professional practice in nursing seeks to promote symphonic interaction between man and environment, to strengthen the coherence and integrity of the human field and to direct and redirect patterning of the human and environmental fields for the realization of maximum health potential."[42]

Jean Watson asserts, "At its most basic level nursing is a human, caring, relational profession. . . . Caring in nursing is a 'human mode of being'; caring is a basic way of 'being-in-the-world' and creates both self and world."[43] One of the tenets of transpersonal caring theory as espoused by Watson is that

---

[40]Virginia A. Henderson, *The Nature of Nursing: Reflections After 25 Years* (New York: National League for Nursing, 1991), 21.

[41]Henderson, *Nature of Nursing*, 22-23.

[42]Martha E. Rogers, *An Introduction to the Theoretical Basis of Nursing* (Philadelphia: F. A. Davis, 1970), 122.

[43]Jean Watson, "Nursing's Caring-Healing Paradigm as Exemplar for Alternative Medicine?," *Alternative Therapies* (1995): 67.

there is unity of mind, body, spirit, and universe as transpersonal caring exists in a unitary field that transcends time, space, and physicality.

Rosemarie Rizzo Parse further expands this approach to nursing: "The nurse centers with the universe, prepares, and approaches the other, attending intensely to the meaning of the moment being lived by the person or family."[44]

The World Health Organization (WHO) provides a more pragmatic definition of nursing to include both autonomous practice and collaborative practice, in all settings, for all people: "Nursing encompasses autonomous and collaborative care of individuals of all ages, families, groups and communities, sick or well and in all settings. It includes the promotion of health, the prevention of illness, and the care of ill, disabled and dying people."[45]

The American Nurses Association (ANA) Scope and Standards of Practice, a valuable resource for standards for professional nursing practice and professional performance, provides the following definition of nursing: "Nursing is the protection, promotion, and optimization of health and abilities; prevention of illness and injury; facilitation of healing; alleviation of suffering through the diagnosis and treatment of human response; and advocacy in the care of individuals, families, groups, communities, and populations."[46]

The ANA Scope and Standards furthermore describe the integration of both the art of nursing (caring, compassion, interprofessional collaboration, and respect for culture and human dignity) with the science of nursing (competency with the nursing process within the professional role).

Note that the last two definitions of nursing offered here include prevention of illness and promotion of health. Also unique to these definitions is the role of the nurse in advocacy and collaboration. These are important distinctions, particularly during the present tumultuous changes in the health care system, as nursing struggles to redefine itself.

We will define Christian nursing through our Christian worldview as *a ministry of compassionate and restorative care for the whole person, in response to God's grace, which aims to promote and foster optimum health (shalom) and*

[44]Rosemarie Rizzo Parse, *Illuminations: The Human Becoming Theory in Practice and Research* (New York: National League for Nursing, 1995), 82.

[45]"Nursing and Midwifery: Overview," World Health Organization, accessed September 23, 2020, who.int/topics/nursing/en.

[46]American Nurses Association, *Nursing: Scope and Standards of Practice*, 3rd ed. (Silver Spring, MD: American Nurses Association, 2015).

bring comfort in suffering and death for anyone in need. We will present the evidence that the concept of nurse grew out of the Christian gospel.

NURSING TODAY

The nursing profession is undoubtedly different today from what it was when Florence Nightingale carried her lamp more than 150 years ago. Nursing has been affected by major health care reform, largely as a result of the changes implemented pursuant to the Affordable Care Act in 2010. The literature cites the high cost of care, changing demographics, lack of quality, variation in health care delivery, and increased incidence of chronic illness as just a few of the drivers of change in the health care system.[47] Nonetheless, nurses are caught in the crosshairs of change. Now, more than ever, nurses need to be committed to caring not only for patients and their families but also for the concerns of the profession. We need to cultivate leadership and develop fluency to discuss the issues of health policy within an interprofessional team to articulate best practice. We need to possess the knowledge and skills that will enable us to appraise and synthesize evidence in order to deliver high quality care that is evidence-based. No one is going to do this work for us. Thus, we assert that an important part of caring includes intentional engagement with the challenges facing nursing today.

Jesus Christ has called us to a bold and refreshing vision for nursing that embraces caring and service. He touched lepers (Lk 5). He applied mud compresses (Jn 9:6). He washed feet (Jn 13). Jesus clearly proclaimed, "Whoever wishes to become great among you must be your servant, and whoever wishes to be first among you must be slave of all. For the Son of Man came not to be served but to serve, and to give his life a ransom for many" (Mk 10:43-45). As Jesus began his ministry he proclaimed,

> The Spirit of the Lord is upon me,
> because he has anointed me
> to bring good news to the poor.
> He has sent me to proclaim release to the captives
> and recovery of sight to the blind,
> to let the oppressed, go free,
> to proclaim the year of the Lord's favor. (Lk 4:18-19)

---

[47]S. W. Salmond and M. Echevarria, "Healthcare Transformation and Changing Roles for Nursing," *Orthopedic Nursing* 36, no. 1 (2017): 12-25.

Throughout the Gospels, physical healing was intimately linked with the proclamation of the gospel. Jesus sent his followers out with instructions to heal the sick and to tell them, "The kingdom of God has come near to you" (Lk 10:9). He underlined our responsibility to provide physical care by explaining in Matthew 25:35-36, 40: "I was hungry and you gave me food, I was thirsty and you gave me something to drink, I was a stranger and you welcomed me, I was naked and you gave me clothing, I was sick and you took care of me. . . . Truly I tell you, just as you did it to one of the least of these who are members of my family, you did it to me."

However, he did not stop there. Throughout the Gospels we see how the ultimate purpose for physical healing was to restore people to a vital relationship with God and the community.

If that is the case, nursing cannot work toward the goal of health without including the clear proclamation of the gospel, as well as providing physical care with a servant attitude. Nursing as a vocation, or *calling*, from God, must return to its roots in the church and Christian faith in order to work toward the goal of true health. Furthermore, if we hope to maintain a strong Christian worldview in nursing, our faith must be nurtured in a Christian community and informed by a clear theology. True nursing cannot be divorced from the Christian story.

FOR FURTHER THINKING

1. What motivated you to become a nurse?

2. What did you learn about nursing history as a nursing student? How does that knowledge shape the way you view nursing?

THEOLOGICAL REFLECTION

Read Matthew 25:31-46, Hebrews 13:1-3, James 1:27, and 1 Peter 2:9.

1. What does each passage say about the relationship between faith and caring for others?

2. To whom should we direct our compassion? For what reasons?

3. How do these passages describe the environment in which we care?

4. What is the nature of health—the goal of our caring?

5. What is involved in providing care?

Case Study: Amy and Flora

Amy, a junior nursing student, was assigned to care for Flora, an eighty-five-year-old woman with bilateral gangrene of the lower extremities secondary to diabetes mellitus. Flora's treatment regimen included maggot therapy. She was on strict contact isolation due to methicillin resistant *staph aureus* (MRSA).

Amy came to clinical well prepared but with some obvious apprehension as she began her day. She donned a gown, gloves, and a mask before entering Flora's room for an initial nursing assessment. The usual morning care followed: breakfast, medication administration, bathing, and tedious dressing changes.

Flora was hearing impaired, so Amy leaned close to her and spoke clearly in her ear. Flora chewed her food slowly, but Amy very deliberately helped her take each bite of breakfast, a process that took over thirty minutes. Flora was afraid and in pain, so Amy touched her gently and combed her hair carefully, gave good skin care, and held her hand.

Flora said she couldn't remember when her family last visited, so Amy read each of her greeting cards to her and listened as Flora reminisced about family. Amy opened the curtains to let Flora feel the warmth of the sun and see the activities outside her window.

Flora was confused due to sleep deprivation, so Amy developed a plan for a soothing bedtime routine. When Flora refused to take her medications, Amy helped her with each pill, calling the pharmacy to get liquid meds where possible. Flora dreaded the painful dressing changes to her lower extremities, but Amy carefully explained each step in the process and used strategies to minimize the pain Flora experienced. When a wandering maggot escaped from under the edge of the dressing, Amy unobtrusively removed it.

Amy was weary as she came out of the room after morning care, sweat matting the hair around her face as she sat down for the first time in two hours to do her charting. When her instructor returned later, she found Amy back in isolation gear, sitting in Flora's room, holding her hand. When her instructor asked Amy why she returned to Flora's bedside, she replied, "I saw Jesus going back into that isolation room to bring comfort to a lonely woman, but I knew Flora would not be able to see him, so I went instead."[48]

---

[48]Adapted from Carol Bence, "I Went Instead," *Journal of Christian Nursing* (2003): 4-5.

DISCUSSION QUESTIONS

1. In what ways does Amy's care for Flora illustrate the principles given in the Bible passages above?

2. How did Amy's personal faith affect her nursing care?

3. What did Amy's care for Flora imply about the way she viewed her patient?

4. How did Amy alter Flora's environment to enhance her care? What seemed to enable Amy to endure the discomfort in her environment?

5. What seemed to be the goal of Amy's care for Flora? How do you think she viewed health?

6. Describe one of your most difficult patients. How could you apply similar approaches in your nursing care for this person?

2

REVOLUTION IN THE NURSING PARADIGM

Purpose: To examine the relationship between shifting worldviews and the changes occurring in nursing practice

Objectives: After reading this chapter and completing the exercises, you should be able to:
1. Describe a paradigm
2. Describe how this struggle between worldviews affects your nursing practice
3. Define the four major concepts of the nursing metaparadigm according to the modern, postmodern, and Christian worldviews
4. Identify the worldview reflected in a nursing theory

Keywords: paradigm, nursing theory, modern, postmodern, Christian

JOANNE FACED A DILEMMA. Working on a large cancer unit over several years, she grew to care deeply for the men and women who were frequently readmitted as their cancer progressed. She grieved when they died, and she recommitted herself to making the lives of other patients as comfortable as possible during their last days. Her sense of being called by the Lord gave her strength for what was often emotionally exhausting work.

Increasingly, however, Joanne began to think that the option of physician-assisted suicide made sense for her patients with terminal cancer. In fact, some patients on her unit were seeking the help of organizations encouraging "the right to die" as a way of ending their prolonged suffering. Some of her colleagues argued that helping these patients end their lives was an act of compassion. Joanne felt confused. According to her Christian worldview, she could not deliberately end the life of anyone in her care. Yet watching her patients suffer moved her to wonder if she should help them contact someone for information about suicide as an option. Although this alternative violated all that she had learned in nursing school about care for the dying, recent articles in nursing journals argued for the right of patients to control their own deaths, dying when they chose to do so. Was Joanne's Christian understanding too narrow?

Maria, on the other hand, faced a different dilemma when she returned to school for a master's degree and took a required course in nursing theory. Like many of her fellow classmates in her undergraduate program, she had viewed nursing theory as one of the subjects to be endured on the way to "real nursing." Now, however, she was trying to see the practical implications of various nursing theories.

The changes in how nurses thought about nursing over the years intrigued her. Florence Nightingale focused on natural laws and the environment; then Virginia Henderson saw nurses acting as substitutes to meet patients' needs when they could not do it themselves. Martha Rogers, a nurse theorist in the 1970s and 1980s, wrote about her view of patients as energy fields within larger energy fields. Because Maria was a deeply committed Christian, she wondered about the connection between the theories she was studying and her faith in God.

One professor suggested that she read the creation story in Genesis, substituting the word *energy* for *God.* Upon trying it she realized that it undermined her understanding of the Christian God, who reveals himself as personal and loving. Over and over throughout the Scriptures, God speaks of wanting to dwell with his people, of wanting to be their God and to have them belong to him. This was the language of love and commitment. Energy, the language of physics, was so impersonal. Was Maria taking the Bible too literally?

Karen, a junior nursing student at a large university, faced yet another dilemma. One of her favorite instructors was teaching a popular elective course in alternative healing, so Karen enthusiastically signed up for it. She hoped to learn new ways to comfort patients. As the weeks went by, however, she began to feel uncomfortable with what she was learning. For example, the professor told the class that she considered herself a witch and that some of the healing methods she taught were "white witchcraft." She encouraged students to chant formulas and burn candles as part of the healing process. She also taught that the Christian church had persecuted witches in order to retain its power over women. During a field trip to a center for therapeutic touch, the instructor encouraged students to take off their clothes as a way to break down barriers between themselves. Karen felt confused but decided not to participate. Was she being too rigid?[1]

Joanne, Maria, and Karen are not alone in their struggles. Nursing—reflecting changes in the larger Western culture—is undergoing major shifts in its thinking and practice. The foundations of nursing itself are being questioned. What is nursing about? What should be the goals of nursing? What is science in nursing? How can these questions be answered?

THE BEGINNINGS OF NURSING THEORY

Until nursing education moved from hospital-based apprentice programs to the academic setting, there was little formal analysis to link theory to practice. Nightingale's concern for a well-ordered environment was taken for granted, and much of nursing focused on keeping things clean. During the early 1900s, hospitals were staffed by nursing students who worked long hours and studied when they could. After graduation, nurses went into either private-duty or public health nursing. Most women in nursing were motivated by Christian values of compassion and service. Nurses saw themselves, for the most part, as assistants to physicians. There was little time or inclination to develop concepts, theories, and philosophies of nursing.

As nursing education moved out of hospital-based schools of nursing into academia, the need developed to establish a body of knowledge unique to nursing. Because nursing entered the academy through science departments, such knowledge was based on research. Scientific research required theories. The purpose of a theory is to describe, explain, or predict phenomena important to the practice of nursing. Serious efforts in theory development began in the 1950s and proliferated in the 1960s and 1970s. Virginia Henderson articulated her famous definition of nursing in 1961 in a pamphlet published by the International Council of Nurses.

Because nursing entered the university through the door of natural science, nursing theories took on characteristics of naturalism.[2] They were couched

---

[1]The three stories are composites of situations the authors have encountered.
[2]Naturalism is the philosophy of science maintaining that natural laws explain everything that we can know for certain. Supernatural or spiritual explanations are ruled out.

in cause-and-effect language, often with elaborate diagrams showing complex relationships between concepts. Many theorists of this era were psychiatric nurses, so their theories focused on the nurse-patient relationship.[3] Even these were framed in naturalistic language of analysis and cause and effect, although in a more personal tone.

Early nursing theories reflected the positivistic philosophy of science prevalent in the university.[4] According to positivism, it is possible to gain true knowledge of reality (what actually exists) through the processes of theory development and testing. The scientific community accepts theories insofar as they seem to correspond with reality. Nurses hoped that through this process of theory testing and refinement they would progressively build the body of knowledge needed for both patient care and academic credibility. Early in this era (1952), the journal *Nursing Research* began to disseminate the findings of researchers. Great optimism among nurses in academia characterized this period as nursing gained recognition as a scientific discipline.

> *A life devoid of the knowledge that theorizing brings us is a poor and paltry thing, short of what God meant our lives to be.*
>
> NICHOLAS WOLTERSTORFF, *EDUCATING FOR SHALOM*

Then in 1962 Thomas Kuhn published *The Structure of Scientific Revolutions*, in which he challenged the prevailing assumption that positivistic science was value-free. Kuhn argued that perception and values shape our understanding of reality, and eventually, the facts no longer fit the theory. When scientific theories no longer explain our experience, a new approach is sought.

SEARCHING FOR NEW NURSING THEORIES

For many years nurses have known intuitively that there was more about our patients and ourselves than could be explained within naturalistic scientific

---

[3]See, for example, Hildegard E. Peplau, *Interpersonal Relations in Nursing* (New York: Putnam, 1952); Joyce Travelbee, *Interpersonal Aspects of Nursing* (Philadelphia: F. A. Davis, 1971).

[4]Positivist science is characterized by three features: presuppositionless objectivity, being empirically testable by experiments, and rationality. Bruce R. Reichenbach and V. Elving Anderson, *On Behalf of God: A Christian Ethic for Biology* (Grand Rapids, MI: Eerdmans, 1995), 16.

theories.[5] Every day we experience life, death, tragedy, birth, and suffering. Often patients press us with questions. "Why did my baby die?" "How can I live with a body that can't move or feel?" How often have we stood dumb before these cries? Our theories were impotent to help us. The naturalistic scientific theories told us about physiology and pathology. The psychosocial nursing theories told us to listen, to feel with, to support and encourage our patients. But we found ourselves powerless in the end. Many of us turned to our faith to help us, and for most nurses that was Christian faith.

Then in 1970 Martha Rogers published her text *An Introduction to the Theoretical Basis of Nursing.*[6] Because her work was so radically different, many dismissed both the book and Rogers herself. Few understood what she was saying, and even fewer grasped the significance of what she was doing for nursing.[7] What she did was open possibilities for new ways of thinking about nursing. Rogers continued using the impersonal language of physics—energy, field theory, simultaneity—to describe the intangible in nursing, but she assigned these words new meaning. Other nursing theorists who followed began to explore new approaches to nursing theory and science, such as phenomenology and existentialism,[8] and to use the language of *spirit, consciousness,* and *goddess.*[9]

In the 1994 edition of her textbook on nursing theory, Barbara Stevens Barnum notes the polarity between the older and the newer nursing theories. The older nursing process theories are associated with taxonomies and quantitative measures, whereas the new, holistic theories use more qualitative measures and softer phenomena.[10]

---

[5]Naturalistic theories assume that reality is only empirical, natural. There is no account of God or spirit in these theories.

[6]Martha A. Rogers, *An Introduction to the Theoretical Basis of Nursing* (Philadelphia: F. A. Davis, 1970).

[7]Rogers's book for nursing is comparable to Kuhn's for the larger scientific community in that both formulated a new way to approach the work of their respective disciplines.

[8]"The discipline of phenomenology may be defined initially as the study of structures of experience, or consciousness. Literally, phenomenology is the study of 'phenomena': appearances of things, or things as they appear in our experience, or the ways we experience things, thus the meanings things have in our experience. Phenomenology studies conscious experience as experienced from the subjective or first person point of view." David Woodruff Smith, "Phenomenology," *The Stanford Encyclopedia of Philosophy* (2018), https://plato.stanford.edu/archives/sum2018/entries/phenomenology.

[9]Jean Watson, *Human Science and Human Care* (New York: National League for Nursing, 1988); Margaret A. Newman, *Health as Expanding Consciousness,* 2nd ed. (New York: National League for Nursing, 1994).

[10]Barbara Stevens Barnum, *Nursing Theory: Analysis, Application, Evaluation,* 4th ed. (Philadelphia: Lippincott, 1994), 251-52.

Both nursing education and practice continue to feel the impact of the shift from the old to the new approaches. This shift—or revolution, according to Kuhn—is what Joanne, Maria, and Karen, who were introduced at the beginning of this chapter, were experiencing. The shift affects not merely our thinking about nursing but also our nursing interventions and the way we make ethical decisions.

The polarity Barnum notes is particularly wide when it comes to how we develop nursing knowledge. Two opposing and irreconcilable ontologies (views of reality) underlie the old and the new theories: realism and conceptualism.[11] Barnum writes,

> In realism, one believes that the world exists "out there," independent of the knower. Research and theory seek to discover and explain the nature of that external reality. . . . In conceptualism, reality does not exist independent of the knower. Invention, rather than discovery, is the dominant mode of knowing reality. The two concepts are the extreme poles, with all sorts of variations on the continuum that spans them.[12]

Some of the newer theories of nursing were very abstract *grand theories* and based on spiritual or even Neopagan worldviews rather than naturalism. Martha Rogers's *Nursing: Science of Unitary, Irreducible, Human Beings*, Parse's *Man-Living-Health*, and Margaret Newman's *Health as Expanding Consciousness* are examples. Over time, however, other more *practice-oriented theories* have replaced them.

While we agree that naturalistic theories alone are much too narrow for nursing, we also think that there are serious problems with many of the newer approaches that were based on Neopagan worldviews. The issue is much more fundamental. It lies with our ultimate view of life, the philosophy of nursing. We appreciate the openness to spirituality, but we believe that there is a far deeper concern than merely adding religion and spirituality, as if they were the missing parts that will slack the hunger for meaning not addressed in naturalistic theories. What is happening in nursing (and in our larger culture) is a major shift in worldviews. It is at the worldview level that we must begin.

---

[11]Ontology is the study of being, of what exists, of ultimate reality. Its investigations concern what exists beyond what is directly observable, and its conclusions are arrived at by logic and speculation.
[12]Barnum, *Nursing Theory*, 269.

Seven Basic Worldview Questions

James Sire defines a worldview as "a commitment, a fundamental orientation of the heart, that can be expressed as a story or in a set of presuppositions (assumptions which may be true, partially true or entirely false) which we hold (consciously or subconsciously, consistently or inconsistently) about the basic constitution of reality, and that provides the foundation on which we live and move and have our being."* He asserts that to understand the concept of worldview, we must answer the following questions:

- What is prime reality?
- What is the nature of the world around us?
- What is a human being?
- What happens to a person at death?
- Why is it possible to know anything at all?
- How do we know what is right and wrong?
- What is the meaning of human history?
- What personal, life-orienting commitments are consistent with each worldview?**

For the Christian nurse, the answers to these questions come from the stories, themes, and patterns found in the Bible. This careful study of Scripture reveals to us the nature of persons, the context in which we live and practice, the meaning of health, and the impetus for nursing care. For Christians, prime reality is God, who created and sustains all things. Thus, this worldview is derived from a Christian theology of nursing.

---

*James W. Sire, *Naming the Elephant: Worldview as Concept* (Downers Grove, IL: InterVarsity Press, 2015), 122.
**Sire, *Naming the Elephant*, 20.

BEGINNING WITH WORLDVIEWS

Until recently the term *worldview* was part of the technical language of philosophers and anthropologists. Philosophers refer to worldview when they mean the basic assumptions that underlie a system of thought. Anthropologists use the term in a broader way to identify not only the wellsprings of our thinking but our way of life as well. "It shapes and integrates our various fields of knowledge from theology, anthropology, and missions to physics and the culinary arts. Worldview governs everyday behavior" (see Mt 6:8; 7:11; Lk 12:32).[13] "Worldviews are the most fundamental and encompassing views of reality shared by a people in a culture. A worldview incorporates assumptions about the nature of things—about the 'givens' of reality" (Heb 4:15).[14] "They are made up of the categories, values, and assumptions we use to examine our world."[15] Worldviews provide the cultural lenses that shape how we see the world, and they give meaning to life, both personally and for humanity as a whole.

Because a worldview is so overarching, it can integrate many theories from different aspects of life and help us see how they may complement each other. But when theories reflect very different worldviews, they will conflict with one another. Ultimately, differing worldviews cannot be reconciled; either one or the other gives us a truer picture of reality.

The modern Western worldview. During the Renaissance (beginning about the fifteenth century), thinkers turned away from the supernatural and a traditional understanding of God's involvement in creation. Instead, they turned to the natural world of humans, animals, plants, and matter. They began to see the world as autonomous, operating according to natural laws. Their hope was that the newly developing science would enable them to understand these laws and use them to solve practical human problems.[16]

Hebrew and Christian thinking have influenced science. The Bible has given the Western world its strong emphasis on the value of the individual person who is not to be lost within the group. The biblical teaching that life has its source in God and that humans are created with the capacity to relate to God in a personal way has supported our respect for each person. The creation story undergirds our belief that creation is orderly and that the "laws" of nature can be discerned by science. Westerners retain the idea of history moving to a climax, rather than in endless natural cycles, from the biblical story of God acting in history and finally bringing it to a conclusion. Biblical values of love and justice have shaped Western ethics.

---

[13]Paul G. Hiebert, *Anthropological Reflections on Missiological Issues* (Grand Rapids, MI: Baker, 1994), 11-12.

[14]Hiebert, *Anthropological Reflections*, 36.

[15]Hiebert, *Anthropological Reflections*, 204.

[16]Bruce R. Reichenbach and V. Elving Anderson, *On Behalf of God: A Christian Ethic for Biology* (Grand Rapids, MI: Eerdmans, 1995), 11. English philosopher Francis Bacon (1561-1626) called himself the "trumpeter of his times." He sought to reform science, which until then had been influenced by Aristotle's search for essences. He advocated empirical science instead. For Bacon, the function of science ultimately was to control nature for human benefit. He believed that science was a form of power. To exercise power over nature we must understand nature and its causes or principles.

While most early scientists saw the world as an orderly creation dependent on God for its existence, eventually people began thinking of God as distant. They saw themselves created for their own destiny.

Today many are dismissing the modern worldview as having been tried and found wanting, seeing it as causing alienation from the world of the spirit. Some see Christianity as part of the problem because it has become so intertwined with the modern worldview. Nevertheless, its themes are still powerful in our culture even though they are reinterpreted on a secular basis.

The postmodern worldview. Many philosophers argue that we now live in a postmodern world.[17] Despite the powerful benefits of science and technology, there is increasing recognition that science cannot give meaning to life. Many scientists are themselves rejecting the dualism that divorces spiritual from material realities and separates values from scientific objectivity. Social scientists and health care professionals are calling for a more holistic view that brings humans into harmony with their environment.

Some nursing theorists reflect this postmodern worldview: Joyce Fitzpatrick, Margaret Newman, Rosemarie Rizzo Parse, Martha E. Rogers, and Jean Watson. Each of these thinkers is quite different in her approach, but each is calling for something beyond the mechanistic, natural-science approach to nursing. Some of these theories draw from various sources in Eastern philosophy, Theosophy,[18] and traditional religions, including shamanism, Native American spirituality, and Wicca.[19]

---

[17]To read more about the development called postmodernism, see Albert Borgmann, *Crossing the Postmodern Divide* (Chicago: University of Chicago Press, 1992); Stanley J. Grenz, *A Primer on Postmodernism* (Grand Rapids, MI: Eerdmans, 1996); Dennis McCallum, ed., *The Death of Truth* (Minneapolis: Bethany House, 1996); Pauline Marie Rosenau, *Post-Modernism and the Social Sciences* (Princeton, NJ: Princeton University Press, 1992); Gene Edward Veith, *Postmodern Times: A Christian Guide to Contemporary Thought and Culture* (Wheaton, IL: Crossway, 1994); Nicholas Wolterstorff, "Does Truth Still Matter? Reflections on the Crisis of the Postmodern University," *CRUX*, September 1995, 17-28.

[18]Theosophy began as a quasi-Christian philosophy that taught that the Divine could be approached by mystical experiences. It was introduced in America by Dora Kunz, a Dutch psychic, who immigrated to America and became president of the Theosophical Society in America. Kunz developed a healing technique called "Therapeutic Touch," along with Dr. Dolores Krieger, a nursing faculty member at New York University. Kunz explained in her writings and lectures that Therapeutic Touch was based on ancient Yogic texts written in Sanskrit, which describe it as a pranic healing method. The practice was adopted by NYU's school of nursing and many other nursing programs in the 1970s and 1980s.

[19]Barbara Blattner, *Holistic Nursing* (Englewood Cliffs, NJ: Prentice-Hall, 1981), 7-16; and Lynn Keegan, *The Nurse as Healer* (Albany, NY: Delmar, 1994), 4-6.

Some advocates of these theories and practices claim the effectiveness of the associated modalities, such as energy therapies and various meditative techniques. Others are attempting to use both quantitative and qualitative research methods to support the effectiveness of these modalities. However, the research methodologies are often problematic.[20] Christian nurses who practice these modalities without understanding their spiritual basis may not recognize that they may be incompatible with Christian faith.

So far in this chapter we have presented the worldviews that have shaped and are shaping nursing theory—the modern worldview and the postmodern worldview. We agree that theories of nursing based on the modern mechanistic worldview are not adequate to undergird the practice of nursing. Theories that reduce people by materialistic explanations and ignore the spiritual realm can never satisfactorily encompass the richness of nursing: caring for people in life and death, in times of high joy and crushing sorrow.

However, we challenge the idea that theories based on Neopagan religions are the answer. Returning to shamanism and Spiritism where we must appease spirits, or to magic where we seek to dominate reality for our own ends through rituals and formulas, will lead to dehumanization, disillusionment, and spiritual oppression. These worldviews undermine the practices and ways of thinking that face Joanne, Maria, and Karen; the worldviews promise much but offer only illusions. Instead we affirm a Christian worldview for nursing. We turn to that worldview in the next chapter. First, to set the context, we present an overview of several nursing theories in table format. Nursing theory often reflects the worldview of the theorist. Because theory guides nursing practice and research, it is important to critique a theory's origins and assumptions and to carefully consider how each theory aligns (or does not align) with a Christian worldview of nursing.

Worldviews in nursing theories. Nursing theories provide a conceptual framework for directing and organizing our work. A theory is a set of interrelated concepts or statements that are meant to either describe or explain a phenomenon or predict an outcome. Nursing theories can be categorized in terms of scope, from grand theory (very abstract, macrotheory) to practice

---

[20]Sharon Fish, "Therapeutic Touch: Can We Trust the Data?," *Journal of Christian Nursing* (1993): 6-7.

theory (situation-specific, microtheory).[21] Nursing theorists who have produced grand theories, or theories that are highly abstract in scope, often organize their theoretical assumptions based on what is called the nursing metaparadigm. The metaparadigm of nursing includes the concepts of person, environment, health, and nurse. For nursing to exist, each element of the metaparadigm must be realized.

As noted, theories guide nursing science but they also reflect each theorist's view of science and of truth. Although at times it is implicit, each theory assumes an underlying worldview. Theories also reflect shifts in the worldview of the larger society. The worldview descriptions of theories in table 2.1 provide beginning examples of how Christian nurses can examine the concepts of the metaparadigm (person, health, environment, and nursing) as they relate to individual nursing theories.

Table 2.1 demonstrates how the four concepts of the nursing paradigm are defined from different worldviews.

FOR FURTHER THINKING

1. What major changes have you encountered since you first entered nursing?

2. What evidence have you seen that worldviews in nursing are shifting?

3. How would you describe your own worldview?

THEOLOGICAL REFLECTION

Read Acts 8:4-24.

1. Compare the ministry of Philip to that of Simon.

2. What outcomes did each of them seek?

3. What motivated each?

4. Describe the worldview of each based on the information given about them.

5. Why did Peter and John judge Simon so harshly?

6. What resulted?

---

[21]Denise F. Polit and Cheryl Tatano Beck, *Nursing Research: Generating and Assessing Evidence for Nursing Practice*, 10th ed. (Philadelphia: Wolters Kluwer, 2017).

Table 2.1. Worldview concepts in selected theories (classification of theories based on Ann Marriner-Tomey, *Nursing Theorists and Their Work*, 3rd ed. [St. Louis: Mosby, 1994]).

Betty Neuman: Neuman Systems Model[a] (Conceptual Model: Grand Theory)				
GOD	**ENVIRONMENT**	**PERSON**	**HEALTH**	**NURSING**
Source of human spirit or soul. Holy Spirit is a gift that combines with the human spirit; the spirit controls the mind that controls the body.	"Consists of both internal and external forces surrounding the client, influencing and being influenced by the client at any point in time, as an open system. The created environment is an unconsciously developed protective environment that binds system energy and encompasses both the internal and external client environments." "*Stressors*; Environmental factors, intra-, inter-, and extra personal in nature, that have potential for disrupting system stability. A stressor is any phenomenon that might penetrate both the flexile and normal lines of defense, resulting in either a positive or negative outcome."	"*Client/Client System*; A composite of variables (physiological, psychological, socio-cultural, developmental and spiritual), each of which is a subpart of all parts, forms the whole of the client. The client as a system is composed of a core or basic structure of survival factors and surrounding protective concentric rings. The rings are composed of similar factors yet serve varied and different purposes in either retention, attainment, or maintenance of system stability and integrity or a combination of these. The client is considered an open system in total interface with the environment. The client is viewed as a system, and the terms can be used interchangeably with the client/client system." "*Basic Structure*; The basic structure consists of common client survival factors, as well as unique individual characteristics. It represents the basic system energy resources." "*Boundary Lines*; The flexible line of defense is the outer boundary of the client system. All relevant variables must be taken into account, as the whole is greater than the sum of the parts; a change in one part affects all other system parts."	"A continuum of wellness to illness, dynamic in nature, that is constantly subject to change. Optimal wellness or stability indicates that total system needs are being met. A reduced state of wellness is the result of unmet systemic needs. The client is in a dynamic state of either wellness or illness, in varying degrees, at any given point in time." "*Stability*; A state of balance or harmony requiring energy exchange as the client adequately copes with stressors to retain, attain, or maintain an optimal level of health, thus preserving system integrity." "*Lines of Resistance*; Protective factors activated when stressors have penetrated the normal line of defense, causing a reaction symptomatology. The resistance lines ideally protect the basic structure and facilitate reconstitution toward wellness during and following treatment, as stressor reaction is decreased and client resistance is increased."	"A unique profession concerned with all variables affecting clients in their environment." "*Prevention as intervention*; Intervention typology or modes for nursing action and determinants for entry of both client and nurse into the health care system. Primary prevention: before a reaction to stressors occurs. Secondary prevention: treatment of symptoms following a reaction to stressors. Tertiary prevention: maintenance of optimal wellness following treatment." "*Goal*; The system goal is stability for the purpose of client survival and optimal wellness."

[a]Betty Neuman, *The Neuman Systems Model*, 3rd ed. (Stamford, CT: Appleton & Lange, 1995), 45–48.

Table 2.1. *(continued)*

Dorthea Orem: Self-Care Deficit Theory[a] (Conceptual Model: Grand Theory)

GOD	ENVIRONMENT	PERSON	HEALTH	NURSING
Not identified. Relevant only to the patient's understanding.	Physical, chemical, biological and social (family, community) features with which the person interacts. Contributes to the person's development.	Human beings are: 1. Persons moving toward personalization (maturation and achievement of human potential) while living a life of faith in respect of things hoped for and to perfect themselves as responsible human beings who raise questions, seek answers, reflect and become aware of the relationship between knowledge and behavior. 2. A unity of structures and functions that actively maintains self-care and/or dependent-care agency by regulating factors affecting life, health or well-being. Seek health care for self-care or dependent-care deficiencies.	A state of being structurally and functionally whole or sound; psychologically, biologically and socially. It includes the individual's view of self as a self-care or dependent-care[b] agent and the freedom with which the individual acts with responsibility in matters of self-care or dependent-care.	Nurses help patients meet or develop their self-care agency—or their dependent-care agency. Includes (1) doing for, (2) guiding, (3) teaching, (4) supporting, (5) providing a developmental environment. Nursing care is therapeutic in sustaining life and health, in recovering from disease or injury, or in coping with their effects (primary, secondary, and tertiary prevention). It contributes to personal development and maturation.

[a]Dorthea E. Orem, *Nursing Concepts of Practice*, 3rd ed. (New York: McGraw Hill, 1985), 55, 136-43, 176-83.
[b]Care of children or others for whom the person is responsible.

Madeline Leininger: Culture Care Theory[a] (Middle Range Theory)

GOD	ENVIRONMENT	PERSON	HEALTH	NURSING
Defined by the culture.	Technology, religion, kinship and society, values and traditions, politics and law, economy, education, language and history of the culture.	Individuals, families, communities as defined by the culture.	Well-being: Culturally defined and reflects the ability of individuals or groups to perform their daily activities according to their culture.	Directed toward assisting, supporting or enabling an individual or group with evident or anticipated needs to maintain or regain their well-being in culturally meaningful and beneficial ways, or to help them face death.

[a]Madeleine M. Leininger, "The Theory," in *Culture Care Diversity and Universality: A Theory of Nursing*, ed. Madeleine M. Leininger (New York: National League for Nursing, 1991), 5-68.

Table 2.1. *(continued)*

Sister Callista Roy: Adaptation Model[a] (Conceptual Model: Grand Theory)				
GOD	ENVIRONMENT	PERSON	HEALTH	NURSING
God is intimately revealed in the diversity of creation and is the common destiny of creation.	All conditions and influences surrounding and affecting the development and behavior of persons or groups. Persons must adapt to positive and negative factors in environment. • All conditions, circumstances and influences surrounding and affecting the development and behavior of persons and groups with particular consideration of mutuality of person and earth resources. • Three kinds of stimuli: focal, contextual and residual. • Significant stimuli in all human adaptation include stage of development, family, and culture.[b]	A biopsychosocial being in constant interaction with a changing environment. A living, complex, adaptive system. A whole made of parts or subsystems that function as a unity for some purpose. • An adaptive system with coping processes. • Described as a whole composed of parts. • Functions as a unity for some purpose. • Includes people as individuals or in groups (families, organizations, communities, nations and society as a whole). • An adaptive system with cognator and regulator subsystems acting to maintain adaptation in the four adaptive modes: physiologic-physical, self-concept-group identity, role function and interdependence.	• *Health*: a state and process of being and becoming integrated and whole that reflects person and environmental mutuality. • *Adaptation*: the process and outcome whereby thinking and feeling persons, as individuals and in groups, use conscious awareness and choice to create human and environmental integration. • *Adaptive Responses*: responses that promote integrity in terms of the goals of the human system, that is, survival, growth, reproduction, mastery, and personal and environmental transformation. • *Ineffective Responses*: responses that do not contribute to integrity in terms of the goals of the human system. • *Adaptation levels*: represent the condition of the life processes described on three different levels: integrated, compensatory and compromised.	Helping persons to adapt to changes in their physiological needs, self-concept, role function, and interdependent functions during health and illness. • Nursing is the science and practice that expands adaptive abilities and enhances person and environment transformation. • Nursing goals are to promote adaptation for individuals and groups in the four adaptive modes, thus contributing to health, quality of life and dying with dignity. • This is done by assessing behavior and factors that influence adaptive abilities and by intervening to expand those abilities and to enhance environmental interactions.

[a]Carolyn L. Blue et. al., "Adaptation Model," in *Nursing Theorists and Their Work*, ed. Ann Marriner-Tomey, 3rd ed. (St. Louis: Mosby, 1994), 246-68.
[b]Callista Roy, Boston College Nurse Theorist website, accessed February 3, 2004, www2.bc.edu/%7Eroyca/.

Table 2.1. *(continued)*

Martha Rogers: Science of Unitary Human Beings[a] (Conceptual Model: Grand Theory)				
GOD	ENVIRONMENT	PERSON	HEALTH	NURSING
Not identified as a distinct being(s). All reality is pan-dimensional, infinite energy fields, characteristics usually associated with God. *Energy field*: the fundamental unit of the living and nonliving; unifying concept. *Energy* signifies dynamic nature of fields; *fields* are infinite.[b] Two energy fields are identified, human and environmental. Energy fields are *open* fields; causality is invalid; change is continuously innovative.[c] "Fields are coextensive with the universe, thus without boundaries, everything is interconnected through energy patterning."[d] *Pattern* is the distinguishing characteristic of an energy field perceived as a single wave; an abstraction; gives identity to the field; changes continuously.[e] *Four-dimensionality/ pan-dimensionality*: a nonlinear domain without spatial or temporal attributes; characteristic of all reality; relative nature of change; a way of perceiving human beings and their world.[f]	An irreducible, pan-dimensional energy field identified by pattern, manifesting characteristics of the whole and integral with the human field.[g] Each environmental field is specific to its given human field. Both change continuously, mutually and creatively.[h] The *patterns* of human and environmental fields are characterized by: *Resonance*—the continuous change from lower to higher frequency wave patterns; *Helicy*—the continuous innovative, unpredictable, increasing diversity of the patterns. *Integrality*—the continuous mutual human field and environmental field process.[i]	The unitary human being (human field) is an irreducible, indivisible, four-dimensional/ pan-dimensional, energy field identified by pattern; manifesting characteristics that are different from those of the parts (specific to the whole) and cannot be predicted from knowledge of the parts.[j] In continuous mutual total process with the environment.[k] Capacity for thought, imagination and emotion.[l] Paranormal and mystical experiences derived from openness, pan-dimensionality and patterning of human and environmental fields.[m] Because there are no boundaries, persons extend beyond their skin.[n]	Passive health symbolizes wellness and absence of disease. Positive health is rhythmic consistency.[o] The life process evolves irreversibly onward along the space-time continuum that may continue after death.[p] Health is a value term defined by the culture or individual. "Health and illness are manifestations of pattern and are considered 'to denote behaviors that are of high value and low value.' Events manifested in the life process indicate the extent to which man achieves maximum health according to some value system."[q]	A science and an art. Promotes symphonic interaction between the environment and man, to strengthen the coherence and integrity of the human being and to direct and redirect patterns of interaction between man and his environment for the realization of maximum health potential.[r]

[a]Martha E. Rogers, *An Introduction to the Theoretical Basis of Nursing* (Philadelphia: F. A. Davis, 1970); Joann Sebastian Daily et al., "Unitary Human Beings," in *Nursing Theorists and Their Work*, ed. Ann Marriner-Tomey, 3rd ed. (St. Louis: Mosby, 1994), 211-30; Martha E. Rogers, "Science of Unitary Human Beings," in *Explorations on Martha Rogers' Science of Unitary Human Beings*, ed. Violet M. Malinski (Norwalk, CT: Appleton-Century-Crofts, 1986).

[b]Rogers, "Science of Unitary," 4-5.

[c]Rogers, "Science of Unitary," 5.

[d]Violet M. Malinski, "Nursing Practice Within the Science of Unitary Human Beings," in *Explorations on Martha Rogers' Science of Unitary Human Beings*, ed. Violet M. Malinski (Norwalk, CT: Appleton-Century-Crofts, 1986), 26.

[e]Malinski, "Nursing Practice," 26.

[f]Malinski, "Nursing Practice," 26.

[g]Daily et al., "Unitary Human Beings," 230.

[h]Rogers, "Science of Unitary," 5.

[i]Daily et al., "Unitary Human Beings," 215.

[j]Rogers, "Science of Unitary," 5.

[k]Daily et al., "Unitary Human Beings," 216.

[l]Rogers, *Introduction*, 67-73.

[m]W. Richard Cowling, "The Relationship of Mystical Experience, Differentiation, and Creativity in College Students," in Malinski, *Explorations*, 131-39.

[n]Malinski, "Nursing Practice," 26.

[o]Daily et al., "Unitary Human Beings," 216.

[p]Malinski, "Nursing Practice," 29.

[q]Daily et al., "Unitary Human Beings," 216.

[r]Daily et al., "Unitary Human Beings," 214.

Table 2.1. *(continued)*

Jean Watson: Philosophy and Science of Caring[a] (Philosophy)

GOD	ENVIRONMENT	PERSON	HEALTH	NURSING
The sacred unconscious, the universal mind. A deeper higher energy source.	The universe is alive, conscious, intelligent and compassionate. Caring consciousness as energy within the human environment field of a caring moment.	Mind-body-spirit oneness; person-nature-universe as oneness. Transpersonal, transcendent, evolving consciousness. Consciousness as energy. Embodied spirit.	Health is consciousness; human-environmental energy field. Phenomenal field/unitary consciousness: unbroken wholeness and connectedness of all.	"Clinical Caritas (Love) Process." Nursing is a transpersonal caring relationship. Transpersonal caring is consciousness. Aims to facilitate individuals gaining "a higher degree of harmony within the mind, body and soul, which generates self-knowledge, self-reverence, self-healing and selfcare processes while allowing increasing diversity."

[a]See Jean Watson, *Postmodern Nursing and Beyond* (Edinburgh: Churchill Livingstone, 1999), 147.

Rosemarie Parse: The Human Becoming Theory[a] (Middle Range Theory)

GOD	ENVIRONMENT	PERSON	HEALTH	NURSING
Not clearly identified. "The universe" seems to fulfill the role of higher power.	"The universe." A pattern and organization of energy. Man and environment interchange energy to create what is in the world. Humans construct what is real for them from choices made from many realms of the universe.	The human is 1. coexisting while coconstituting, rhythmical patterns with the universe; 2. an open being, freely choosing meaning in situation, bearing responsibility for decisions; 3. a living unity continuously coconstituting, patterns of relating; and 4. transcending multidimensionally with the possibles.	Health is a synthesis of values, a way of living. A process of being and becoming. Becoming is 1. an open process, experienced by the human; 2. a rhythmically coconstituting human universe process; 3. the human's pattern of relating value priorities; 4. an intersubjective process of transcending with the possibles; and 5. human evolving.	Directed toward illuminating and mobilizing family interrelationships in light of the meaning given to health. "True presence," including: 1. Illuminating meaning. 2. Synchronizing rhythms. 3. Mobilizing transcendence.

[a]Rosemarie Rizzo Parse, ed., *The Human Becoming Theory in Practice and Research* (New York: National League for Nursing Press, 1995), 5-8, 81-83, and Rickard E. Lee et al., "Man-Living-Health," in *Nursing Theorists and Their Work*, ed. Ann Marriner-Tomey, 3rd ed. (St. Louis: Mosby, 1994), 445-59.

Case Study: Rachel and the Class She Couldn't Take

As a junior nursing student, Rachael was required to attend a weekly student-led seminar. During one class session, several students presented Therapeutic Touch (TT) as an alternative pain management technique. Rachael knew nothing about TT but felt uneasy about it. Later she learned that TT would be covered more thoroughly in an upcoming nursing lab.

Rachael began to discuss her concerns with several other students and to seek more information about TT. After reading articles in the *Journal of Christian Nursing* about the occult and Eastern religious roots of TT, she became increasingly concerned. She compiled the information she had collected and distributed it among her classmates. Rachael and one classmate decided to skip the lab.

Upon discussing the lab with classmates afterward, she discovered that not only had information about TT been presented, but students had also been required to practice it on each other. Many of the students who attended the lab were outraged by it. When one of the students brought up the subject in a clinical postconference, a heated discussion arose between the students and their instructor. Rachael explained what she had discovered in her research and offered to write a letter to the faculty about her concerns. The instructor urged her to do so.

Rachael's letter elaborated the points she had brought up in the postconference but also discussed the negative effects of TT (which were not mentioned in the lab) and the ethical issues regarding informed consent. She gave the letter to her instructor, who presented it to the faculty curriculum committee. The faculty complimented Rachael on her work. They decided to discontinue the lab and set restrictions on the way TT could be presented to students in the future.[22]

DISCUSSION QUESTIONS

1. Why do you think Rachael felt troubled by the presentation on Therapeutic Touch?

2. Describe your own experience with Therapeutic Touch, Reiki, and other alternative therapies. What troubles you? What intrigues you?

---

[22]Adapted from Rachael Foster, "The Class I Couldn't Take," *Journal of Christian Nursing* 15, no. 1 (1998): 8.

3. How has your school or work situation addressed alternative therapies? How have you responded?

4. Examine Rachael's responses. What did she do well? How would you handle the situation?

5. Worldviews not only affect spiritual issues but also ethics, economics, physical care, and interpersonal relationships. How do you see this reflected in your own nursing environment?

3

A CHRISTIAN VISION
FOR NURSING

Purpose: To determine the characteristics of a Christian worldview for nursing

Objectives: After reading this chapter and completing the exercises, you should be able to:
1. Explain a Christian view of nursing
2. Define *truth* according to Christian, modern, and postmodern worldviews
3. Describe each concept of the nursing metaparadigm according to a biblical worldview (person, environment, health, nursing)
4. Describe the implications of your own worldview on your vision for nursing practice

Keywords: theory, theology, holism, truth, worldview, Christian, Bible, Creator, Redeemer, Holy Spirit, modern, postmodern, metaparadigm, vision, person, environment, health, nursing

THE WAY THAT ORGANIZED NURSING began in Norway illustrates a common pattern for how nursing became established around the world. Ingeborg Gjersvik tells the story:

> Around 1850 Norway experienced a spiritual awakening which motivated an important social awakening. People began to see the need to care for the sick and the poor. The very thought of women caring for sick people outside of their own families, and furthermore establishing a training course to do so, was unheard of and unacceptable in Norwegian society at that time. However, many prayer groups were formed, asking for God's guidance in this matter.[1]

---

[1] Ingeborg Gjersvik, "A Heart of Compassion: How Nursing Started in Norway," *Journal of Christian Nursing* (1997): 12.

The answer to their prayers came through Cathinka Guldberg, a pastor's daughter who often made home visits to the sick with her father. One night Cathinka discovered that a homeless woman, who had been going from door to door begging for shelter, had been found frozen to death in the snow. Deeply convicted, Cathinka prayed about how she could make a difference. Soon afterward, she found a leaflet about the Kaiserswerth deaconess community in Germany and considered it an answer to her prayers. She studied nursing in Kaiserswerth, and then returned to begin a nurses' training program for deaconesses. The school expanded to include lay nurses. Soon, additional nursing schools were established, and nursing spread throughout Norway.

The beginning of nursing in Norway continues a long tradition of care for the sick that began in the early Christian church. This was a radical change from the pre-Christian society. Second-century theologian Tertullian noted, "It is our care of the helpless, our practice of loving-kindness that brands us in the eyes of many of our opponents. 'Only look,' they say, 'how they love one another! Look how they are prepared to die for one another.'"[2]

During a devastating third-century plague, historian Eusebius of Caesarea recorded, "The Christians were the only people who amid such terrible ills, showed their fellow-feelings and humanity by their actions. Day by day some would busy themselves by attending to the dead and burying them; others gathered in one spot all who were afflicted by hunger throughout the whole city and give them bread."[3]

Nursing grew out of a Christian worldview, in response to Jesus' teaching and example of caring for the sick. What was it about the Christian worldview that motivated the early church to reach out to the poor, the sick, and the marginalized?

While other worldviews of the time focused on gaining control of the physical elements and spiritual powers, the early Christians looked instead to God as one who deserved love and obedience and who inspired loving service to others. As we have seen, that tradition of caring for others in the form of nursing has continued throughout church history and shapes our vision for Christian nursing today.

---

[2] Quoted in Josephine Dolan, M. Louise Fitzpatrick, and Eleanor Krohn Herrmann, *Nursing in Society: A Historical Perspective*, 15th ed. (Philadelphia: W. B. Saunders, 1983), 43.
[3] Dolan, Fitzpatrick, and Herrmann, *Nursing in Society*, 43.

Nursing from a Christian Worldview

What we believe about God shapes our understanding of human persons and the environment in which we find ourselves. That, in turn, informs our concept of health and directs us to the means by which we nurture one another toward health and healing (see figure 3.1). So as Christians, we begin with a *theology* of nursing more than a philosophy or theory. By theology of nursing, we mean a biblically informed, God-centered view of nursing. If we truly believe what we say we believe about God, we cannot help but act in obedience to him, which means communicating the good news of salvation, health, and healing through word and deed.

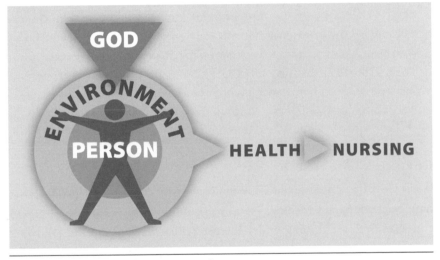

Figure 3.1. Nursing from a Christian perspective

The Christian worldview affirms good empirical science and the appropriate use of technology. They are gifts from God to be used for the benefit of creation. The methods of science give us knowledge of the physical aspects of creation. However, science has its limits. The personal, spiritual aspects of creation are veiled, and, while manifested in the physical world, they cannot be explained by science. The meaning of the personal and spiritual are seen only in the context of a larger worldview.

Christians also affirm many of the concerns and goals of nursing theorists described in chapter two, although our understanding of the concepts involved may differ. We share the concern for a more personal approach to health care, including the use of touch. We hold a holistic view of the person and recognize the need to provide comfort in human suffering. The Christian worldview includes the reality of the spiritual and unseen and the importance of faith and prayer. We recognize that there may be forms of physical energy that we cannot yet measure, and we reject the scientism that reduces all reality to physical or material phenomena.

The uniqueness of Christ-inspired nursing lies in its emphasis on caring for the whole person as embodied, respecting each person as created in the image of God. It is both a science and an art, but primarily it is a response to God's grace and a reflection of God's character.

The Nursing Metaparadigm

In the Christian worldview, the nursing metaparadigm begins with God. God created the world (environment) and everything in it. God created human beings (persons) and placed them within this created environment, to live in shalom (health). This kind of health allows the person to live at peace in a God-centered human community with a sense of physical, psychosocial and spiritual well-being. Nursing, then, works toward wholeness, or shalom among individuals and the community.

CHRISTIAN UNIQUENESS

While Christian values such as unconditional love and compassionate caring have been widely appreciated, even by postmodern nurses, other aspects of Christian faith are coming under intense criticism. Consider the following discussion that took place with a group of nursing faculty members.

"With increased diversity and the rapid proliferation of other religions in our society, nursing has to become more inclusive," one professor explained, then continued. "We have to be more open-minded and approach spirituality from a broader perspective."

Another added, "It is presumptuous for Christians to think they can know God better than people of other religions. Although the Christian faith is right for me, I think we have to respect their traditions as well."

"All truth is God's truth," interjected another. "If alternative therapies work, we should use them, regardless of the worldview behind them."

While all of these nurses are Christians, they are also postmodern in their understanding of spirituality. Their comments mirror the views of many in our society today. A Christian worldview cannot simply be superimposed on any other worldview. One of the unique features of Christianity—the one that grates most on the postmodern conscience—is that there is only one way for all people to know God. The Bible teaches that God singled out one people (the Hebrews) at a particular time and place in history to whom he revealed himself as the only true God. He drew firm boundaries, requiring absolute faithfulness. Any worship of other gods he labeled idolatry or spiritual adultery. He then took on human flesh in the one person of Jesus Christ, who said, "I am the way, and the truth, and the life. No one comes to the Father except through me" (Jn 14:6). You can't get much more exclusive.

However, Jesus also said, "I am the bread of life. Whoever comes to me will never be hungry, and whoever believes in me will never be thirsty. . . . This is indeed the will of my Father, that all who see the Son and believe in him may have eternal life; and I will raise them up on the last day" (Jn 6:35, 40).

God's offer of salvation is, in reality, the most *inclusive* belief system. He calls all of creation into relationship with himself. It is a free gift, but it is on his terms. When Job, in the Old Testament, questioned God's design, the Lord responded by charging, "Where were you when I laid the foundation of the earth? Tell me, if you have understanding" (Job 38:4). When we presume to know a better way than what God has revealed to us in Scripture, we are like children crying, "Everybody else is doing it!" Every wise parent knows that what "everybody else" is doing is not necessarily right or good. The call to be spiritually inclusive sounds virtuous but ends in practical rebellion against God. Furthermore, the kind of tolerance advocated by many people in our society is merely indifference, not kindness and compassion. This tolerance can be compared to nurses allowing patients to remain in bed too long because it hurts for them to move.

To see the effects of our belief systems on nursing practice today, we will first look at what we know about God, then briefly compare the concepts of the nursing metaparadigm in the Christian worldview to the other worldviews that prevail in our culture today, modernism and postmodernism. The chapters that follow will further explore the practical implications of the biblical worldview and other worldviews in the nursing metaparadigm. In the process we will discover some of the reasons why the present health care system has evolved into the impersonal, highly technological approach to care, while at the same time it has turned to a widening array of often unproven alternative therapies. We aim to propose a more satisfying alternative.

A Biblical View of God

A theology of nursing must be centered in Christian doctrine as contained in the Scriptures and affirmed by the historic Christian creeds. Although some Christian traditions would like to avoid referring to creedal formulations, preferring instead to claim "Christ alone" as their only creed, in today's religious climate the terms *God, Jesus,* and *Christ* mean many different things. The historic creeds of the church provide a definitive summary of essential theological understandings.

Theologian Timothy Lull explains:

> The early church discovered it could not live by Scripture alone in the simple sense of settling every question on the basis of biblical teaching. Some rule of faith was needed to distinguish true Christians from those many others who used Christian writings—and even the person of Jesus Christ—as a character in a very different story. The ancient world was full of competing religious groups, almost any one of which could incorporate the Jesus story in some way and use him for their own purposes.
>
> The three Creeds specify the precise Jesus story which is the authentic witness of the Bible. They speak with increasing precision and length about the God who loved the world, and about his coming among us in Jesus Christ. They speak of one God who made the world, but did not stand afar off when human beings fell into sin. Rather, "for us and for our salvation he came down from heaven and . . . was made man."[4]

The three creeds Lull references are the Apostles', Nicene, and Athanasian Creeds. The Apostles' Creed was developed in the second century out of a baptismal liturgy used by the church in Rome. The Nicene Creed was constructed by the Council of Nicea in 325 and revised to its present form in 381, to counter the heresy of Arianism (which denied the divinity of Christ). The Athanasian Creed developed in about the fifth century.

The trinitarian nature of God—Father, Son, and Holy Spirit—forms the basic structure for each of the historic creeds. God is described as Creator of the universe, who established both time and eternity; redeemer of the world, who entered history in human form to suffer and die for our sins; and sanctifier of his people, who continues to dwell among and within us. We can

---

[4]Timothy F. Lull, *Called to Confess Christ* (Philadelphia: Parish Life, 1980), 37.

The Apostles' Creed

I believe in God, the Father almighty,
creator of heaven and earth.
I believe in Jesus Christ, his only Son, our Lord.
who was conceived by the Holy Spirit
and born of the Virgin Mary,
suffered under Pontius Pilate,
was crucified, died, and was buried;
He descended to the dead.
On the third day he rose again.
He ascended into heaven,
and is seated at the right hand of the Father,
and he will come again to judge the living and the dead.
I believe in the Holy Spirit,
the holy catholic church,
the communion of saints,
the forgiveness of sins,
the resurrection of the body,
and the life everlasting. Amen.

know God personally, but we cannot become God or force him to do our bidding. Furthermore, we can know God only as he reveals himself to us. We cannot merely shape God into whatever we want him to be. The Bible calls that *idolatry*.[5]

God requires our obedience and faithfulness, and he cannot be manipulated or controlled (Job 38:4–40:1; Is 43:13). He is both transcendent (beyond us) and immanent (with us). The prophet Isaiah tells us, "Thus says the high and lofty one who inhabits eternity, whose name is Holy: I dwell in the high and holy place, and also with those who are contrite and humble in spirit, to revive the spirit of the humble, and to revive the heart of the contrite" (Is 57:15). We are to worship God in spirit and in truth (Jn 4:23), not turn to him as a good luck charm or try to bargain with him. He is not a celestial candy machine, ready to churn out treats if we insert the right coins.

---

[5]See Isaiah 44 for a graphic description of how God views our idolatry.

Just as the Christian creeds were developed in times of upheaval and controversy, when many conflicting views of God vied for adherents in the church, we need to clearly identify the essential components of Christian theology today. We believe that truth exists, as opposed to everyone creating their own truth. The problem of heterodoxy, or false doctrine, is not new. Many old heresies simply reappear in new forms, but as our culture moves from modernism to postmodernism, the lines may once again need to be drawn in new places. Jesus warned that false doctrines would develop and that his followers would need discernment:

> Not everyone who says to me, "Lord, Lord," will enter the kingdom of heaven, but only the one who does the will of my Father in heaven. On that day many will say to me, "Lord, Lord, did we not prophesy in your name, and cast out demons in your name, and do many deeds of power in your name?" Then I will declare to them, "I never knew you; go away from me, you evildoers." (Mt 7:21-23)

At strategic points in history, ecclesiastical councils, reformations, and revivals developed to root out heresy and reform the church. The reformers knew that the way people viewed God not only affected their worship and personal salvation but also shaped their ethics and morality—the way they related to one another, and their use and abuse of power. These results are evident in church history as it relates to nursing history. With a few exceptions, during times when the church remained faithful to Scripture and orthodox in beliefs, nursing flourished. When the church grew weak and corrupt, nursing suffered and declined.[6]

God the Creator. When Saint Paul preached to Greek philosophers in Athens, he commended them for being very religious and even erecting an altar to an unknown god. He claimed to know who this god was: "The God who made the world and everything in it, he who is Lord of heaven and of earth . . . he himself gives to all mortals life and breath and all things. From one ancestor he made all nations to inhabit the whole earth . . . he is not far from each one of us" (Acts 17:25-27). Paul then quoted two of their poets, "For 'In him [God] we live and move and have our being'; as even some of your own poets have said, 'For we too are his offspring'" (Acts 17:28). Paul was asserting what Jews

---

[6]Ann Bradshaw, *Lighting the Lamp: The Spiritual Dimension of Nursing Care* (London: Scutari, 1994), 97-169.

and Christians believe, that God alone is the only uncreated reality, the only being who is eternally self-existent. All else that exists, living and nonliving, is created and sustained by the Creator.

We are God's offspring in the sense that he created us. By asserting that all humanity descended from one ancestor, Paul affirmed the unity of the human race as well as the source of our life in God. Paul meant that we are totally dependent upon God for our life, *even if we do not recognize it.*[7]

While all created things are dependent upon the Creator, God, on the other hand, has life in himself. He is self-existent. Jesus said, "For just as the Father has life in himself, so he has granted the Son also to have life in himself" (Jn 5:26). Jesus, the Son, was both God and human (a mystery indeed), and here he was claiming to have the same self-existent life as God the Father. He spoke these words in the context of teaching about the resurrection of all who have ever lived and died. Saint Paul wrote of Jesus Christ, "He is the image of the invisible God, the firstborn of all creation; for in him all things in heaven and on earth were created, things visible and invisible, whether thrones or dominions or rulers or powers—all things have been created through him and for him. He himself is before all things, and in him all things hold together" (Col 1:15-17).

A loving heavenly father. Our knowledge of God is not something we can use to gain power over others. If we try it, we risk God's rejection (see Mt 7:21-23). Knowing God doesn't convey social status; instead it gives us a family identity. We understand God in terms of relationship—a relationship of faithfulness and trust. The Bible provides several vivid analogies. We relate to God as a child to a parent, as a bride to her husband, a sheep to its shepherd, and as a branch to the vine. These are intimate and essential relationships, necessary to create, sustain, and nurture life itself.

We understand God as Creator most clearly when we see him as our loving heavenly Father. While many people struggle with the idea of God as Father because their relationship with an earthly father was marred, that does not

---

[7]A word picture from the Old Testament envisions people being "bound in the bundle of the living under the care of the LORD your God" (1 Sam 25:29). Another picture is that of being held in God's hand: "In his hand is the life of every living thing and the breath of every human being" (Job 12:10). God is seen as a life-giving fountain of water: "For with you is the fountain of life; in your light we see light" (Ps 36:9). God is like a protective trail guide: "Bless our God, O peoples, let the sound of his praise be heard, who has kept us among the living, and has not let our feet slip" (Ps 66:8-9).

negate the imagery. For it is in looking at God that we see how a father should relate to his children.

We can learn a great deal about God from parenthood. In many ways we are all like two-year-olds who have broken away from our parents in a toy store. Surrounded by delightful playthings, we assume that they have been put there for us. We do not realize that they belong to someone else and will cost our parents dearly if we break them. Neither do we see the dangers that surround us. We cannot read the labels that say "Not safe for children under three." Nor do we realize that pedophiles may be lurking in the aisles waiting to abduct children. Furthermore, it does not occur to us that our parents may be frantically looking for us, while we wander gleefully among the goodies.

The love and pain that parents sometimes feel is nothing compared to the great love our heavenly Father has for us. Jesus tells us, "If you then, who are evil, know how to give good gifts to your children, how much more will your Father in heaven give good things to those who ask him!" (Mt 7:11). God faces the same tensions in his relationship to us, yet he remains absolutely faithful. The psalmist tells us, "As a father has compassion for his children, so the LORD has compassion for those who fear him" (Ps 103:13).

The fact that God is our Creator and Father indicates that we owe him our full allegiance and gratitude. Although we represent him in all that we do, we can never impersonate him, much less become God. However, the relationship we experience with God is intended to be one of joy and delight.

The implications of this fatherly relationship with God for nursing are abundant. We serve a loving God who truly cares for us—and for our patients. He knew us before we were formed in our mother's womb (Ps 139). He is concerned about our nutrition, hydration, and appearance (Mt 6:25-34). He knows us intimately, even the number of hairs on our heads (Mt 10:30); he calls us by name (Is 43:1). Not only is he aware of human suffering, he walks with us through it (Ex 3:12; Is 43:2) and suffers with us (Heb 2:9). We can trust him in the midst of our suffering, just as young children trust their parents, because we know he is faithful. First Peter 4:19 tells us, "Therefore, let those suffering in accordance with God's will entrust themselves to a faithful Creator, while continuing to do good."

While the biblical understanding of God certainly does not answer all the *why?* questions, it puts them into perspective. Children don't understand why they have to eat their vegetables, or struggle through learning to read and write, or suffer the pain of immunizations, but parents know what is best for them. In the same way, we do not know why our patients suffer and die, but we can be assured that God loves them and cares for them far more than we do. What a contrast to the modernist worldview that sees God (if he exists at all) as dispassionate and uninvolved with creation. The contrast is even starker when we compare the biblical view of God with an impersonal energy served by an array of amoral spirits who must be manipulated and appeased.

God in human form. God's relationship to his people is most clearly demonstrated in Jesus Christ. Jesus is not just a good example or cosmic consciousness. He is Almighty God himself who came to live among us as fully human. He shared our struggles, experienced excruciating pain, suffered and died so that we could be restored to full relationship with God, our heavenly Father.

> Since, then, we have a great high priest who has passed through the heavens, Jesus, the Son of God, let us hold fast to our confession. For we do not have a high priest who is unable to sympathize with our weaknesses, but we have one who in every respect has been tested as we are, yet without sin. Let us therefore approach the throne of grace with boldness, so that we may receive mercy and find grace to help in time of need. (Heb 4:14-16)

In Jesus we see God's presence with us in concrete terms. We know God is concerned about human illness and suffering because we can read about how Jesus healed the sick, cast out demons, and even raised the dead. Furthermore, his whole earthly life was ordered around the ultimate purpose of going to the cross to suffer *for* us so that we could escape eternal suffering. First Peter 2:24 tells us, "He himself bore our sins in his body on the cross, so that, free from sins, we might live for righteousness; by his wounds you have been healed."

It is through Jesus that we receive the motivation and power to care for others. He is the clear demonstration of God's love for us (Jn 3:16; 1 Jn 3:1), and it is because he first loved us that we can love others (1 Jn 4:19). Furthermore, he has blessed and commissioned us to go out in his name, continuing his works of caring, healing, and deliverance (Mt 28:19-20; Mk 16:17; Lk 10:9). In John 14:12 Jesus tells us, "The one who believes in me will also do the works that I do and, in fact, will do greater works than these."

Spirit of the living God. We experience God's ongoing intimate involvement in our lives through the work of the Holy Spirit. The Holy Spirit is not an energy field we can transmit, as practitioners of touch therapies sometimes claim, nor is it the spark of divinity inherent in human beings as might be claimed by some new religious movements. The Holy Spirit is God's personal presence.

Soon before his death, Jesus said that he would send the Holy Spirit as Counselor (Advocate) to be with us forever (Jn 14:16). This Spirit teaches us all things and guides us into truth, who comes from God the Father and bears witness to Jesus (Jn 14:25; 15:26; 16:13). The apostle Paul tells us, "Likewise the Spirit helps us in our weakness; for we do not know how to pray as we ought, but that very Spirit intercedes with sighs too deep for words. And God, who searches the heart, knows what is the mind of the Spirit, because the Spirit intercedes for the saints according to the will of God" (Rom 8:26-27).

The Holy Spirit bestows gifts upon us and produces godly fruit in our lives. The *gifts* are those things that empower us to serve others in Christ's name—wisdom, knowledge, faith, service, giving aid, acts of mercy, healing, working miracles, teaching, prophecy, exhortation, discernment of spirits, and tongues (Rom 12:6-8; 1 Cor 12:8-10). Through these gifts we are able to participate in the work of God's kingdom. We are not left on our own to try to conjure up the power and ability to face the weight of suffering and death in nursing; the Holy Spirit gives us all that we need. Once we realize that we do all good things in partnership with God, we can relax and allow God to work through us. Life—including nursing—becomes an amazing adventure where we are constantly surprised by God's great goodness.

The *fruit* of the Spirit is the character of God demonstrated in our lives—love, joy, peace, patience, kindness, generosity, faithfulness, gentleness, and self-control (Gal 5:22-23). Again, these are not personal accomplishments we have to strive toward. They simply result from the Holy Spirit living within us. Jesus said, "I am the vine, you are the branches. Those who abide in me and I in them bear much fruit, because apart from me you can do nothing" (Jn 15:5). As we spend time with God in prayer and live our lives in obedience to him, we will demonstrate the fruit of his Spirit and experience his power in our daily lives—while at the same time becoming intensely aware of our own inadequacy and sinfulness.

The only appropriate response to an encounter with this true God is a humble recognition of our own sinfulness and powerlessness. John tells us that the Holy Spirit will "prove the world wrong about sin and righteousness and judgment" (Jn 16:8). When we stand before our Holy God, we lose any of our culture's pretensions about being "basically good" or having "a basically positive direction."[8] The prophet Isaiah vividly described his response to an awesome encounter with God: "And I said: 'Woe is me! I am lost, for I am a man of unclean lips, and I live among a people of unclean lips; yet my eyes have seen the King, the LORD of hosts!'" (Is 6:5).

Our culture tends to view this recognition of human sinfulness as negative and goes to great lengths to avoid it. However, the biblical understanding of sin is one of the most liberating theological concepts in Christian doctrine. How else can we explain the ravages of war, illness, accidents, natural disasters, and all the abuse and violence in human relationships? Even those who do not acknowledge God insist that we must recognize our problems before we can do anything about them. It is our confession of sin that drives us to Jesus Christ as Savior to find forgiveness and redemption. It restores our perspective to see that God is on his throne; his kingdom is secure. Confessing our own sinfulness and experiencing God's forgiveness frees us to delight in the joy of his salvation.

This relationship of grace overflows into praise to God and a life of service to humanity. Nursing, as a public ministry of the church, developed out of this understanding of sin and redemption.

THE SEEN AND UNSEEN

The Christian worldview includes a spiritual dimension—things that we cannot see. In our own culture, scientism has blinded us to the reality of the spiritual world. The Bible affirms that the personal, spiritual, unseen world is real and was created by God (Eph 6:12). The Nicene Creed affirms, "We believe in one God, the Father, the Almighty, maker of heaven and earth, of all that is, *seen and unseen.*"

Spiritual beings are not merely psychological projections. They are personal, intelligent beings, and they have intentions toward us (Lk 22:31; 1 Pet 5:8-9;

---

[8]Carl R. Rogers, *On Becoming a Person* (Boston: Houghton Mifflin, 1961), 26. Rogers asserts that this understanding of persons as having strongly positive directional tendencies was basic to his personality theory.

Jas 4:7). One form of spiritual beings, angels, are God's servants under his authority (Col 1:16; Heb 1:14). God often directs them to protect and shelter his people (Gen 19:15; 1 Kings 19:5-7; Mt 4:6; Lk 1:30; 4:10; 22:43).

Another form of spiritual beings, evil spirits or demons, were also created by God but rebelled against him (Rev 12:9). They are beings who intend to deceive us about God and to control us, ultimately destroying us (1 Pet 5:8). We are not to worship angels or evil spirits or enter into collusion with them (Ps 91:11; Mt 26:53; Lk 4:10; Col 2:18).

Because demons deceive and destroy and because they are spiritually powerful and crafty, we are to have no dealings with them (1 Cor 10:20-21; 2 Cor 2:11; 1 Tim 4:1). Christians are protected from demons' power by being in Christ Jesus, but they constantly tempt us (Mt 28:18; Jn 8:31-32; Acts 19:11-20; Eph 6:11).

As we have noted previously, the four basic concepts that shape the nature of nursing are the *person, environment, health,* and *nursing.* We have found it necessary to begin with the concept of God to make sense of the concepts that follow. In the following chapters we will provide some basic definitions and understandings of these concepts based on a Christian worldview. They are summarized in table 3.1. Each concept will be more fully explored in the following chapters.

FOR FURTHER THINKING

Summarize what you believe about the following in one or two sentences:

God	
Person	
Environment	
Health	
Nursing (caring)	

Table 3.1. Worldviews in brief

Concept	Modern	Christian	Postmodern
PRIME REALITY/GOD	Higher Being may be acknowledged but is not involved in the world. Not important in human life.	Personal, triune (Father, Son, Holy Spirit), Creator and Sustainer, sovereign Lord of the universe, present with us. Jesus Christ is the way, the truth and the life. We worship God alone (Is 57:15).	May be impersonal energy (*ch'i, ki, prana, life force*), one with all things. Sometimes explained by quantum physics. May be personal and include gods or spirits. Manipulated for human desires.
ENVIRONMENT	Physical matter we control by science and technology. Exploited for human gain.	All things, seen and unseen, distinct from God but under his nurture and control, created good but polluted by sin, redeemed and to be re-created by God. Under human stewardship.	May be viewed as god(s), *energy* with no distinctions (only graded intensities), spiritual, and/or conscious. Physical matter may be considered illusion. Nature worshiped.
PERSON	Autonomous, body-soul dualism, biochemical processes, genetically or socially determined.	Created in image of God, sinful, integrated being, relational (to God and others), loved and redeemed by God, responsible and accountable.	*Human energy field*, related by collective unconscious, not distinct from the environment. Transpersonal body. The body is illusory. Divine spark within.
HEALTH	Absence of disease—aging and death are diseases to be cured.	Shalom—God-centered community characterized by peace, prosperity, rest, safety, security, justice, happiness, health, welfare and wholeness.	Expanded consciousness, balanced energy, wholeness, self-actualization, harmony with nature.
NURSING	Conquering illness through technology and scientifically determined care (*medical model*).	A ministry of compassionate care for the whole person in response to God's grace, which aims to foster optimum health (shalom) and bring comfort in suffering and death.	*Holistic*, "transpersonal caring" primarily in the mind, moves away from caring for the body. Manipulation of energy. May include ritual and contacting spirits.

THEOLOGICAL REFLECTION

Read Colossians 1, and fill in the chart again, using the information in this passage to define each of the concepts in the nursing metaparadigm:

God	
Person	
Environment	
Health	
Nursing (caring)	

1. How do the definitions according to Colossians 1 compare with your earlier definitions?

2. What would nursing look like, in practical terms, if it were based on these definitions?

3. How do the worldviews demonstrated in your own nursing environment compare with a Christian worldview?

4. What tensions arise from the differing worldviews of your employer, colleagues, and those in your care?

Case Study: A Spiritual Journey

Although JoAnn grew up in a Catholic family and attended a Baptist school of nursing, faith came hard for her. As a child, she explains, "I looked for him at church, through the Mass and the music, but I was never sure I had really discovered him." Sometimes she would challenge God to make a candle flicker at her command, but saw no response. She relates, "When I was a teenager, my view of Christianity was rather nebulous. I knew I was a sinner and felt guilty in God's presence, fearing his punishment. I didn't think much about Jesus' resurrection or his love for me. . . . Christianity wasn't too useful to me." However, because of her family's strong faith, she kept seeking God.

In high school she became intrigued with the transcendentalism of Emerson and Thoreau, which introduced her to Buddhist philosophy. She pursued Buddhism in college and volunteered to go to Vietnam as an Army nurse, hoping to learn more about Buddhism there. "Buddhism was attractive to me because it paralleled my own work ethic. Buddha is not a loving, interfering god, but is rather dispassionate and inaccessible. Thus the only love you find is what you create with your good works, what you do for yourself and others.

"I didn't want to rely on a god; I wanted to do things myself, get myself out of my own jams, and fix undesirable things in my life through meditation. I liked the idea that human beings can learn to become Buddha, able to take care of all problems. In fact my approach to nursing was to help people help themselves."

After returning from Vietnam she worked on a master's degree then began teaching nursing in a university program. Eventually her life began to unravel. Vietnam left lingering questions. Then a relationship with a man she loved ended. She explains, "At this point, I began to realize that Buddhism was not fulfilling my needs. It seemed as if my whole world had turned upside-down. I didn't know who I was or where I was going and could find nothing but futility in my life.

"My inner emptiness came clear to me one night in the hospital." A patient she had worked with for almost a year became seriously ill and asked JoAnn to pray for her. Feeling unable to pray, she replied, "I'll have to get somebody else to do it."

JoAnn explains, "That cut me to the core. I knew this woman and wanted to help her. But I had nothing to offer. I felt completely inadequate. I couldn't pray; I couldn't help her at all.

"I didn't realize that the Lord was working on me, pestering me! As it turned out, a whole group of students was praying for the faculty and specifically for me."

The students often talked about Jesus within JoAnn's hearing, gave her tracts, and offered to talk further with her. Eventually JoAnn read some of the tracts and was struck by a personal God who loved her enough to send his Son. She began frequenting a Christian bookstore and reading the Bible and books recommended by the store clerk. From her reading, she decided that she wanted to become a Christian. She then looked up the student who had offered to talk to her about Jesus to tell her of her new commitment. The student drove weekly to JoAnn's home to meet for Bible study and prayer.

JoAnn continues, "I had become a Buddhist for the security of being able to do everything for myself. Now I came to the Lord, gratefully letting go of that burden. The Lord gave me inner healing and understanding of who I am. He gave me knowledge that I am really loved, that I belong to him, that I can relinquish my feelings of inadequacy. I can just come to the Lord and say, 'You are completely able; my adequacy comes from you.' For me this is a whole new identity. . . . In fact I have become an agent of his healing. Several years ago my students were praying and reaching out to me. Now after experiencing God's love, forgiveness and healing, I'm eager to reach out to others."[9]

DISCUSSION QUESTIONS

1. What did JoAnn seem to be seeking as a teenager?

2. How does JoAnn describe her worldview as a Buddhist?

3. How did Buddhism affect her nursing practice?

4. How did her worldview change when she became a Christian?

5. What changed in her relationships with others? In her nursing practice?

6. In what ways does Christian faith foster excellence in nursing practice?

---

[9]Adapted from JoAnn Rollings, "My Search for God," *Journal of Christian Nursing* (1988): 14-17.

PART TWO

•••

THE PERSON

CARING IN
RELATIONSHIP

4

WHAT DOES IT MEAN
TO BE HUMAN?

Purpose: To describe the practical implications of our humanity

Objectives: After reading this chapter and completing the exercises,
you should be able to:

1. Explain the implications of the *imago Dei* (image of God)
for nursing care
2. Describe human nature from a Christian perspective
3. Explain the significance of human multidimensionality
for wellness and health care
4. Apply a Christian understanding of the person to
specific ethical dilemmas

Keywords: person, human, relational, multidimensional, sexual,
moral, mortal

ALICE WASN'T SURE WHAT TO EXPECT when she walked into her maternity patient's room after hearing morning report. During the night, the patient, an unmarried eighteen-year-old, had given birth to a baby with anencephaly. Alice had heard the pediatrician's rage that the mother had refused to terminate the pregnancy when the scan revealed the defect. Alice knew from the night shift nurse's report that the young mother had instead chosen perinatal palliative care for the baby. Nervous about what to say and even more anxious about what she would see, Alice whispered a quiet prayer and entered the room. She watched as the mother gently lifted baby Morgan out of his crib and held him close. Immediately, his high-pitched crying stopped, and his body relaxed. Alice took in the sight of a perfectly formed face, a blue stocking cap covering the anencephalic head, and she thought of the joy she had felt when her own children were born. "He's beautiful, isn't he?" asked the mother. Deep in her being, Alice realized that this child, though physically imperfect, was created in the image of God. "Yes," she answered. "He is beautiful."

THE IMAGE OF GOD

The Christian understanding of human beings as created in the image of God bestows dignity and honor on every person, regardless of social, mental, or physical status. The *imago Dei* (image of God) forms the basis of Western society's understanding of human rights and undergirds our legal system as well as our health care and social service agencies. But challenges from both modernism and postmodernism threaten to change this basic assumption, that all human beings are created in the image of God.

Consider this introductory statement in a textbook on family systems theory: "[Bowen] believed that a major obstacle to the acceptance of human behavior as a proper subject for scientific inquiry is that, traditionally, humankind has tended to consider itself a unique form of life, one with a special place in God's plan. Such self-glorification precludes our seeing the myriad ways we act just like other forms of life."[1]

The postmodern argument against viewing persons as the *imago Dei* takes a different tack. Drawing from an eclectic array of ancient and newly constructed religions and philosophies, as we have seen, many are beginning to view the earth as a living organism. Kleffel explains, "Humans are one functioning part of the totality and act in harmony within the organism."[2] In other words, human life is no more valuable than a rock or a raccoon. The philosophy reveals itself in the T-shirt slogan borne by Margie, a junior nursing student: "Save the rats, experiment on people."

Recognizing the *imago Dei* in each human being does suggest that we have a special place in God's plan, with serious moral consequences. We can own dogs, cats, and cattle, but not human slaves. We eat chickens and pigs for dinner, but not people—not even our enemies. We shoot lame horses, but not disabled veterans.

It was the *imago Dei* that drove Mother Teresa to care for the sick and dying in Calcutta, as it has motivated Christians throughout the centuries to care for the poor, the sick, and the disenfranchised. Whenever a society ceased to recognize the image of God in human beings, whether in the name of science,

---

[1]Roberta M. Gilbert, *Extraordinary Relationships: A New Way of Thinking About Human Interactions* (Minneapolis: Chronimed, 1992), viii. Despite Bowen's apparent dislike for the doctrine of the *imago Dei*, his theory is actually quite compatible with Christian thought.

[2]Dorothy Kleffel, *Exploring Our Environmental Connections* (New York: National League for Nursing Press, 1994), 9.

political ideology, religion, or simply greed, serious moral decay soon followed. We have only to look at the Nazi Holocaust, the decline of compassionate health care under the Communist regimes, and our own profit-driven health care system for vivid illustrations.

What is the *imago Dei?* The concept begins in Genesis 1:26: "Then God said, 'Let us make humankind in our image, according to our likeness; and let them have dominion over the fish of the sea, and over the birds of the air, and over the cattle, and over all the wild animals of the earth, and over every creeping thing that creeps upon the earth.'"

This single verse delivers a powerful threefold message. First, we are *created* and thus distinct from God, our Creator. Second, we somehow reflect the nature of God. And finally, God gives us a position of responsibility and authority over the rest of creation.

To be created in the image of God means that we must look to God for our meaning, purpose, value, and direction. It also makes us thinking, feeling, willing, relational creatures who reflect these attributes of our Creator. In order to understand ourselves in any depth, we must first look to God to know what he intended us to be. The late theologian Paul Jewett explained:

> The truth that we have our being as human only in a fellowship of an *I* and a *thou* in no way impugns the distinction between them. True, I cannot rightly understand myself apart from God who gave me my existence and my neighbor with whom I share that existence. But the boundary between the self and the other is an ineluctable one. Hence Christian theology rejects all pantheistic, mystical merging of the creature with the Creator and recognizes, at the human level, the uniqueness and worth of the personal self over against all other selves.[3]

It is not presumptuous to see ourselves as unique, valuable individuals with a delegated authority over creation. God has given us what every human being so desperately seeks. Each of us wants to be loved and recognized as significant. As Christians, we believe that our value and significance come from a loving God who sent His son to die for us while we were yet sinners. As the apostle Paul said, "In Him we live and move and have our being" Acts 17:28.

---

[3]Paul K. Jewett, *Who We Are: Our Dignity as Human* (Grand Rapids, MI: Eerdmans, 1996), 23.

Isaiah 43:1-3 reveals the extent to which God meets the human need for significance:

> But now thus says the LORD, he who created you, O Jacob, he who formed you, O Israel: Do not fear, for I have redeemed you; I have called you by name, you are mine. When you pass through the waters, I will be with you; and through the rivers, they shall not overwhelm you; when you walk through fire you shall not be burned, and the flame shall not consume you. For I am the LORD your God, the Holy One of Israel, your Savior.

In the face of sickness, death and other forms of distress, such an understanding of human existence provides the only satisfying explanation and offers the only real hope for the future. If we view ourselves merely as naturalistic beings who can control the physical environment at our will, we very quickly reach the limits of our powers. Science and technology bring us amazing capabilities, but they have yet to conquer death or rid the world of social or environmental problems. On the other hand, if we view ourselves as one with the universe, we are at the mercy of fate and the natural elements, with no basis for hope or for personal relationships.

The Genesis account tells us that God created everything good—in fact, *very* good (Gen 1:31). But something happened to mar that image. It happened soon after creation itself. For in creating us in his image, God also gave us the freedom to choose our own way over God's. By the third chapter of Genesis our first ancestors had already exercised that prerogative in a self-destructive way. We have been dealing with the consequences of sin ever since and repeating the same dysfunctional patterns generation after generation.

Hence, we cannot fully understand ourselves by empirical means alone. Nor can we know our true nature intuitively. Our observations and experience will always be colored by our fallen human nature. Not even science can be "value free." The only way we can know what God intended us to be is to look at Jesus Christ. Hebrews 1:3 tells us that "he [Jesus] is the reflection of God's glory and the exact imprint of God's very being." Theologian Jürgen Moltmann asserts, "Christian anthropology is an anthropology of the crucified Lord: it is in relation to this 'son of man' that man recognizes his truth and first becomes true man."[4]

---

[4]Jürgen Moltmann, *Man: Christian Anthropology in the Conflicts of the Present* (Philadelphia: Fortress, 1974), 20.

So what can we learn about ourselves and the persons entrusted to our care by looking at Jesus? First, we should be impressed that Jesus was a relational being. His relationship to God the Father is clearly described in Scripture, but he was also born into a very human family and community, and he saw himself as a citizen of both the kingdom of God and the political kingdom in which he resided. Second, Jesus demonstrated our multidimensional nature. By taking on human flesh, God reaffirmed the goodness of our physical bodies and human emotions without downplaying the importance of the spiritual aspect of our nature.

Third, Jesus showed us that we are sexual beings. He came as a man, "who in every respect has been tempted as we are, yet without sin" (Heb 4:15 RSV). Yet he also raised the status of women and was not afraid to use female metaphors for God's actions toward his people (see, for example, Mt 23:37).

Furthermore, Jesus demonstrated that God made us moral creatures who are to share God's love with our fellow creatures through ethical conduct and compassionate actions. Finally, Jesus showed us that we are mortals destined for eternal life. Even Jesus died, but he rose again in a new body that could not be destroyed.

Each of these characteristics of human existence holds profound implications for nursing. From them we draw our motivation for being nurses in the first place, but, more than that, they shape the nature of nursing itself. Em Olivia Bevis recognizes this fact by asserting, "Nursing works with people . . . and as such it is concerned with human welfare. To be concerned with human welfare is to act out of a belief in the worth of the individual and the worth of life."[5]

Seeing and Finding Ourselves in Jesus

- Relational
- Multidimensional
- Sexual
- Moral
- Mortal
- Destined for eternal life

---

[5]Em Olivia Bevis, *Curriculum Building in Nursing: A Process* (New York: National League for Nursing Press, 1989), 43-44.

What we believe about human beings and ultimately about God will determine how we treat one another. The Christian understanding of the person is that we are physically, psychosocially, and spiritually integrated sexual, moral, and mortal beings, created in God's image to live in relationship with God and others and as responsible stewards of the environment. If nurses lose sight of this understanding of human worth, human dignity, and human life, our profession will cease to exist, for there will no longer be any reason to provide nursing care. With this in mind we will investigate each of these aspects of human nature more carefully from a Christian perspective.

Relational Beings

The next two stories, based on actual events, illustrate the power of relationship for human beings. Joe Blevins, age eighty and in relatively good health except for minor short-term memory loss, was admitted to the same-day surgical unit for a stapedectomy. He expected to go home that same day, but an unexpected drop in his blood pressure led to an overnight hospital stay. When his son Bob arrived to get him the next morning, he explained to his father that the family could no longer care for him. So Joe would be going to an assisted living unit in a local retirement community instead of his familiar room at Bob's house. Joe reeled and stumbled into a nearby wheelchair, holding his head in his hands. "I don't feel good—get the nurse!" By the time the nurse arrived, only a few minutes later, Joe had spiked a fever of 104.6 degrees and seemed disoriented. He died of pneumonia three days later.

Mary Evans cared for her husband, Ken, as he grew increasingly debilitated from amyotrophic lateral sclerosis (ALS). Although exhausted from long hours of hard work, she maintained excellent health. After Ken's death, however, she began to catch every virus that went around. One Sunday morning during a blood pressure check, Mary told Susan, her faith community nurse, that she didn't have any reason to live now that Ken was gone. Susan told Mary that she could use her help teaching a class for the youth group about living with disabilities. Mary didn't think she had the energy, but she agreed to try. Three weeks into the course she was a different person. The teenage class members appreciated Mary's listening ear and soon began to drop by her house just to talk. Some deep friendships began to develop. Mary eventually became involved with a local support group for people with ALS and their families.

God created human beings to live in community. Consider Adam. God created Eve because he deemed that "it is not good that the man should be alone" (Gen 2:18). When people lose that sense of love and belonging, they lose their meaning and purpose in life. Without this sense of hope, they lose their will to live, and they may even die without apparent cause. Most experienced nurses could tell too many stories like the ones above. On the other hand, most could also tell stories about terminally ill patients who seemed to hang on against all odds until a son could return from military service or a strained relationship could be repaired.

The most basic unit of relationships is the family. The family was God's idea, and it holds a high place throughout the Bible. Psalm 68:5-6 (NIV) tells us, "A father to the fatherless, a defender of widows, is God in his holy dwelling. God sets the lonely in families." A cursory look at the book of Genesis reveals that these families were far from perfect. The family is marred by the same sin that pervades every human heart. Adam and Eve established the world's first dysfunctional family, where sibling rivalry eventually escalated to murder. The generations that followed continued in patterns of conflict, deceit, manipulation, and abuse. The Bible is strangely silent about how to deal with these dysfunctions. In fact, it almost seems as if God chose people we might label as narcissistic or borderline personalities for special honor and responsibility![6]

The biblical understanding of family went far beyond the nuclear family of today's North American culture. Ruth, who became an ancestor of Jesus, was taken in by a distant relative of her late husband (Ruth 4). The Old Testament makes it very clear that the people of God were to care for those people who did not have families. For example, God expresses his concern for those who have no families in Deuteronomy 10:17-18, saying, "For the LORD your God is God of gods and Lord of lords . . . who executes justice for the orphan and the widow, and who loves the strangers, providing them food and clothing." In Deuteronomy 27:19 he instructs, "Cursed be anyone who deprives the alien, the orphan, and the widow of justice." This theme is repeated throughout the Old Testament.[7]

---

[6]Consider, for example, Abraham, who twice allowed his wife to be taken into a foreign king's harem because he feared for his own life (Gen 12; 20). Lot offered his virgin daughters to an angry local mob to be raped (Gen 19). Jacob deceived his brother out of his birthright to become a patriarch of the nation of Israel (Gen 27).

[7]See, for example, Isaiah 1:17; Psalm 82:3; Job 31:18-22; Jeremiah 7:5-6; Ezekiel 22:7; Zechariah 7:9-10.

The New Testament expands the understanding of family to include the whole believing community. Jesus told his disciples, "For whoever does the will of my Father in heaven is my brother and sister and mother" (Mt 12:50). This theme of love and relatedness within the Christian community resonates throughout the New Testament. Jesus said, "I give you a new commandment, that you love one another. Just as I have loved you, you also should love one another. By this everyone will know that you are my disciples, if you have love for one another" (Jn 13:34-35).

However, throughout the New Testament we also see a clear recognition that this love will not come easily. The Gospels record how Jesus dealt with jealousy, prejudice, doubt, greed, abandonment, power ploys, and abuse from both his friends and his enemies. He suffered greatly in the process: in the end he was executed by those who felt threatened by his love. The rest of the New Testament gives detailed instructions to Christians about how we are to live in loving relationship with one another, including how to deal with strained and broken relationships.

This love expanded beyond the Christian community to also include the neighbor. When asked by a skeptical lawyer, "Who is my neighbor?" Jesus replied with the story of the good Samaritan (Lk 10:25-37). The neighbor in this case turned out to be a man of a different race, religion, and social status who willingly provided compassionate care for an injured man.

What this means for us as nurses is that we cannot adequately care for people if we see them only as isolated individuals. We view each one in the context of families, communities, and cultures. From this vantage point we can observe patterns that may contribute to illness or provide strength for healing. As we will see in chapter ten, human relationships are basic to a Christian understanding of health.

MULTIDIMENSIONAL BEINGS

Brothers Fred and Wayne hardly spoke to one another. Both were active members of the same church. Both spoke easily of their deep faith to friends at work and in the neighborhood. But mention one brother's name to the other and you could see his face flush and his neck veins stand out. Always competitive with one another, their rivalry had grown ugly when Fred accused Wayne of taking more than his share of their parents' estate. Their pastor tried to encourage them to forgive each other, but each replied, "Never!" Within ten years both developed serious coronary artery disease and hypertension. They died of myocardial infarctions within a year of each other.

The psalmist described a similar interrelationship between spiritual and physical problems: "While I kept silence, my body wasted away through my groaning all day long. For day and night your hand was heavy upon me; my strength was dried up as by the heat of summer. Then I acknowledged my sin to you, and I did not hide my iniquity; I said, 'I will confess my transgressions to the LORD,' and you forgave the guilt of my sin" (Ps 32:3-5).

Central to both the Old and New Testaments is the understanding of the person as an integrated whole. There is no body-mind dualism. Instead there is a vibrant sense of the person in relationship to God and the world through the bodily senses and functions.

First let's look at the Old Testament. In order to understand Hebrew terms, we must get inside the Semitic mind, keeping in mind two significant points. First, concepts like "heart," "soul," "flesh," and "spirit" are often interchangeable in Hebrew thought. Second, Hebrew thinking is stereometric, simultaneously presupposing "a synopsis of the members and organs of the human body with their capacities and functions."[8] In other words, often when a part of the body is mentioned, its function is implied.[9]

The Hebrew term *nepeš* refers to the person in need and encompasses everything from throat and neck to desire, soul, life, and the person as a whole. *Basar,* while referring to the body or flesh, essentially means the person in relationship and the person in weakness. *Rûaḥ,* referring to wind, breath, vital powers, spirit, feeling, and will, describes the person as empowered. Hence, the individual does not *have* a body, soul, or spirit, but *is* all of these things at once. *Leb* is the reasonable, thinking person, and it is tied to the heart. Ultimately the individual is always viewed in relationship.

The Hebrew concept of the human being provides a solid foundation for nursing theory and practice. Nursing is concerned about the whole person and how persons interrelate to maintain and restore health. For the Hebrew, health was found in a dynamic relationship with Yahweh. Sickness was both

---

[8]Hans Walter Wolff, *Anthropology of the Old Testament* (Philadelphia: Fortress, 1974), 8.
[9]For example, Isaiah 52:7, "How beautiful upon the mountains are the feet of the messenger who announces peace," refers not to the appearance of the feet but to their function in bringing the message.

a physical and a spiritual problem that warranted not only hygienic practices but also self-examination, confession, and prayer.

The New Testament also views the person in relationship to God as a total being. For instance, Paul closes his first letter to the Thessalonians by praying, "May the God of peace himself sanctify you entirely; and may your spirit and soul and body be kept sound and blameless at the coming of our Lord Jesus Christ" (1 Thess 5:23). Here he is speaking in the common Hebrew form of parallelism, repeating the same thought in different words. Rather than suggesting that people have three distinct parts (spirit, soul, body), he is simply referring to the sanctification of the whole person.

The most comprehensive New Testament term characterizing the person's total existence is the Greek word *sōma* (body).[10] A person does not have a *sōma* but is *sōma*, just as in the Old Testament a person does not have a *nephesh* but is *nephesh*. In a similar way, the terms *psychē* (soul, or life itself) and *pneuma* (spirit) are used by Paul to designate the person as a whole. When the terms are used in conjunction with one another, such as in 1 Thessalonians 5:23, they are intended to summarize the totality of a human being.[11] Furthermore, the terms *kardia* (*heart*) and *nous* (*mind*) are largely synonymous and designate the person as a "willing, planning, intending self."[12]

The body, soul, mind, spirit, and even the various body parts are expressions of the wholeness that is the human self. They designate the whole person as seen from different perspectives. All of these aspects are summed up in the term *zōē*: life that is given by God and makes the person the subject of his or her own actions.[13]

While this view does not divide the person into unrelated parts, it does allow for distinctions. A corpse is not a person because the *psychē* (in this case *life*) has departed from it. Our bodies are the way we experience life and relate to the world. But we are embodied spirits (or souls), and, to some degree, the spiritual takes preeminence over the physical. After death we will not be left disembodied but raised in "spiritual bodies" (1 Cor 15:35-57). Jewett explains: "When used of the human creature, 'spirit' refers to that vital principle which

---

[10]Here *Greek* refers to the Greek language, not Greek philosophy.

[11]Rudolf Bultmann, *Theology of the New Testament* (New York: Scribner's, 1951), 205.

[12]Bultmann, *Theology of the New Testament*, 220-21.

[13]Raymond E. Brown, Joseph A. Fitzmyer, and Roland E. Murphy, *The Jerome Biblical Commentary* (Englewood Cliffs, NJ: Prentice-Hall, 1968), 820.

animates the body and enables one to feel, think, will, and desire. As such, it is the seat of psychic experience and has essentially the same meaning as 'soul' (*psychē*). Being the seat of psychic experience, the human spirit is especially engaged as one relates to God."[14]

This view of the person is quite different from that of New Paradigm theorists who describe the person as an energy field. In the New Paradigm the body is merely an illusion or a lump of "congealed energy." It assumes that the spiritual is the only reality. Thus spiritual cultivation—mindfulness, meditation, and certain spiritual disciplines—become the means of escaping bodily ills and healing the physical body.

In the biblical view, spirit is personal, and each person's spirit is distinct from others'. On the other hand, the New Paradigm assumes that everything that exists is essentially energy; therefore, there are no real distinctions between the universe, people, or God. Hence, some New Paradigm theorists claim that we are really gods and goddesses—but at the same time, we are one with the frogs and rocks and trees.

The Bible teaches that God is not just an energy field, and neither are we. Although God creates people in his image, we remain creatures: we are not divine; we are not part of God. The body is the temple of the Holy Spirit.[15] God enters his people to enliven and inspire them, but we are not God and cannot become gods. However, God is both transcendent and immanent. In Isaiah 57:15 God says,

> For thus says the high and lofty one
>   who inhabits eternity, whose name is Holy:
> I dwell in the high and holy place,
>   and also with those who are contrite and humble in spirit,
> to revive the spirit of the humble,
>   and to revive the heart of the contrite.

God relates to us as a Father to his children (Mt 6:8; 7:11; Lk 12:32). In fact, through Jesus Christ, God became human in order to "sympathize with our weaknesses" (Heb 4:15).

---

[14]Jewett, *Who We Are*, 38.

[15]1 Cor 6:19. The temple was viewed as the dwelling place of God by the Jewish people. In Christianity this was expanded to realize that God dwelt among and within his people.

SEXUAL BEINGS

Scripture presents us as created sexual beings and even uses the sexual relationship in marriage as an analogy for God's relationship with us. Perhaps it is not surprising that human sexuality would hold such a lofty position. Because this aspect of our humanity is so essential to our identity, we experience our human weakness most acutely in this area. Most of us know sexual temptation; we must deal with sexual discrimination; all too often we see the broken lives that result from sexual abuse. But by creating us as male and female and declaring that *good*, God blesses sexuality as good.

Genesis 1:27 tells us, "God created humankind in his image, in the image of God he created them; male and female he created them." It is no accident that humans are both male and female. They are two complementary aspects of God's nature. His image is not complete in one gender alone. We need each other. That does not mean that everyone has to be married to be complete. Instead, we need to think and work together. Both all-male and all-female living or working situations tend to lead toward distortions of the way God intended us to live.

Mystics in past centuries extoled the sexual images of God, seeing God as a divine Lover. Our understanding of sex has been warped by sin, just as our relationship with God is marred by sin. Studying sexuality can teach us more about God's love for us.

Paul uses an analogy in Ephesians 5: "For no one ever hates his own body, but he nourishes and tenderly cares for it, just as Christ does for the church, because we are members of his body. 'For this reason a man will leave his father and mother and be joined to his wife, and the two will become one flesh.' This is a great mystery, and I am applying it to Christ and the church" (vv. 29-32).

Here we see that, just as the marriage relationship brings a man and a woman together in full unity, so Jesus draws us to himself and cares for us completely. We are not his individual lovers, but part of a body (the church) that is called "the bride of Christ." We must be a functioning part of that body in order to relate to God fully. But then, we see that our relationship with God naturally should be charged with passion and emotion (Ezek 16). It should be characterized by a deep desire to please him and to enjoy him. There is a sense of permanence and exclusivity. Nothing should be able to woo us away from our loving God.

God is deeply hurt by our unfaithfulness. He vividly demonstrated his pain in the book of Hosea when he told the prophet Hosea to marry a prostitute named Gomer. Gomer did not change her ways, and Hosea constantly grieved over her unfaithfulness and its disastrous effects on their family. When he had Hosea's full attention, God explained how the pain and destructiveness of Gomer's behavior related to Israel's and Judah's idolatry.

The analogy works the other way around too. We can learn about good sex from examining God's relationship with us. It is based on unselfish love. He is willing to sacrifice anything for us, even his own Son. His commitment does not waver, despite our weak faith and roaming eyes.

Later in Genesis we read, "Now the man knew his wife Eve, and she conceived" (4:1). The verb *to know* is not just a Hebrew euphemism for sexual intercourse. In Hosea 13:5 (RSV) God says, "It was I who knew you in the wilderness." Then he describes his commitment to love, nourish, and heal. "It is I who answer and look after you. I am like an evergreen cypress, from me comes your fruit" (Hos 14:8 RSV). Genital sexuality should always be placed in the context of absolute commitment. And the fruit of that union brings further commitment to care for it properly.

Because God created us as sexual beings, good nursing care must include working toward sexual health. Sexual function cannot be divided into a separate compartment, any more than nutrition, hydration, or exercise can. Sexual behavior affects not only a person's physical health but also self-image, interpersonal relationships, and relationship with God. Choosing to have sex outside of God's design of one man and one woman for life may affect a person's health and even their entire future. An unplanned pregnancy may result in unfulfilled dreams. A woman who ends her pregnancy in abortion may suffer a lifetime of guilt and shame. Sexually transmitted diseases may result in a lifetime of anguish or even death.

Sexuality encompasses the physical, emotional, and spiritual aspects of our being. Therefore, simplistic campaigns such as "safe sex" (advocating condoms to prevent venereal disease) or encouraging birth control to prevent pregnancy in single women do not truly promote sexual health. Sexual health involves engaging a person's total being in expressing sexuality—with or without sexual activity—according to God's plan in creation. It also includes an understanding of the role of gender in human relationships and an appreciation of the differences between men and women.

What does good nursing care include for people who because of disability or illness cannot experience genital sex? First of all, we need to acknowledge that this is a painful loss. Second, we can help such people to find their ultimate meaning and significance in God rather than in the sexual experience. However, all people still need human intimacy. We can offer and encourage appropriate caring touch and also give practical counsel on how to deal with sexual feelings.

Just as nurses will care for people from all cultures and religions, they will also care for people who identify as lesbian, gay, bisexual, transgender, or queer (LGBTQ). All people must be respected and treated with kindness and understanding. Assessing the sexual health and well-being of an LGBTQ patient may present challenges to some nurses, but that is also part of our nursing responsibility.

MORAL BEINGS

As sexuality only too clearly reminds us, God also created us to be moral beings. The fact that there are some boundaries around our sexual behavior implies that we must make moral choices. While the boundaries seem to be shifting much faster in today's world and the expanding choices may feel overwhelming, the problem is not new. The human struggle with morality began in the Garden of Eden.

> The LORD God took the man and put him in the garden of Eden to till it and keep it. And the LORD God commanded the man, "You may freely eat of every tree of the garden; but of the tree of the knowledge of good and evil you shall not eat, for in the day that you eat of it you shall die." (Gen 2:15-17)

> Now the serpent was more crafty than any other wild animal that the LORD God had made. He said to the woman, "Did God say, 'You shall not eat from any tree in the garden'?" The woman said to the serpent, "We may eat of the fruit of the trees in the garden; but God said, 'You shall not eat of the fruit of the tree that is in the middle of the garden, nor shall you touch it, or you shall die.'" But the serpent said to the woman, "You will not die; for God knows that when you eat of it your eyes will be opened, and you will be like God, knowing good and evil." So when the woman saw that the tree was good for food, and that it was a delight to the eyes, and that the tree was to be desired to make one wise, she took of its fruit and ate; and she also gave some to her husband, who was with her, and he ate. (Gen 3:1-6)

Played out right here in the very beginning, we can see the same tensions that we face today. God set a moral boundary. The serpent challenged it and convinced the woman to cross it. In the process, she moved from ethical absolutism to ethical relativism. But even then she did not reject morality entirely. She used an ethical decision-making process based on what was *good*. She rationalized that the good she saw through her own reasoning outweighed the good that God intended, and then she acted on her decision.

That moral sense is a key factor that separates human beings from the rest of the animals. Although the perception of what is good or just may differ from culture to culture and even from person to person, we are all born with some sense of fairness and a need for rules. Those who refuse to live by those moral boundaries are considered immoral.

Dogs, frogs, and amoebas cannot be immoral. If I leave my sandwich within range of my cocker spaniel and turn my back, she will grab it and disappear. I may yell "Bad dog!" at her, and she will sulk in a corner because she has displeased me, but she is not immoral. However, if I leave my wallet on the table, and my friend steals a twenty-dollar bill while I am not looking, she has committed an immoral act. We even use different language for human behavior. We don't accuse horses of lying, cheating, stealing, jealousy, murder, idolatry, or unfaithfulness. That is the language of human moral codes, including the Ten Commandments (Ex 20:1-17).

The problem of good and evil has occupied philosophers from the beginning of time. What makes the question so consuming is that the problem is not just in the external world—it is within us. The apostle Paul describes the dilemma this way: "So I find it to be a law that when I want to do what is good, evil lies close at hand. For I delight in the law of God in my inmost self, but I see in my members another law at war with the law of my mind, making me captive to the law of sin that dwells in my members. Wretched man that I am! Who will rescue me from this body of death?" (Rom 7:21-24).

The question of morality looms large for nurses, because our profession claims to be doing good for others. Nursing puts us face to face with issues and situations that demand a moral response. We have to know what the good is before we can do it, and the answers are not always clearly evident.

For example, during a rather intense ethical discussion, a frustrated nursing student shouted, "Don't give me alternatives; just tell me the Christian position!" She was not the first one to feel that way. Ethical decision making always puts us in an awkward situation. We are usually forced to choose the least-worst alternative, for there are seldom purely good solutions.

It would be nice if there were a clear Christian position on all the questions we face about life, death and morality. We wouldn't have to wrestle with gut-wrenching decisions or study ethics. We could just check out the manual on Christian positions, find the answer and go about our business. Some Christians have tried to make the Bible into such a manual, but it doesn't really provide us with clear directions about when to remove a ventilator, or the morality of altering human genes, or even an absolute definition of death.

The Bible does give us some absolutes by which to make ethical decisions. The Ten Commandments lay down the basics: honoring and remaining faithful to God, keeping the Sabbath, honoring our parents, protecting life, maintaining sexual faithfulness, respecting private property, practicing honesty and being content with what we have. Jesus summarized the commandments by saying, "'You shall love the Lord your God with all your heart, and with all your soul, and with all your mind.' This is the greatest and first commandment. And a second is like it: 'You shall love your neighbor as yourself.' On these two commandments hang all the law and the prophets" (Mt 22:37-40).

Being a moral Christian in the real world is not easy. The line between life and death is often blurred. New technology makes old definitions of death obsolete. The twentieth century has compounded the problem with the frantic pace of technological development, but the problem is not new. The poet James Russell Lowell (1819–1891) put it well:

> New occasions teach new duties;
> time makes ancient good uncouth;
> they must upward still and onward,
> who would keep abreast of truth.[16]

Truth doesn't change, but the context does. Our moral nature makes us strive to do good.

In a society lost in a sea of relativism, people are desperate for absolutes. Even those without a strong Christian faith are beginning to be alarmed by

---

[16]James Russel Lowell (1819–1891), "This Present Crisis," accessed at https://poets.org/poem/present-crisis.

the "if it feels good, do it" philosophy that has guided American ethics for the past several decades. When voters must decide whether physicians should be permitted to kill their patients, something is drastically wrong!

Many Christians are grasping for a solid dividing line between the morally acceptable and the unacceptable, fearing the slippery slope into antinomianism (lawlessness).[17] In the process, we have sometimes alienated or excommunicated one another, refusing to respect one another's decisions or methods of decision making. However, ethical decision making involves complex moral issues that may not have a perfect solution. We choose to act based on good thinking, Scripture, and prayer, and the Holy Spirit helps us discern the right alternatives. Ultimately, though, we have to trust that God knows our intentions are to please him and desire the best for those in our care.

MORTAL BEINGS

We are both moral and mortal. We struggle with questions of life and death. The preacher in Ecclesiastes tells us, "For everything there is a season, and a time for every matter under heaven: a time to be born, and a time to die" (Eccles 3:1-2).

We don't like to face our mortality. People have been seeking the "Fountain of Youth" from the beginning of time. Most of us deny our own mortality. Recently, a friend close to my age and I (Judy) struggled to stand up after sitting on the floor to watch a video. As I reached to assist her, she remarked, "I guess we're just feeling the effects of middle age." Suddenly the irony of her statement struck me. Although the definition of "middle age" seems to be getting progressively older as I age, I seriously doubt that I will live to be over a hundred!

Middle-class American culture clings to the hope in "progress" when it comes to death. If diet, exercise, and cosmetics can't hold death at bay, certainly medical technology will save us. We hide people who are dying in medical centers or long-term care facilities, and we bury those who have "passed on," their appearances improved by makeup, in what are sometimes called "memorial gardens." We thereby lose sight of our personal mortality— the fact that we will one day die. In this we tend to be an anomaly in human history and culture.

---

[17]Lawlessness was the charge that Martin Luther faced from his critics when he insisted that we are saved by grace alone.

In former times, and in many cultures today, people died at home, surrounded by family and friends. As a teenager I (Judy) remember my great uncle Otto lying in state in the parlor of his home. We sat around eating meals, telling family stories, even laughing. My aunt shuddered as she confided, "Every time I walk into this room I think of death." I had to agree that it felt a bit strange to be enjoying ourselves with Uncle Otto's body laid out in the open casket, but is it so bad that we were forced to think about death?

My own church building was constructed because the farmers in a rural area wanted a place to bury their dead. Today we complain that there is no room to expand because we cannot move the graves. But there is also a sense of continuity with the saints who have died in the Lord. Some of the older members have already erected their tombstones in anticipation of their own deaths. That is a healthy sense of human mortality.

We are mortals, but God has given us eternal life in Jesus Christ. We die, and yet we live. That is but one of the tensions that we embrace as Christians. We will explore the concept of death more fully in chapter twelve, but here let us briefly summarize the implications of this mortality for nursing. First, all human beings will die. Many of our patients will die in our care, but those deaths do not necessarily mean we have failed. Freed from the anxiety to preserve physical life at all costs, we can offer comfort, care, and hope in the face of death.

On the other hand, poor stewardship of the life God has given us may well exacerbate the death and decay that surround us. Poor diets, lack of exercise, substance abuse, environmental pollutants, dysfunctional relationships, and a host of other irresponsible human actions may hasten death. But God has instructed us: "I have set before you life and death, blessings and curses. Choose life so that you and your descendants may live, loving the Lord your God, obeying him, and holding fast to him; for that means life to you and length of days" (Deut 30:19-20).

As nurses who are mortal human beings, we have committed ourselves to choosing life in its fullness for ourselves and those in our care. We work toward health and healing. We fight death as an enemy. At the same time, we recognize our limitations, knowing that we are not able to control all circumstances, but remaining confident that we can know and trust the One who does.

Being human makes us glorious beings who reflect the nature of God. We are thinking, feeling, willful beings, embodied spirits who are moral and mortal. Although God created us to live in relationship with himself, we struggle with sin and are constantly rebelling against God and wounding our neighbors. Yet God restores us to himself through Jesus Christ. In Jesus we find our true humanity, freeing us to love and care for others.

FOR FURTHER THINKING

1. If someone asked you to describe who you are, what would you say?

2. What makes us human?

THEOLOGICAL REFLECTION

Read Genesis 1:26-31, Psalm 8:3-6, Psalm 32:3-5, Isaiah 43:1-7, John 3:16, and Ephesians 4:1-3.

1. What do each of these passages tell us about God's purpose for human beings?

2. How do they describe the physical dimension of persons?

3. How does the psychosocial dimension affect the physical?

4. What is sin? What role does sin play in human health and illness?

Case Study: Is It Gonna Leave a Scar?

A winter storm resulted in a busy night in the emergency room. Accident victims were arriving two to an ambulance. Then a message came that a rescue unit would be arriving with an injured four-year-old child and her father, who was also injured. Another crew was on the way with John (twenty-two), the driver of the other car, who appeared to be intoxicated.

The trauma team was ready for the child, but her injuries were too severe. She died. Her father was mildly injured, but he would be okay physically. The question among the staff was, "Who's going to take care of the drunk that killed the little girl?"

John arrived strapped to a spine board and yelling about his pain. His face was cut from hitting the windshield. Significant head and neck injuries were ruled out with a CT scan and x-rays. His only injuries appeared to be the facial lacerations.

Upon returning from x-ray, he was still noisy, obnoxious, and reeking of alcohol. His blood level was greater than 0.1, legally drunk. He continued to yell, voicing concerns about himself but never asking about those in the other car. All he wanted to know was, "Is it gonna leave a scar?" Is it going to leave a scar? We were incredulous. How could he think only of that?

The ER began to quiet down, and it became apparent that Sara, a nurse practitioner, would sew up John's cut face. As she gathered the needed supplies, some of the staff suggested that she use 2-0 silk suture, certain to leave a scar, and forego any anesthetic.

As John lay on the gurney with his head draped, he continued to ask, "Is it gonna leave a scar?"

Sara worked efficiently and quietly, trying to avoid conversation with him. She took tiny stitches with small caliber nylon suture. John remained uncooperative throughout, periodically sitting up and demanding a mirror.

The ER staff specialized in difficult patients, especially the late-night crew. They were used to dealing with the drunk and the drugged, the homeless, the helpless, the hopeless, the mentally ill, the physically injured, those near death and those wishing they were, child abuse, sexual abuse, elder abuse, those whose hearts were failing and those whose hearts were breaking. As a staff, they cared for all of these and more.

Sara cared deeply for the child John killed and for her family, but she also began to feel compassion as she cared for John. Sara reflected, "Could I have cared more? Yes, I am certain of that. In a similar situation, would I care more now, some twelve years later? I hope so. I hope that I have grown in my faith over the ensuing years, so my compassion and kindness for John would come more graciously.

"At some level that night, I understood that John was created by God. God loved him, even though his actions had taken the life of a child. I believe that I grew a little in my understanding of God's love and grace and what it is to be an instrument of God's peace. I chose not to inflict more pain on John in the way I sewed up his face. I supposed that someday, on some level, he would have to deal with the pain he had caused others, so it wasn't for me to cause him any more than necessary."[18]

---

[18]Adapted from Sara P. Campbell, "Is It Gonna Leave a Scar?," *Journal of Christian Nursing* 15, no. 2 (2003): 6-7.

DISCUSSION QUESTIONS

1. Who was more "human" in this story: the dead child or John?

2. How would you feel if you were assigned to care for John?

3. What would you be thinking as you cared for him?

4. In this situation how did sin affect human health?

5. Describe the person you found the most difficult to care for in your nursing practice.

6. How did you handle the situation?

7. What could you have done better?

8. How does viewing a person as created in God's image help you to care for those who seem hard to love?

5

THE PERSON AS
A SPIRITUAL BEING

Purpose:	To describe the spiritual dimension of personhood
Objectives:	After reading this chapter and completing the exercises, you should be able to:
	1. Identify three critical attributes of spirituality found in nursing literature
	2. Compare mysticism in Christian and monistic traditions
	3. Articulate an understanding of Christian spirituality
	4. Describe the relationship between spirituality and health care
Keywords:	spiritual, spirituality, religion, belief, prayer, mysticism, monism, *ruah*, occult, energy-based therapies

ANNA MOANED IN PAIN. She was three days post-op from removal of abdominal adhesions, and everything indicated that she was healing well, but the pain continued. Nothing seemed to help. I (Judy) had given her all the PRN analgesics she could have and called her physician to have the dosage increased. He refused. I tried rubbing her back, bringing her a cup of tea, and turning her radio to some soothing music. Still her muscles tightened in agony. "Why does God allow me to suffer so?" She moaned, "He must hate me!"

From her clenched fist dangled a rosary. An idea struck me. "Do you think God hated *him*?" I asked, pointing to the crucifix.

"Of course not—he *was* God!" Anna replied.

We continued to talk about God's love for us being demonstrated in the cross of Christ. Then I offered to pray for her. Afterward Anna's muscles slowly relaxed, and the pain eased. She slept through the night.

While most nurses would quickly acknowledge that Anna's pain stemmed from more than physical causes at this point, they would probably attribute it to psychological factors. However, Anna's problem was spiritual. Further discussions with her revealed a complicated web of broken family relationships and a painful estrangement from her church. Anna harbored a deep anger toward her former husband, her son, the church, and God. She figured that God must hate her as well.

My friend Martha would have a different approach, although her assessment of the problem would be similar. I met Martha at a nursing convention and liked her immediately. A devout Roman Catholic, Martha taught a course on therapeutic touch and other alternative therapies in her church-related college nursing program. She enthusiastically described how these energy-based therapies brought marked relief almost every time she used them.

After listening for several minutes, I finally asked her about the source of the energy she believed she was channeling. "Oh, it's the Holy Spirit!" she said happily. As I probed further, it became apparent that she was working from an eclectic worldview. In typical Western fashion she had put her Christian beliefs into the category of "religion" but somehow reserved a pragmatic area for what she called "spirituality," which she could relate to her nursing practice. For Martha, spirituality dwelt in the worldview of monistic energy fields, which she envisioned as the Holy Spirit.

"It makes me kind of nervous to think of trying to manipulate God," I replied, trying to gently move her toward thinking about the implications of what she was doing.

"But we are *supposed* to be channels of the Holy Spirit," she continued. "It's just the laying on of hands with another name."

It soon became apparent that our conversation might quickly degenerate into a fruitless argument, so we changed the subject. However, Martha kept coming back to talk more. By the end of the week we were friends. Although we respected each other, neither of us changed the other's mind.

What differentiates the spiritual from the physical or psychological? We have already established that these aspects are not separate parts of a person, but that they can be distinguished. Our dualistic Western culture would like to see the spiritual as either nonexistent or irrelevant. It would say that Anna's pain should be controlled with the proper medical or surgical intervention, or at least a psychiatric consultation if all else failed. In this worldview, reality is essentially physical or material. However, in the face of Anna's very real pain, the spiritual dimension had to be addressed in order to bring relief.

On the other hand, Martha and other proponents of new spiritualities would argue that the heart of *all* Anna's problems was spiritual, and that they could be corrected by techniques to balance her universal energy flow. Although most advocates of the new spiritualities also use Western allopathic remedies, they do so with reluctance. In this worldview, reality is essentially spiritual.

In the Christian worldview, spirituality is essentially relationship—a relationship of the whole person to a personal God and to other people (or other spirits). The spiritual is always personal. It is not an impersonal energy force. The personal nature of spirituality imbues it with deep moral and ethical implications. The late theologian Dallas Willard explains, "Spirituality is simply the holistic quality of human life as it was meant to be, at the center of which is our relation to God."[1] He further elaborates, "The spiritual is a homogeneous aspect, part and parcel of the biological (and therefore social) nature of human beings."[2]

The spiritual is always personal.

SPIRITUALITY IN NURSING

The nursing literature reflects our culture's changing understanding of spirituality. Although earlier definitions attempted to differentiate spirituality from religion, most saw spirituality as involving a person's relationship with God, while later references began to view it as an impersonal life principle.

Joan Haase and others attempted to synthesize the definitions of spirituality in the nursing literature. They came to the conclusion that while spirituality was consistently seen as a basic or inherent quality of all human beings, what differed was spiritual perspective, which they defined as "a highly individualized awareness of one's spirituality and its qualities." They found three critical attributes of spiritual perspective: (1) connectedness (with others, nature, the universe or God), (2) belief (in something greater

---

[1]Dallas Willard, *The Spirit of the Disciplines* (San Francisco: HarperSanFrancisco, 1988), 77.
[2]Willard, *Spirit of the Disciplines*, 78.

than the self), and (3) creative energy "that is in constant, yet dynamic, evolutionary flux."[3]

Based on these attributes, they defined spiritual perspective as "an integrating and creative energy based on a belief in, and a feeling of interconnectedness with, a power greater than self." Their literature review also found three apparent outcomes of spirituality: (1) purpose and meaning, (2) guidance of human values, and (3) self-transcendence.[4] However, the worldviews inherent in the articles they surveyed were not differentiated, so that they merely combined and summarized incompatible spiritual perspectives.

Using concept analysis, Emblen investigated the terms *spiritual* and *spirituality* in the nursing literature, comparing them with the concept of *religion*. In definitions of *religion*, six terms appeared most frequently: *system, beliefs, organized, person, worship,* and *practices*. On the other hand, *spirituality* was associated with the terms *personal, life, principle, animator, being, God (god), quality, relationship,* and *transcendent*. By using these terms to form consensus definitions, Emblen concluded that *spirituality* is a broader term that may include some aspects of religion. However, she also notes that "the term *spiritual* is rapidly acquiring new and varied definitions."[5]

In a concept analysis aimed to define spirituality, Buck asserts that while nurses view the term *spirituality* as a concept that transcends religion, patients see spirituality as synonymous with religion. Such a divergence in conceptual meaning may make spiritual assessment challenging. Furthermore, Buck cites fear of offending a patient or feelings of inadequacy as barriers to delivering spiritual care. She proposes a "Model of Integrated Spirituality" as a theoretical guide for nurses in their holistic assessment of patients' spiritual needs. The model illustrates the domains of spirituality as concentric circles, with the inner most layer as the intrapersonal, the middle layer as interpersonal, and the outer layer as transpersonal connectedness. She describes the criteria of spirituality as intrinsically human, both ontological and teleological, self-transcendent, connecting with others, nature, and a Supreme Being, and the

---

[3]Joan E. Haase, Teri Britt, Doris D. Coward, Nancy Kline Leidy, and Patricia E. Penn, "Simultaneous Concept Analysis of Spiritual Perspective, Hope, Acceptance and Self-Transcendence," *Image* (1992): 143.

[4]Haase et al., "Simultaneous Concept Analysis," 143.

[5]Julia D. Emblen, "*Religion* and *Spirituality* Defined According to Current Use in Nursing Literature," *Journal of Professional Nursing* (1992): 41.

optional presence of religious traditions. Upon review of the concept in the nursing literature, Buck assigns the following conceptual meaning to spirituality: "that most human of experiences that seeks to transcend self and find meaning and purpose through connection with others, nature, and/or a Supreme Being, which may or may not involve religious structures or traditions."[6]

An earlier study by Burkhardt summarized definitions of terms related to spirituality, showing a wide variation but concluding that "spirituality goes beyond a focus on religiosity" and "spiritual care needs to be based on a more universal concept of inspiriting rather than religion or religiosity."[7] She further concludes, quoting from Viktor Frankl, "The concept of spiriting has no antecedents. Spiriting is 'a thing in itself. It cannot be explained by something not spiritual; it is irreducible. It may be conditioned by something without being caused by it.'"[8]

If such is the case, the idea of a generic, broadly defined spirituality raises serious concerns for the Christian nurse. The spiritual world is not neutral, as most nursing authors seem to imply. The Bible makes it quite clear that when we seek a spirituality apart from the Spirit of God, we open the way for the work of evil spirits (Mt 12:43-45; Col 2:8; Eph 5:6-17; 1 Tim 4:1).

Willard explained that there are two directions that spirituality can take in today's culture, Christian or "general human interest." He further clarified,

> Much of modern thinking views spirituality as simply a kind of "interiority"— the idea that there is an inside to the human being, and that is the place where contact is made with the transcendental. In this view, spirituality is essentially a human dimension.
>
> Christian spirituality is centered in the idea of a transcendent life—"being born from above," as the New Testament puts it. This idea of the spiritual life carries with it the notions like accountability, judgment, the need for justice, and so on. These concepts are less popular, and they are certainly more difficult, than a conception of spirituality that simply focuses on one's inner life.[9]

---

[6]Harleah G. Buck, "Spirituality: Concept Analysis and Model Development," *Holistic Nursing Practice*, November–December 2006, 289-90.

[7]Margaret A. Burkhardt, "Spirituality: An Analysis of the Concept," *Holistic Nursing Practice*, April 1989, 71.

[8]Burkhardt, "Spirituality," 73-74.

[9]Dallas Willard, "What Makes Spirituality Christian?," *Christianity Today*, March 6, 1995, 16.

In other words, secular spirituality is an aspect of human nature to be nurtured. It may include human relationships, but it is usually an inner experience. According to Steve Turner, "As used in secular discourse, *spiritual* can refer to anything that cannot either be tested in a laboratory or bolted to the floor."[10] On the other hand, the Bible presents spirituality as an encounter with a spiritual being separate from ourselves—either God or an evil spirit. Christian spirituality is essentially a personal relationship with God. Turner explains,

> Christian conversion is not a case of fanning that little spiritual spark in the human soul into a flame. It is a case of invading a dark and doomed soul with spiritual light from above.
>
> Christian spirituality does not originate in a small area of the human brain. It is a transference of God's personality into the human life, and it can only happen on the basis of repentance, faith, and discipleship. It cannot be coaxed, kick-started, or chanted into being. The original temptation is that we can become divine through a mechanical act.[11]

Martin Luther reacted strongly against the mystics of his day, believing that "enthusiasm" (in its technical sense of being inspired or possessed by a god) was the essence of original sin.[12] Salvation must come from outside ourselves.

THE CHRISTIAN SPIRITUAL TRADITION

The Christian church does have a rich mystical tradition, which receded during the Enlightenment and the rise of empiricism. Mysticism refers to "the immediate experience of a divine-human relationship, and in particular to the experiences of oneness with a divine . . . being or state."[13] We affirm that there is much in this tradition that should be restored and enjoyed. Mysticism unchecked, however, frequently leads to serious heresy and corruption in the church and blurs the uniqueness of the Christian gospel. Psychologist Elizabeth Hillstrom points out that mystical writers from Maharishi Mahesh Yogi to Christian mystics like Saint John of the Cross all warn about the dangers of "madness, demonic deception or possession for those who venture into the

---

[10]Steve Turner, "Lean, Green, and Meaningless," *Christianity Today*, September 24, 1990, 26-27.
[11]Turner, "Lean, Green, and Meaningless," 26-27.
[12]Gerhard O. Forde, "A Lutheran Response," in *Christian Spirituality*, ed. Donald L. Alexander (Downers Grove, IL: InterVarsity Press, 1988), 192.
[13]Irving Hexham, *Concise Dictionary of Religion* (Downers Grove, IL: InterVarsity Press, 1993), 153.

mystical path."[14] Richard Foster describes the goal of true Christian mysticism: "In meditative prayer there is no loss of identity, no merging with the cosmic consciousness, no fanciful astral travel. Rather, we are called to life-transforming obedience because we have encountered the living God of Abraham, Isaac, and Jacob. Christ is truly present among us to heal us, to forgive us, to change us, to empower us."[15]

The Bible is the central reference point in Christian mysticism. The mystical experience must always be tested by the Scriptures, not the other way around. When mysticism moves beyond biblical limits, it ceases to be Christian, even when Christian terminology is retained.

> *The mystical experience must always be tested by the Scriptures, not the other way around.*

In reviewing the history of Christian spirituality, George Lane defines spirituality as "man's possession by God in Christ through the Holy Spirit."[16] We first see this understanding of spirituality demonstrated by Jesus as he prays in John 17: "And for their sakes I sanctify myself, so that they also may be sanctified in truth. I ask not only on behalf of these, but also on behalf of those who will believe in me through their word, that they may all be one. As you, Father, are in me and I am in you, may they also be in us, so that the world may believe that you have sent me" (vv. 19-21).

In this context Jesus is not referring to "oneness" as a monistic merging with God but as a dynamic personal relationship that results in a oneness of purpose and a reflection of Christ's character in his followers. This understanding of "union" or "oneness" with God is what separates Christian spirituality from all others.

Monism, the belief that "all is one," has challenged Christian faith from the very beginning. The early church faced attacks and subtle corruption by Gnosticism (teaching that salvation was obtained through a secret knowledge) and Platonic philosophy (which sought salvation through ascetic practices

---

[14]Elizabeth L. Hillstrom, *Testing the Spirits* (Downers Grove, IL: InterVarsity Press, 1995), 132.

[15]Richard J. Foster, *Prayer: Finding the Heart's True Home* (San Francisco: HarperSanFrancisco, 1992), 149.

[16]George A. Lane, *Christian Spirituality—An Historical Sketch* (Chicago: Loyola University Press, 1984), 2.

and mystical experiences). Both of those influences taught a spiritual monism—that each person had a "divine spark," or a pure soul, that was imprisoned by a corrupt body. The goal of each divine spark was to shed the confines of the evil body to be rejoined with God. Both the Gnosticism of New Testament times and the later Neoplatonism (third through sixth centuries) incorporated magic and sorcery. The early church fathers were unanimous in pointing to Simon the Magician in Acts 8 as the first Gnostic.[17] We see further evidence of these influences in many of the concerns that New Testament writers express to first-century churches in the Epistles.

Monism is an assumption that there is one eternal principle in the cosmos. It therefore denies a Creator above and separate from creation. It began around the sixth century BC in India and China, gradually spreading to Persia and later to Europe.[18] It appeared in various forms, such as Hinduism, Taoism, Buddhism, Gnosticism, and Neoplatonism. Today, we see it reappearing in New Age religions.

The appeal of monism comes from its assumption that all is One, and therefore all is God. This makes everyone God, removing all external ethical constraints. It is also highly experiential, seeking mystical union with God through meditation, dreams, and visions. This experience then becomes the source of truth for the monist.

Historically, when Christians practiced mysticism, monism often followed; church leaders from Paul to Luther made strong efforts to control it. Prophecy, in the sense of delivering an inspired message from God, is a form of mysticism. The New Testament and early Christian writings, such as the *Didache* (second century) set firm limits on the authority of anyone claiming to have gained knowledge through mystical means (Mt 7:15; 24:24; 1 Cor 14:37-40; 2 Pet 2:1-3; 1 Jn 4:1-6).

Several significant periods in church history produced outbreaks of mysticism—what many Christians would call spirituality today. The first evidence came in the book of Acts and continued through the second and early third centuries. It was a time of intense persecution, and God seems to have provided powerful experiences to give the young church the encouragement and

---

[17]E. M. Yamauchi, "Gnosticism," in *New Dictionary of Theology*, ed. Sinclair B. Ferguson, David F. Wright, and J. I. Packer (Downers Grove, IL: InterVarsity Press, 1988), 272.

[18]Robert Brow, *Religion: Origins and Ideas* (Downers Grove, IL: InterVarsity Press, 1966), 33-36.

sense of mission to survive and grow in a hostile environment. Outstanding mystics from this period included Origen (AD 185–254), an influential teacher in the early church, and Montanus, founder of a prophetic movement that began about 170. Origen was a brilliant scholar who struggled to reconcile his Christian faith with Greek philosophy. He was strongly influenced by Neo-platonism but tried to use it in the service of Christian doctrine. The flam-boyant cult leader Montanus, along with his female disciples Prisca and Maximilla, claimed to speak for the Holy Spirit while in ecstatic states.[19] Both met with strong criticism from the church, yet both also contributed to the rich history of the church's mystical tradition.

In the fourth century a new type of spirituality developed. Christianity had become the state religion with the conversion of Constantine. The church was corrupt, politicized, and spiritually weak. The "desert fathers," including Anthony the Hermit, sought union with God by fleeing to the Egyptian desert to escape the distractions of the world. These monks lived alone in the desert, often exhibiting bizarre behavior (extreme fasting, refusing to bathe, living at the top of tall pillars), but they were often visited by Christians seeking divine guidance, healing, or deliverance from evil spirits. Some of these monks moved away from orthodox Christian teachings and into monism as they became consumed with mystical experiences and the contemplative life.

As life in the desert grew increasingly difficult, many of the monks began to cluster in monasteries. By the sixth century these monastic orders, under the influence of Benedict, became less focused on personal sanctification and more concerned about community life and reaching out to the world in charity and evangelism. One shining light for nursing in the twelfth century, Hildegard of Bingen, came from the Benedictine community. A spiritual leader and visionary who was also an expert in the use of herbs and midwifery, she wrote two books on healing.[20] By the thirteenth century the mendicant orders, led by the Dominicans and Franciscans, lived a common life with the explicit purpose of going out into the world to serve and to preach the gospel. They attempted to balance spirituality and service.

Overshadowed by the horrors of the Black Death, the Hundred Years War, and scandalous corruption in the church, the fourteenth and fifteenth

---

[19]Henry Chadwick, *The Early Church* (Grand Rapids, MI: Eerdmans, 1967), 52.
[20]Linda E. Sabin, "Hildegard of Bingen: A Woman of Vision," *Journal of Christian Nursing* (1987): 8-9.

centuries produced a new round of mystical spirituality. The most famous Rhineland mystic of this period, Meister Eckhart, taught a mystical union with God in the Neoplatonic tradition and was condemned by the church for "pantheism."[21] A bright light in this period was Julian of Norwich, an English mystic with a vibrant relationship with God. Her deep faith led her to reach out in compassion to others. Although Julian, as an anchoress, was not allowed to leave her "anchorhold" (a room attached to the Church of Saint Julian in Norwich, England), she would pray with and counsel local people through her window from behind a curtain.[22]

The sixteenth century was a time of tremendous turmoil in the church. It produced activist reformers like Martin Luther, John Calvin, Thomas Cranmer, Ulrich Zwingli, John Knox, Thomas Müntser, and Conrad Grebel. This period also produced some of the most influential mystics, such as Ignatius of Loyola, Teresa of Ávila, and John of the Cross. The new Protestants and the contemplatives did not understand each other. While Luther ranted against enthusiasm, Teresa of Ávila prayed for him, asking God to "give light to the Lutherans."[23]

This rift between the Reformers and the mystics resulted in a long suspicion of the contemplative tradition in most Protestant churches. Their reasons for concern were not without cause. Many of the mystics, such as the Spanish Illuminati, believed that once they had reached mystical union with God, they no longer had to heed any other authority. Ignatius countered that the union one should seek with God was not a matter of cosmic merging that rendered a person ethically autonomous, but a correspondence to the divine will. His spiritual disciplines and the writings of Teresa of Ávila and John of the Cross provide great inspiration to Christians today who are seeking a deeper spirituality.

SPIRITUALITY IN THE BIBLE

Postmodern people today are reacting against the emptiness of modern religion. Too often liberal Christianity has taught that true religion is doing the

---

[21]Lane, *Christian Spirituality*, 34.

[22]Monica Furlong, *The Wisdom of Julian of Norwich* (Grand Rapids, MI: Eerdmans, 1996), 7.

[23]Teresa of Ávila, *Interior Castle*, ed. and trans. E. Allison Peers (New York: Doubleday, 1989), 35. The original version of this book was written in 1588.

right things.[24] Evangelicals have tended to focus on believing the right doctrines.[25] Neither has fed the deep hunger most people feel for intimacy with God, leaving seekers disillusioned and often angry. The postmodern alternative to organized religion is a free-floating experiential spirituality—what we are calling *generic spirituality*. Interestingly, the term *spirituality* does not appear anywhere in the Bible, nor does the abstract concept of spirituality. However, several Hebrew and Greek terms are translated as *spirit* or *spiritual* in the Bible. If we consider spirituality to be that which pertains to the spiritual realm, then a brief study of these words should inform our definition of Christian spirituality.

The first appearance of the word *spirit* in the Old Testament comes in Genesis 1. It is the Hebrew term *ruah*, which the NRSV translates in this case as "a wind from God." The same term is used in Genesis 2:7: "then the LORD God formed man from the dust of the ground, and breathed into his nostrils the breath of life; and the man became a living being." According to Old Testament scholar Hans Walter Wolff, *ruah* is used in six different ways in the Old Testament: wind, breath, vital powers, spirit(s), feelings and will.[26] When used in relation to humans, *ruah* refers to the person as empowered by God. It is always under God's control, not something humans possess. However, it is the *ruah* of God that communicates with the human *ruah* in dynamic relationship. Wolff explains, "A man as *ruah* is living, desires the good and acts as authorized being—none of this proceeds from man himself."[27]

The equivalent term for *ruah* in the New Testament is the Greek word *pneuma*. It can mean wind, breath, or "that dimension of the human personality whereby relationship with God is possible."[28] It may also refer to disembodied created beings, as well as to God himself. In two cases Paul refers to those who are *spiritual* as Christians who are mature in Christ (1 Cor 3:1; Gal 6:1), but nowhere do we see him urging his followers to develop

---

[24]Liberal Christianity taught this with good biblical reasons! See, for example, Luke 10:25-37; Ephesians 2:10; James 1:26-27; 2:14-26.

[25]Believing the right doctrines, while important, has less biblical precedent. See, for example, Matthew 23:2-3; James 2:19.

[26]Hans Walter Wolff, *Anthropology of the Old Testament* (Philadelphia: Fortress, 1974), 32-39.

[27]Wolff, *Anthropology of the Old Testament*, 39.

[28]J. D. G. Dunn, "Spirit, Holy Spirit," in *New Bible Dictionary*, ed. I. Howard Marshall, A. R. Millard, J. I. Packer, and D. J. Wiseman, 3rd ed. (Downers Grove, IL: InterVarsity Press, 1996), 1125.

their *spirituality*. Instead the New Testament focuses on seeking God through Christ and doing his will. Jesus taught his disciples the importance of prayer, and the spiritual gifts certainly play an important role throughout the New Testament; however, their purpose is centered in restoring humanity's broken relationship with God. They are evidence of God's in-breaking kingdom (Lk 4:18), preparing his people to move out into the world proclaiming good news to the poor, liberty to the captives, sight to the blind and freedom for the oppressed.

The Bible takes for granted that an unseen spiritual world exists. Throughout the Old Testament, God warned his people to avoid any dealings with spirits other than himself (Ex 20:1-6; Lev 19:31; Deut 18:9-14; 1 Sam 28:3-19; 1 Chron 10:13-14). The entire history of Israel provides graphic stories of the personal disintegration and national corruption that resulted when God's people violated this command. In the New Testament, Jesus began his ministry by going into the wilderness, where he was tempted by Satan and attended by angels (Mt 4:1-11; Mk 1:12-13; Lk 4:1-13). Throughout his ministry he confronted evil spirits; furthermore, he commissioned his followers to teach, preach, and cast out demons (Mk 16:17). In his letters to the churches, the apostle Paul gave clear guidelines for dealing with the principalities and powers of this unseen world (Rom 1:18-23; 8:37; 1 Cor 10:20-22; Eph 1:20-23; 6:10-20; Col 1–2; 1 Tim 4:1-5; Jas 2:19).

Most people today—even many Christians—are biblically illiterate. With the loss of biblical knowledge in our culture, people do not know God or the spirit world as the Bible portrays them. Rationalist thinking taught us that we could know and conquer the natural world, using it for our purposes. Such thinking extended even to the social world, where we attempted to learn the laws that govern society, and to the inner world, where we mapped the psyche. Many of the social and psychological scientists early in the twentieth century had great hopes for remaking both human beings and society.

That quest for utopia clearly failed, with a resultant loss of faith in science. At the same time, Christianity has long been viewed as having been tried and found wanting; in fact, many modern problems are attributed to it by its critics. God, if he exists at all, is considered too far off to care about our problems; thus the return to pre-Christian religions (or new religions) with their rituals and occult practices.

LIVING IN A SPIRITUAL WORLD

Even the church in the Western world has contributed to the problem of functional skepticism by not teaching and practicing the reality of God's daily involvement in our lives or the reality of eternal life. While people in difficult circumstances will talk of heaven, for many middle-class American Christians life here is good, and we want to keep it that way. We often think we don't need God to help us. After all, water comes out of the spigot when we turn it on. People in more traditional cultures pray for rain. If we are sick, we take medicine or have surgery, and we pray as a last resort. However, even prayer is now being investigated scientifically. Christians, as well as skeptics and Neopagans, are conducting research to see if prayer and other spiritual techniques "work." Despite the postmodern disenchantment with science, we can't help thinking like modernists. We want to know how things work—and we want to control them. Therefore, we insist our nursing care be "evidence-based."

Few Christians would overtly contradict the reality of the biblically in-formed worldview. But most of us function as if angels and demons were merely a vestige of primitive superstition. Many would go so far as to say that the Bible uses spiritual terminology to describe what we can now explain scientifically. For instance, in Matthew 17:14-20 a man came to Jesus with his son who apparently was having seizures and falling into fires. In other records of this story (Mk 9:14-29; Lk 9:37-43) the father attributes the problem to a demon, but in this account he says the boy is "moonstruck" (from the Greek *selēniazomai*) or, as the KJV translates it, "a lunatic." Interestingly, newer translations struggle with this. The NIV is merely descriptive—the boy "has seizures"—but the NRSV and CEV come right out and diagnose the con-dition as "epilepsy." However, in all accounts Jesus deals with the problem by rebuking "the demon," and the boy is cured.

While many in our culture today talk freely about angels and other sup-posedly benign spiritual forces, even many Christians do not acknowledge the reality of demons. Others see them behind every bush and live in fear. However, as many people, including nurses, begin to flirt with the occult in some alternative therapies and healing modalities, we believe that demonic activity will become much more evident. We have seen evidence of this hap-pening, in the United States as well as in other countries.

ARLENE'S STORY

I (Arlene) lived in Zambia among people who were not only aware of spirits but sought to use and placate them. They attributed sickness and accidents to spirit activity. People who knew how to deal with spirits prescribed the rituals and formulas necessary to remove their evil influence. Unlike many Americans, who naively view spirits as helpful, these people feared them. Observing those under the influence of evil spirits was a terrifying experience. Two examples have stayed etched in my memory for many years.

One afternoon a woman was admitted to the hospital glassy-eyed and hyperventilating. She was brought from a local healer who dealt with spirits. Every woman in the forty-bed ward sat up as she was put in one of the beds. I sensed what they knew: this woman was under powerful spirit influence. Being an outsider to the culture, I wanted to confirm my impression with the hospital chaplain. After a bit of probing on my part, he agreed with my assessment, though indirectly. The word about this poor woman spread among patients, staff, and nursing students.

The next morning, I asked the students if they wanted to pray for this woman. We had been reading in the Gospel of Mark about how Jesus delivered people from the power of evil spirits. I was a novice in such matters, but the issue seemed to be clearly before us. Many gathered at my home that evening and we prayed that Jesus would drive the evil spirit away. During the night, the woman died! The next morning both the students and I were subdued. It seemed as if the evil one had warned us to stay out of his territory. I decided that I would never try this again, at least not with such apparently difficult cases.

There were several times, however, when things went better. Once a young student complained for months of pain in one side of her body. Finally, after aspirin proved useless, I asked her what she thought the problem was. As I suspected, she thought that spirits were bothering her. She agreed to bring a friend with her to my office, and feeling somewhat foolish, I prayed she would be freed in Jesus' name. The pain went away! A short time later she was called home to attend a funeral. Because funerals involved rituals to drive spirits away, I feared that she might return to school with the old problem. But she did not, and never again did she come to the morning clinic complaining of pain in one side of her body.

Another story concerns a schoolteacher admitted to our hospital because she could not walk and refused to eat, a rather strange combination of symptoms. She had consulted but received no help from the local traditional healer. Once again, I sensed that spirit activity was part of the problem, but after the obvious failure with the woman who died, I resolved to stay uninvolved.

But one day, while supervising students in the unit, I watched this woman. She looked directly at me with eyes that I can only describe as burning. Surely there was help for this young woman. Since she was not eating, I wondered if she could be tempted with special foods.

She was! For a while I brought her tasty food and talked to her. She would not talk but with encouragement began to walk. Finally, I asked others to pray with me for her healing. We gathered around her, asking Jesus to drive out the spirit. She began to sing in a loud voice. Her mother, who had joined us, said that the spirit was singing. After that she was not noticeably improved but did continue to eat. Later we transported her to the nearest psychiatric hospital.

Undoubtedly this woman was psychotic, but demonic spirits also were involved. I have since thought that the combination of loving care, prayer for deliverance, and psychiatric care were all part of her recovery.

Judy's Story

Early in my experience as a campus minister, I (Judy) met with a new group of students. Ben, the group leader, told me beforehand that he was having difficulty leading Bible discussions and wanted help. As the meeting started, a strange phenomenon occurred. Whenever Ben would ask the group a question after reading a Bible passage, his face would contort. One side would be smiling and calm, the other side would scowl and twitch. The students on either side of him also responded in opposite ways. Those on the scowling side would sit in utter silence. Those on the smiling side would all talk at once.

After the meeting, Ben and I went for a walk to discuss what had happened. Ben was a good student and proud of his scientific objectivity, but finally he told me, "I think it's demons." As he spoke, his face contorted again, and his voice became uncharacteristically gruff. Surprised, I asked him what made him think so. He went on to tell me of a long family history of Spiritism. His grandmother regularly presided over séances in their dining room when he was a child. Before becoming a Christian, he had consulted Ouija boards, smoked marijuana, and often binged on alcohol. "I think I let evil spirits into my life. I know I'm a Christian, but there is still something that's not right," he confessed.

I knew nothing about demons then. My first inclination was to suggest he see a psychiatrist, but he replied that he had been in therapy for years. Finally, I talked with a colleague who had some experience with deliverance from evil spirits. He and another colleague met with Ben and cast out the demons. I was not present, but I could tell he was different. Ben experienced a radical change. From that point on he began to mature into a strong Christian leader. He never again suffered from his strange malady.

More recently I encountered the bizarre demonic world in a graduate course at a secular university. Trying to investigate the concepts being taught by the postmodern theorists, I enrolled in a course on "The Body—East and West." It was almost entirely East, after the West had been soundly maligned in the first three classes. The professor spoke freely of his own experiences in meditation, where he willingly entered the "demonic realm." He explained that during the early stages of meditation the demons would appear as serpents and monsters so frightening that "you could go crazy without a spiritual guide." However, in the later stages they would become "your friends." These friends often appeared to him as knights in shining armor and told him what to teach in class.

My classmates were almost all seekers or adherents of Eastern religions. Most were also practicing various forms of Eastern meditation as well as an eclectic assortment of spiritual exercises. I became increasingly uncomfortable in that class and began to literally shake as I drove home, so I desperately sought prayer support. My Sunday school class and my husband prayed daily. Arlene would call me to pray over the phone before I left for class each week. With the prayer support I felt much calmer and more confident, but the professor became much more aggressively anti-Christian. My classmates, however, grew increasingly interested in knowing more about Christianity.

One week we were to discuss the demonic realm in class. The readings had been bizarre and vulgar. I enlisted more people to pray. When the professor came into the classroom that day, he walked over to me and bowed, which seemed strange to me and to several of my classmates sitting nearby. Then he told us that he couldn't teach what he had prepared for class because he "had a dream." He asked if anyone had any questions about the readings, but received only blank stares in return. Finally he just started rambling on with a series of anti-Christian stories. I decided that this was not the time to retort, and so I sat calmly listening. Then he suddenly stopped and said, "I can't keep criticizing Christianity like this anymore, because Judy is going to get a gun and shoot me."

I laughed and said, "That wouldn't be very Christian!"

The woman to my left elbowed me and said, "That's his dream! He dreamed you shot him!"

But the ultimate test came when I turned in my final paper on the biblical view of the body (a topic he had approved). He gave it back to me and said, "You can't use this methodology. You've cited both the Old and New Testaments. You can't do that—those are two different gods. This is a B- paper unless you fix that." I did not "fix" it, but amazingly, I got an A- in the course.

SPIRITUALITY AND HEALTH CARE

Although our experiences with the spirit world may seem bizarre and unconvincing, we can see strong parallels with the worldview expressed in the Scriptures. Western culture has been so strongly influenced by scientific "objectivity" that we have difficulty recognizing what people from the beginning of time have acknowledged and exploited.

Testing Mystical Experiences

1. Are they initiated by human effort and techniques?
2. Do they lead to pride?
3. Do they lead to claims of secret knowledge that contradicts Scripture?
4. Do they lead to mental and emotional disturbance?
5. Do they lead to a more godly life?
6. Is the person humble about them and hesitant to discuss them?
7. Do they lead to greater love for God and others?

People in almost every culture have developed various systems for relating to the spiritual realm, especially in regard to healing. Shamans—healers who gain their powers from the spirit world while in a trance-like state—have appeared indigenously on almost every continent. Attempts to appease malevolent spirits and attract familiar spirits through rituals and spiritual exercises are common around the world. Magicians try to compel gods, demons, or spirits to do their bidding. They follow a pattern of occult practices to bend psychic forces to do their will. Even societies with atheistic philosophies, as well as those with strong monotheistic religions, including Christianity, have provided fertile soil for occult beliefs and practices. An undercurrent of paganism seems to lie dormant, even in Christianized cultures, only to resurface periodically. We are seeing just such resurgence in many of the postmodern nursing theories and therapies today.

Our primary concern in discussing spirituality is to look specifically at its relationship to health and health care. Probably the greatest contribution of the postmodern nursing theorists to nursing is their strong emphasis on viewing the person holistically with a focus on the spiritual. However, as we have seen, spirituality cannot be generic or neutral. Practicing energy-based therapies, praying to other gods, or encouraging a person toward any spiritual beliefs and practices contrary to Christ only courts disaster. Even evidence that a particular alternative therapy appears to "work" does not necessarily make it permissible for the Christian nurse.

When nurses come upon patients who seem to be troubled by demonic spirits, resources for help are available. Look for legitimate sources of help as many are manipulative and self-promoting. Some persons, knowledgeable and specially gifted with spiritual discernment and wisdom, have ministries of healing prayer for deliverance.[29] Some churches have clergy trained and authorized for exorcism. Erich Junger, an exorcist in the Anglican Church of North America, "advises fellow believers to 'put on the full armor of God, so that you can take your stand against the devil's schemes'" (Eph. 6:11).[30] The Catholic Church has priests authorized for this ministry.[31]

If we view Christian spirituality as the whole person in dynamic relationship with God through Jesus, then our definition impels us to nurture that relationship in contemplation, community, and compassion for others. Rather

---

[29]Francis MacNutt, *Healing* (Alamonte Springs, FL: Creation House, 1993). Also, Heather Davediuk Gingrich, *Restoring the Shattered Self: A Christian Counselors Guide to Complex Trauma* (Downers Grove, IL: InterVarsity Press, 2013) offers some important perspective on complex trauma, which can manifest in ways that look similar to demonic influence but requires certain kinds of trained psychological care.

[30]Griffin Paul Jackson, "The Protestant Exorcists," *Christianity Today*, October 2019, 53-56.

[31]Mike Mariani, "Why Are Exorcisms on the Rise?," *The Atlantic*, December 2018, theatlantic.com /magazine/ archive/2018/12/catholic-exorcisms-on-the-rise/573943/.

than seeking a vague inwardness or manipulation of the spirit world, spirituality leads us to a mature faith and a life of service.

FOR FURTHER THINKING

1. How would you define *spirituality*?

2. What does it mean to be a *spiritual being*?

3. In what ways have you experienced the spiritual realm?

THEOLOGICAL REFLECTION

Read Psalm 16:9-11, Psalm 32:1-7, Romans 12:1, and 1 Corinthians 2:6-16.

1. According to these passages, how are the physical, spiritual, and psychosocial aspects of our lives interrelated?

2. How do these passages describe what is spiritual?

3. How does that differ from the ways spirituality is commonly described in the nursing literature?

4. Based on these passages, what are spiritual needs?

5. Read Ephesians 6:10-20. According to this passage, how are we to deal with the spiritual realm?

Case Study: I See Glory!

Sally Jones, ninety-three, was admitted to the hospital after a stroke. A frail woman with coarse white hair, her knees moved toward her chest and her arms tightened against her body. She came to the hospital from a nursing home. Her chart indicated that she had one son who lived nearby, but she was alone.

In the days after she was admitted to the hospital, she never spoke a word. She didn't respond to painful stimuli or gentle touch. However, one night as her nurse, Sue, hummed "Amazing Grace," she thought she saw the corners of Sally's mouth turn up.

Sue made sure that Sally received excellent physical care. She bathed her gently, rubbed lotion into her dry skin, attempted to maintain range of motion, and turned her frequently. Whenever she had extra time, Sue would spend it with Sally so she would not be alone. However, Sally did not improve.

One evening, when Sue made her rounds, she found Sally diaphoresing. Her eyes were open and glassy, her pulse and respirations irregular.

Suddenly Sally straightened herself and sat up in bed. Her withered arms stretched toward the heavens. Her eyes seemed transfixed but did not focus on anything in the room. She spoke in a crackly voice just above a whisper, "I see glory—it's so *beau*-ti-ful!" She fell back on the pillow as the monitor alarm blared. Her heart had stopped beating. She had entered the glory of heaven.[32]

DISCUSSION QUESTIONS

1. What indications did the author have that Sally had spiritual needs?

2. How did she meet those needs?

3. In what ways did her physical care meet spiritual needs?

4. What spiritual perceptions did the author express?

5. What did she learn from Sally?

---

[32]Adapted from Sue Henley, "I See Glory!" *Journal of Christian Nursing* (2004): 31-32.

6

THE PERSON AS A CULTURAL BEING

Purpose: To examine the relationship between culture and spiritual care

Objectives: After reading this chapter and completing the exercises, you should be able to:
1. Define culture
2. Contrast *ethnocentrism* and *cultural humility*
3. Assess spiritual and cultural influences in health practices
4. List guidelines for Christian crosscultural nursing in a pluralistic world

Keywords: culture, diversity, pluralism, enculturation, supracultural realm, ethnocentrism, multiculturalism, crosscultural

A VISIBLY DISTRAUGHT MOTHER rushed into the emergency room clutching a small child. Although the child appeared acutely ill, the mother spoke only Russian and could explain the problem only by making gestures. No one in the emergency room spoke Russian. Finally, someone remembered the nurse on another unit who was also an Orthodox priest. When he arrived and spoke words of greeting in Russian, the mother calmed down. At last here was someone who would understand her plight. The physician diagnosed the child's illness, and treatment began.

As we have cared for people from other cultures in the course of our long nursing experience, we have seen all kinds of unusual (to us) practices—pans of water and pots of burning paper under beds, bags of herbs or amulets tied around necks, copper bracelets on arms and bottles of foul-smelling potions at the bedside—all purported to ward off various illnesses or evil spirits. Along the way we have learned some key words in other languages. Patients from various ethnic backgrounds and their families have enriched our nursing and introduced us to a wide variety of foods and customs. Health-related practices that may seem unusual to us are often long practiced cultural traditions, passed on through generations, intended to heal and protect. Although many cultural practices may be harmless, some traditional interventions, particularly those related to childbirth, are potentially harmful. For example, feeding a newborn baby honey and herbal tea, covering a baby with salt, bathing a newborn in cold water, or coating an umbilical cord with butter can be detrimental. Other practices, such as expressing colostrum and discarding it before putting the baby to breast are indicative of cultural traditions that are not explicitly harmful, but are based on lack of accurate information.

Consider the following scene. I (Arlene) visited an African American home in Pennsylvania with a Cambodian student. The grandmother was dying from congestive heart failure. The family had moved the living-room furniture into the dining room to make room for the grandmother's bed. While we were there, the pastor came to give Communion. Then the grandson stopped in to see his parents and his grandmother. The dying woman's son was handicapped. The student and I were concerned about the weary daughter-in-law, who was the primary caregiver. It was a cluttered, people-filled environment. Yet everyone present focused on the well-being of the dying woman.

My student from Cambodia, who was the only Christian in her Buddhist immigrant family, attempted to assess the needs of this multigenerational African American family. My own Swiss-German ancestry added another flavor to the mix, my father having been raised in the Amish church. I felt acutely aware of the cultural diversity. Yet we were joined in our common concern for the welfare of a dying woman.

Both of us (Arlene and Judy) have lived in other cultures outside the United States. We have been honored as guests in Asian, European, and African homes. Returning this kindness to international guests has been our privilege. We have attended international conferences where nurses from many countries shared common concerns and also faced unique issues. The different cultural perspectives have broadened our thinking and enriched our lives.

Most nursing texts today include information about cultural aspects of health and illness. Dr. Madeleine Leininger developed a nursing theory she called Culture Care Theory. In her book she relates the story of how she came to see the importance of educating nurses in cultural theory to improve nursing care.[1] Dr. Rachel Spector spent years teaching and researching the rich cultural diversity in American society. Her book *Cultural Diversity in Health and Illness*, first published in 1985, is now in its ninth edition.[2] A literature search reveals a rapidly expanding body of material about cultural health practices in general nursing journals. Furthermore, a growing number of organizations and journals focus entirely on cultural perspectives in nursing.

The renewed interest in complementary, or alternative, health practices has caused the interest in cultural health practices to explode. Nursing and medical texts now include modalities from Native American, Chinese, Indian, Tibetan, Japanese, Latin American, African and pre-Christian European cultural traditions. In most instances these practices are presented as complementary to scientific medicine, not as replacements. In a postmodern worldview the only criterion given for judging these practices from widely divergent cultures is whether or not they bring comfort and healing to the patient.

What Is Culture?

"Culture" is anything that humans produce when they interact with each other and with God's creation. When we interact with each other and with God's creation, we cultivate the ground (grain, vegetables, livestock), produce artifacts (clothes, housing, cars), build institutions (governments, businesses, schools), form worldviews (theism, pantheism, atheism), and participate in religions (e.g., Christianity, Hinduism, Buddhism, Islam, Animism, atheism). We produce culture, and at the same time our cultural context shapes us, affecting who we are, what we think and do, and how we feel.[3]

Culture is learned, passed on from one generation to another through a process of *enculturation*. It is the *nurture*, not *nature*, aspect of human behavior. Enculturation is both deliberate and conscious, when we are taught by parents, teachers, and clergy. Yet it also happens unconsciously, when we imitate elders and peers and absorb their values and ideas. Because culture is acquired, not inherited, it is constantly changing—sometimes rapidly and at

[1]Madeleine Leininger and Marilyn R. McFarland, *Transcultural Nursing: Concepts, Theories, Research, and Practice*, 3rd ed. (New York: McGraw-Hill, 2002).
[2]Rachel E. Spector, *Cultural Diversity in Health and Illness*, 9th ed. (New York: Pearson, 2017).
[3]B. R. Ashford, *Every Square Inch: An Introduction to Cultural Engagement for Christians* (Bellingham, WA: Lexham, 2015), 13.

other times more slowly. Even traditional cultures that are not exposed to outside influences change.

Several models help us to understand the various aspects of culture and how they relate to one another. One model pictures culture as a series of four layers.[4] The deepest layer consists of the cultural worldview, assumptions that answer questions about people and the world. (See chapter two.) The second layer, closely related and largely derived from the worldview, is that of values, particularly ethical and moral values. Based on both the worldview and values, the next layer of culture is social institutions such as marriage, law, education, and so on. Finally, at the surface but growing out of the layers below, there is the layer of material artifacts (technology, art, clothing) and observable behavior and customs. This surface layer is more easily described and more easily changed. It is this layer where nurses see health-related practices. (See figure 6.1.)

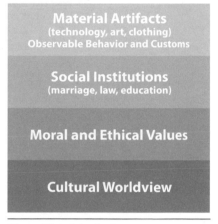

Figure 6.1. Levels of culture

Nicholls suggests that the interaction between the layers of a culture can be viewed as a pyramid with the worldview as an unseen hidden base. The values, institutions, and observable behavior form the three sides interacting with each other. (See figure 6.2.)

Anthropologists consider religion integral to culture—a *human factor* influencing and influenced by each aspect of the culture. *Religion* is a slippery term and hard to define. It can be applied to the assumptions of a worldview, even if the culture claims to be secular, because worldviews are based on faith, not only empirical observations. Secular societies like North America relegate religious practices to people's private lives. In many societies—such as tribal groups, some Islamic countries, and Hindu societies—religion permeates all levels of the culture and strongly influences health practices.

From a Christian perspective, religion is far more than a human factor. Throughout this book we have referred to reality as both seen and unseen.

---

[4]Bruce Nicholls, *Contextualization: A Theology of Gospel and Culture* (Vancouver: Regent College Publishing, 1979), 11.

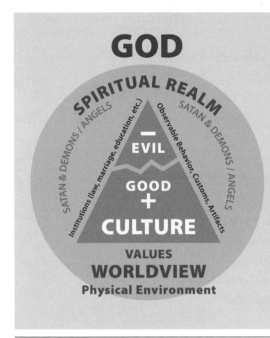

GOD

Everything inside the circle is part of creation. God is above creation and sustains it. He is bringing people of all cultures into his kingdom. The three sides of the pyramid represent the three interacting aspects of culture: Institutions, Customs and Behavior, and Values. The values are the base of the pyramid. The values come from the worldview on which the pyramid sits. Cultures live within spiritual and physical environments that also influence their values, institutions, and practices. Some spiritual influences are good, and others are evil. Every culture has both good and evil aspects. God has left his "footprints" in every culture.

Figure 6.2. Culture and worldview

Nicholls refers to unseen reality as the *supracultural realm*—"the phenomena of cultural belief and behavior that have their source outside of human culture."[5] The biblical writers assume the reality of a spiritual realm that includes God, angels, Satan, and demons. In contrast, secular anthropologists assume that all the factors that determine religion are contained within the culture itself. Christians accept the biblical view that the unseen reality—the supracultural realm—interacts with the culture.

A CHRISTIAN UNDERSTANDING OF CULTURE

The diversity of human cultures shows many complex ways in which people have organized their social relationships and their response to their environment. When God told the first people to multiply and fill the earth, the development of various human cultures began.[6] However, because humans decided to turn away from God's authority, sin corrupted every culture.

---

[5] Nicholls, *Contextualization*, 13.

[6] Genesis 1:28 reminds us that part of creation order is to go forth and create life, families, social systems, and cultures. See Soong-Chan Rah, *Many Colors: Cultural Intelligence for a Changing Church* (Chicago: Moody, 2010), 28-29.

The Bible itself reflects a diversity of cultures. Its writings were collected over a period of at least fifteen hundred years by people from a wide range of social backgrounds. Customs are recorded from a diversity—eastern, Judaic, and Hellenistic cultures. There were many shared ideas and practices between ancient Israel and the different people groups among whom they lived. However, God's covenant with them at Sinai gave them beliefs and ways of living and worshiping that distinguished them from others. Some biblical stories are of godly persons living comfortably within this covenant people. Others, however, are of persons who resist cultural pressure where they are living. Daniel and his friends provide an example of protesting food that violated their beliefs, refusing to worship a statue, and refusing to stop praying to the God of Israel when ordered by law to do so (Dan 1:8-17).

Followers of Jesus live in two worlds, the physical world we can see and touch and the spiritual unseen world. Jesus Christ entered into this world with the good news that "the Kingdom of Heaven" was already present in himself, he was the King. Those who accepted the invitation to follow him and become members of the heavenly kingdom began to live by his example of life and his teaching. He taught that in the future, heaven and earth would eventually be joined and his way of life and teachings would characterize all life.[7] Until that time, Jesus' followers would seek justice, reach out to the poor and outsiders, and pursue peace and reconciliation. They would live lives of humble service. They would work for the betterment of each culture in which they lived. Followers of Jesus are found in every culture on earth each living out the kingdom life in differing ways.

God manifests his goodness in every culture. Human beings bear God's image, both as individuals and as a social group. The gift of language enables people to create culture and to pass on traditions. All cultures have some idea of the family as the foundation for social organization. All cultures have respect for human life. All persons show God's gift of creativity when they create institutions, art, and music—all things beautiful. At the same time, because of human rebellion against the Creator, humans look to their own

---

[7]"We await the return of Jesus Christ, the arrival of the new heaven and the new earth, the dawning of the resurrection, the glory of perfection, the beauty of holiness. Until that day, we are a people in tension. On the one hand, we belong to the broader culture in which we find ourselves; on the other, we belong to the culture of the consummated kingdom of God, which has dawned upon us." Ashford, *Every Square Inch*, 32–33.

creations to save them. Paul wrote, "They exchanged the truth about God for a lie and worshiped and served the creature rather than the Creator" (Rom 1:25). This is the essence of idolatry. God works in human history to establish his rule in the hearts of those who accept the gospel.

We see many examples where Christians are different from and yet identify with their larger culture. Navajo Christians retain the strong Navajo sense of family and their keen awareness of the spirit world. Instead of calling the hand-trembler and medicine man for the traditional healing "sing," they substitute Christian prayer at community camp meetings. Zambian Christians reject the traditional practice of polygamy and teach monogamous marriage instead. But they retain the culture's concern for support and help within the extended family. In North America, Christians struggle to free themselves from the rampant individualism of our culture and yet retain a strong sense of personal responsibility. Korean Christians maintain their deep respect for the elderly. At the same time, they gather for daily early-morning prayer meetings instead of practicing traditional shamanistic rituals.

The boundary line between what is Christian and what belongs to the culture can be exceedingly difficult to draw. Only Christ's lordship and the illumination of the Holy Spirit on Scripture can guide the individual Christian and the church to make this distinction. It is usually best done by those within the culture itself, rather than by outsiders. At the same time those from other cultures often see things about beliefs and practices to which insiders are blind. For example, African and Asian Christians help North Americans to see the way we neglect our elders. Christians from poor countries help us to see how often we equate God's blessing with affluence.

Each culture contains evidence both of evil and of God's goodness. On one occasion, when Paul and Barnabas healed a man in Jesus' name, the crowd wanted to worship them. The people thought these men were appearances of the gods Zeus and Hermes, and the priest was prepared to sacrifice to them. Paul and Barnabas barely restrained them with these words:

> Friends, why are you doing this? We are mortals just like you, and we bring you good news, that you should turn from these worthless things to the living God, who made the heaven and the earth and the sea and all that is in them. In the past generations he allowed all the nations to follow their own ways; *yet he has not left himself without a witness in doing good—giving you rain from heaven*

and fruitful seasons, and filling you with food and your hearts with joy. (Acts 14:15-17, italics ours)

Paul recognized the gratitude of the crowd for healing the man, but he was deeply pained by their misguided understanding of its true source, the Creator God who gives everything to sustain earthly life.

Theologian Charles Sherlock suggests three general approaches for thinking about culture.

1. We should put away the idea that any one culture embodies Christian faith (this is especially true for those of us who live in Western cultures that have been most influenced by Christianity).

2. We should use crosscultural relationships to reflect on our own culture— both to identify our prejudices and to be enriched by others' experiences and ways of thinking.

3. We must recognize the effects of sin on all human cultures: the outworking of human pride, self-centeredness and the desire to be in control are present in every culture.[8]

CULTURAL PLURALISM

Nurses are experiencing the cultural diversity of our society and, even more, the cultural pluralism of the world. We are forced out of cultural isolation by modern communication and travel. We live in each other's neighborhoods: we see each other in health care settings. We work with nurses and caregivers from cultures different from our own. For the most part, we view this diversity as a positive development. Yet there is also trouble in the global village. Hatred between cultural and ethnic groups spills over into violence and war.

---

[8]Charles Sherlock, *The Doctrine of Humanity* (Downers Grove, IL: InterVarsity Press, 1996), 135-37. "Customs such as human sacrifice, female circumcision, widow-burning, foot-binding, prostitution, slavery and torture are clearly opposed to God's will for human life. Others are less obviously wrong, but reinforce sinful attitudes such as selfishness, greed or lust; television commercials provide plenty of evidence in the highly ambiguous culture of consumerism. Even in those aspects of a culture which embody the highest ideals to which human beings aspire, or which celebrate the goodness of God that pervades everyday life, sin is present. Consider birth, retirement, setting up a new home, or beginning a meal: a child can be seen only as evidence of a parent's achievement, whether in fertility or child-rearing; retirement as boasting or escaping to laziness; a new home can provide the chance for ostentatious display; and even grace at the table can be a means of controlling behavior. Indeed, the worst idols are precisely the best things set in the place of God, and it is their God-given goodness which makes them attractive" (137-38).

Multiculturalism is the widely used term describing North American society today—there are many cultures and subcultures.[9] Pluralism and multiculturalism are related terms, describing the plurality of beliefs and practices in our world. However, multiculturalism is only one aspect of pluralism. We encounter differing economic systems, political systems, philosophical systems, and religions as well.

In the postmodern worldview, the philosophy of pluralism and multiculturalism foregoes making judgments about the relative goodness of any one culture. Our culture's conventional wisdom views tolerance as the virtue to resolve cultural conflict—tolerance for diversity in ideas and lifestyle.[10] Tolerance, even approval, for all points of view and ways of living is advocated. Stan Gaede, however, asks the question, "Is tolerance based on a commitment to truth and justice, or is it merely indifference?"[11]

Jesus Christ, the Only Way to God

In the present climate of cultural pluralism, saying that the Christian worldview is right and that Jesus is the only way to God offends many. How can all other religions be wrong? We do not claim that *everything* taught and practiced in other religions is wrong. Some aspects of other religions are true. They may be understood as expressions of the longing for communion with God, an essential human characteristic. We were created to worship and serve God. An example is the Temple of Heaven in Beijing, where the emperor would offer yearly sacrifices for the blessings of heaven. The architecture of the circular buildings is beautiful, and the many altars with images of sacrificial cattle surrounding the main temple speak of human awareness of the need for sacrifice.

Yet even though traces of truth and beauty can be seen in other religions, Christians believe "there is salvation in no one else, for there is no other name

---

[9]Multiculturalism is "the presence of, or support for the presence of, several distinct cultural or ethnic groups within a society." Lexico.com (Oxford: Oxford University Press, 2020), s.v. "multiculturalism," https://www.lexico.com/en/definition/multiculturalism.

[10]Theologian Adam Johnson argues that tolerance is not a virtue because it cannot deal with intolerance. It becomes *intolerant* of intolerance. "What we need is sustained reflection on the kinds of virtues which enable us not merely to embrace tolerance, but grapple with intolerance with love, honor and dignity." "The Virtue of Tolerance," *The Scriptorium Daily*, November 8, 2016, http://scriptoriumdaily.com/the-virtue-of-tolerance.

[11]S. D. Gaede, *When Tolerance Is No Virtue* (Downers Grove, IL: InterVarsity Press, 1993).

under heaven given among mortals by which we must be saved" (Acts 4:12). While such a claim is indeed exclusive, we would note that, when taken seriously, all other religions are also exclusive. Those who argue that all religions are the same, or that they are only different paths to the same God, have only a superficial understanding of what each of them teaches. Each religion has unique beliefs about salvation, for instance, and the existence of God or gods. To argue this point is beyond the focus of this chapter. We only want to say that it is the very nature of religion to make exclusive claims. So, we make no apology for the exclusive claims of Christianity.

At the same time, Christianity is the most inclusive of religions. Many other religions are ethnic in nature, including only people of a certain tribe or race. Christianity encompasses people worldwide in every culture. The last book in the Bible describes a heavenly scene of all the people gathered around the throne of God. "After this I looked, and there was a great multitude that no one could count, from every nation, from all tribes and peoples and languages, standing before the throne and before the Lamb, robed in white, with palm branches in their hands. They cried out in a loud voice, saying, 'Salvation belongs to our God who is seated on the throne, and to the Lamb!'" (Rev 7:9-10).

Approach to Crosscultural Nursing Practice

We now return to the concerns nurses have for practicing in crosscultural settings. The Transcultural Nursing Society was founded in 1974.[12] Nursing texts are replete with lists of how culture affects health care. Most include discussions about cultural views of birth, health, illness, death, and behaviors associated with each of these. Spector identifies the following health domains: health traditions, healing traditions, familial health traditions, and health and illness in modern health care.[13] Nurses need to recognize how each of these are shaped by their own culture and the culture of those they serve.

Each of us must recognize that we are members of our own culture. Our worldview and cultural practices are where we begin and determine what seems like the right way to do things. We are naturally ethnocentric— "evaluating other peoples and cultures according to the standards of one's own

---

[12]Joyceen S. Boyle, "An Early History of the Journal of Transcultural Nursing," *Journal of Transcultural Nursing* 30, no. 6 (2019): 537.

[13]Spector, *Cultural Diversity in Health and Illness*.

culture."[14] Many of those among whom we practice nursing are enculturated quite differently. They may see us as misunderstanding and wrong in our approach. What is our attitude? If they need our services for health concerns, do we see ourselves as having all the answers? If we are there to teach others good health practices, do we consider them ignorant or wrong? Might it be possible that we could learn from those we teach? Do we see them as the persons they are, loved by God and created in his image? As Christian nurses we are with them as the hands and feet of Jesus, to serve them as he would.

We begin as learners, desiring to know and understand those among whom we practice nursing. Cultural competence, an ability to interact effectively with people of different cultures, is viewed as essential for nurses and other health care professionals. The NCLEX Exam for Registered Nurses includes questions related to cultural difference and health practices. The US Department of Health and Human Services provides a free e-learning program, "Culturally Competent Nursing Care: A Cornerstone of Caring," from the HHS Office of Minority Health.[15] HHS also defines the National Standards for Culturally and Linguistically Appropriate Services (CLAS) in Health and Health Care.[16]

Cultural competency includes four components among others: (1) awareness of one's own cultural worldview, (2) attitude toward cultural differences, (3) knowledge of different cultural practices and worldviews, and (4) crosscultural skills.[17] Some nurses, however, view competency as too narrow, because it implies that a person can totally understand another culture. It becomes a goal to be achieved. A more suitable approach is *cultural humility*, according to an article by Melanie Tervalon and Jann Murray-García in 1996.[18]

A comparison of the two approaches shows the distinctives of each. While the aim of cultural competency is to understand minority cultures in order to

---

[14]Lexico.com (Oxford: Oxford University Press, 2020), s.v. "ethnocentrism," www.lexico.com/en/definition/ethnocentric.

[15]"Culturally Competent Nursing Care," https://ccnm.thinkculturalhealth.hhs.gov.

[16]"National CLAS Standards," https://thinkculturalhealth.hhs.gov/clas.

[17]Centers Health Care, "FIDA Provider Training: Cultural Competence," https://centershealthcare.com/share/pdfs/CPHL_Uploads/fidaculturalcompetencytraining.pdf.

[18]Melanie Tervalon and Jann Murray-García, "Cultural Humility Versus Cultural Competence: A Critical Distinction in Defining Physician Training Outcomes in Multicultural Education," *Journal of Health Care for the Poor and Underserved* 9, no. 2 (1998): 117-25, https://ncbi.nlm.nih.gov/pubmed/10073197.

provide services more effectively, cultural humility focuses on service providers' personal reflection and growth related to culture in order to increase their awareness. Cultural competency promotes building skills and achieving goals. Cultural humility is defined "not by a discrete endpoint but as a commitment and active engagement in a lifelong process." This process entails developing mutually respectful and beneficial relationships with clients, communities, and coworkers, while seeking to reduce harmful power imbalances.[19]

We think there are benefits in each approach. Nurse theorist Josepha Campinha-Bacote describes a synergistic relationship between cultural humility and cultural competence. She describes it as *cultural competemility*.[20] Campinha-Bacote says that nurses must have the *desire* to become culturally competent. In other words, to care.[21]

Professor of nursing Dr. Wanda Thuma-McDermond spent her childhood in Zambia, where her father was a physician. In a conversation with the author, she affirmed the approach of cultural humility, saying that "it fits with my theology." While she knows the local language and culture, she is always learning. She takes nursing students each year to Zambia to participate in the local hospital and clinics.

Even those of us living and working in "our own" culture should be aware there are vast differences. For example, author Colon Woodward has identified eleven subnations in America, each with distinct attitudes and values.[22] As nurses we will find differences within families, generations, social classes, genders, and so on. Thus, we are always listening and learning.

EVALUATING CULTURAL PRACTICES AND VALUES

Being open and adapting to the culture of those for whom we care demonstrates respect and honors them as persons created in God's image. Such an approach also increases our appreciation of the creativity and wisdom of the wonderful humanity God has created. However, there are some distinctions

---

[19]Tervalon and Murray-García, "Cultural Humility Versus Cultural Competence," 118.

[20]Josepha Campinha-Bacote, "Cultural Competemility: A Paradigm Shift in Cultural Competence Versus Cultural Humility Debate—Part 1," *Online Journal of Issues in Nursing* 24, no. 1 (2019), doi:10.3912/OJIN.Vol24No01PPT20.

[21]Campina-Bacote, "Spiritual Key to Cultural Competence."

[22]Colin Woodward, *American Nations: A History of the Eleven Rival Regional Cultures of North America* (New York: Penguin Random House, 2012).

that we need to make. This is even true for our own culture. We noted earlier that as Christians our ultimate citizenship is in God's kingdom, not the earthly one in which we live. So, in one sense, we are living crossculturally at all times. There are some practice and values in our own culture as well as others which we are called to avoid. How do we make these decisions? Here are some guidelines that have helped us in our practice.

First, not everything labeled *spiritual* is good. For example, there is a long and continuing history of spiritual or metaphysical movements in America that promise access to secret knowledge, to angels or spirit guides, or to giving mental or mystical power over disease among other things.[23] We are indeed spiritual beings, and we relate to God through Jesus and the Holy Spirit. In Scripture God has revealed to us what we need to know. We are cautioned to not go beyond that. "The secret things belong to the LORD our God, but the revealed things belong to us and to our children forever, to observe all the words of this law" (Deut 29:29). "He reveals deep and hidden things; he knows what is in the darkness, and light dwells with him" (Dan 2:22).

Another guideline is to question any practice that accesses a universal mystical energy often referred to as *life force*. One website, "Higher Awareness," gives an extensive list of names for this energy.[24] This energy is sometimes referred to as bioenergy and claimed to be an as-yet unmeasurable energy produced by the human body. Others clearly refer to it as spiritual energy. One modality based on this so-called energy is *Reiki*.[25] Nurses who are also Reiki healers direct this universal energy toward the patient to heal, relieve pain, and reduce anxiety. An article by George Smith, available on the Christian Medical Fellowship website, concludes:

> From a Christian perspective, there certainly are spiritual dangers, which cannot be ignored. The concept of Rei as the invisible source of all being and

---

[23]Metaphysical movements are "groups that share a common definition of metaphysics as a practical religious philosophy and that seek to relate spiritual and psychic phenomena to everyday life." They include spiritualism and theosophy and "tend to blend an occult with a metaphysical stream of thought." "Metaphysical Movements," *The Concise Oxford Dictionary of World Religions*, Encyclopedia.com, August 11, 2020.

[24]See "Invisible Life Force—A List of Choices," Higher Awareness, www.higherawareness.com /manifesting-abundance/life-force-energy.html. Accessed September 25, 2020.

[25]Susan Thrane and Susan M. Cohen, "Effect of Reiki Therapy on Pain and Anxiety in Adults: An In-Depth Literature Review of Randomized Trials with Effect Size Calculations," *Pain Management Nursing* 15, no. 4 (2014): 897-968.

of Ki as the Universal Life Force are completely at variance with the Christian belief in God as Creator and Heavenly Father. Reiki claims to be independent of any religious belief systems but Buddhist, Hindu and Taoist influences can be clearly identified.[26]

The Scriptures tell us, "Beloved, do not believe every spirit, but test the spirits to see whether they are from God; for many false prophets have gone out into the world. By this you know the Spirit of God: every spirit that confesses that Jesus Christ has come in the flesh is from God, and every spirit that does not confess Jesus is not from God" (1 Jn 4:1-3).

Further, we need to evaluate the quality of research being done on these modalities. Are the researchers themselves unbiased? Does the protocol meet the highest standards? Are the published conclusions accurate? (See appendix, Guidelines for Evaluating Alternative Therapies.)

Finally, can the observable practices and behavior be separated from the underlying worldview and values? Sometimes people do the right thing for the wrong reason. For example, some forms of massage are based on the theory that it balances the flow of *chi*. However, the benefits of massage can be explained physiologically through processes of muscle relaxation and blood flow. For centuries, people learned things that promote health through trial and error, long before they could explain them scientifically. Much of even present-day health care practice remains empirical; we know it seems to work but not exactly how and why. The scientific fields of psychoneuroimmunology (PNI) and psychoneuroendocrinology (PNE) have described many of the physiological responses associated with psychological states.[27]

As an example, consider *mindfulness-based stress reduction*, a practice increasingly recommended for anxiety. According to the Mayo Clinic website,

> Mindfulness is a type of meditation in which you focus on being intensely aware of what you're sensing and feeling in the moment, without interpretation or judgment. Practicing mindfulness involves breathing methods, guided imagery, and other practices to relax the body and mind and help reduce stress. . . .

---

[26]George Smith, "Reiki," *Triple Helix*, Summer 2004, cmf.org.uk/resources/publications/content/?context=article&id=1263.

[27]Psychoneuroimmunology is the study of the effect of the mind on health and resistance to disease. Psychoneuroendocrinology is the study of the interaction of the brain and nervous system with the release of endocrines.

Meditation has been studied in many clinical trials. The overall evidence supports the effectiveness of meditation for various conditions, including: stress, anxiety, pain, depression, insomnia, high blood pressure (hypertension).[28]

Put this way, mindfulness seems a positive way to slow down and calm oneself. However, it is not without its critics. Sahanika Ratnayake, who grew up as a Buddhist, had a long, tangential history with meditation. As a graduate student at Cambridge she turned to meditation to deal with the stress of the academic environment. She writes,

> I have been instructed to observe my breath, to scan my body and note the range of its sensations, and to observe the play of thoughts and emotions in my mind. . . . At the end of the Cambridge study, I found myself to be calmer, more relaxed and better able to step away from any overwhelming feelings. . . . Yet I'd also become troubled by a cluster of feelings that I couldn't quite identify. It was as if I could no longer make sense of my emotions and thoughts. . . . Something about the mindfulness practice I'd cultivated, and the way it encouraged me to engage with my emotions, made me feel increasingly estranged from myself and my life.[29]

Ratnayake concludes that mindfulness is "'metaphysically loaded.' . . . In particular, mindfulness is grounded in the Buddhist doctrine of *anattā*, or the 'no-self.' *Anattā* is a metaphysical denial of the self, defending the idea that there is nothing like a soul, spirit or any ongoing individual basis for identity."[30] She continues, "Its roots in the Buddhist doctrine of *anattā* means that it sidelines a certain kind of deep, deliberative reflection that's required for unpacking which of our thoughts and emotions are reflective of ourselves, which are responses to the environment, and—the most difficult question of all— what we should be doing about it."[31]

Ute Kreplin, a lecturer in psychology at Massey University in New Zealand, asks regarding mindfulness, "Does research into its efficacy meet scientific standards?" Most of the researchers were also teachers of the practice and were biased toward positive results. Because mindfulness is hailed as the panacea for everything from cancer to war, it is very hard to say anything against it.[32]

---

[28]"Mindfulness Exercises," Mayo Clinic, September 15, 2020, www.mayoclinic.org/healthy-lifestyle/consumer-health/in-depth/mindfulness-exercises/art-20046356.

[29]Sahanika Ratnayake, "The Problem of Mindfulness," *Aeon*, July 25, 2019, https://aeon.co/essays/mindfulness-is-loaded-with-troubling-metaphysical-assumptions.

[30]Ratnayake, "The Problem of Mindfulness."

[31]Ratnayake, "The Problem of Mindfulness."

[32]Ute Kreplin, "Does Meditation Work?," *Aeon*, July 9, 2018, https://aeon.co/essays/can-meditation-really-make-the-world-a-better-place.

Some of the mindfulness exercises are indeed helpful, such as stopping to take a deep breath when feeling overwhelmed or going for a walk outside. There are other things as well that nurses can encourage for dealing with stress and anxiety. Elizabeth Moyer suggests worship, prayer, asking for help, seeking community, meditating on Scripture, and reducing your work load.[33] The Psalmist encourages us with "Be still, and know that I am God! I am exalted among the nations, I am exalted in the earth" (Ps 46: 10). Knowing that God is managing the world assures us that he will be with us and help us with managing our world.

> ### Relating Crossculturally
>
> 1. Be aware of ethnocentrism.
> 2. Seek to identify transcultural truths.
> 3. Learn from other cultures.
> 4. Be humble and tolerant of differences.
> 5. Accept people where they are.
> 6. Respect people's freedom.
> 7. Evaluate beliefs underlying customs and rituals.
> 8. Practice cultural humility.
> 9. Pray continually.

GUIDELINES FOR FINDING OUR WAY

Be aware of ethnocentrism. Judging other cultures by the standards of our own is wrong. Scripture, rightly interpreted, is the only standard by which cultures are to be judged.

Seek to identify transcultural truths. The view that truth, ethics, and standards for health care can be defined only from within each specific culture is not a valid position. There *are* transcultural truths, ethics, and standards for nursing. Nurses should work to define these in intercultural conferences and research.[34]

---

[33]Elizabeth Moyer, "Six Biblical Methods for Handling Stress," The Institute for Faith, Works and Economics, March 30, 2016, https://tifwe.org/six-biblical-methods-for-handling-stress.

[34]Cultural relativism is the view that all beliefs, customs, and ethics are relative to the individual within his own social context. In other words, "right" and "wrong" are culture-specific; what is considered moral in one society may be considered immoral in another, and, since no universal standard of morality exists, no one has the right to judge another society's customs.

Learn from other cultures. Appreciation for the many cultural practices that make sense only within specific cultures is the best approach. It brings joy, and often frustration, to crosscultural relationships. Taking off one's shoes makes a lot of sense in Korean homes where people traditionally sit on the floor to eat and roll out mats for sleeping. We can learn much from the health practices of other cultures. Congenital hip displacement in children is not seen in rural Zambia. Infants may have been born with shallow acetabula, but the way mothers carry them on their backs for two years provides a natural corrective splint.

Be humble and tolerant of differences. Humility will keep us from being closed-minded about what seems negative in others' ways of doing things. Much of what seems senseless or wrong is simply our misunderstanding. We begin by learning, observing, inquiring, and trying to understand. Tolerance will help us to love in spite of differences that annoy or offend. It is a tolerance based not on indifference but on commitment to God's honor and his grace extended both to us and to others.

Accept people where they are. God takes a long time to work out his purposes in our lives. This is true both in individuals and within a culture. Practice kindness and courtesy, even when health practices are clearly in conflict with the scriptural teaching. If the person is a Christian, you can give reasons for why you think the practice is wrong and then trust the Holy Spirit to convince the person in his time. If the person is of another religion or says he or she has no religion, you can simply explain that you see things differently because you are a Christian.

Respect people's freedom. Remember that the freedom to make choices and accept the consequences reflects God's image in us. Letting people make decisions about their own health care is not the same as condoning what they are doing. Learning the language of those among whom we work is the highest form of respect. Having culturally appropriate literature is essential. Do those things that bring comfort and security to patients and families, even if they seem senseless to you, as long as they are not actually harmful to their health.

Evaluate beliefs underlying customs and rituals. Those customs connected to non-Christian religions or worldviews can be tied to demonic powers. If rituals involve spirits, angels, demons, gods, or goddesses, Christians should not be involved. Sometimes, in order to learn, observing such rituals and practices may be helpful.

Practice cultural humility. Campinha-Bacote wrote the following:

Christ's love for the church motivates a person to want to be culturally sensitive. Spiritual caring and spiritual love are intrinsic qualities in the nurse-client relationship that cannot be directly measured. However, clients perceive these qualities positively, sensing that they are being cared about and valued. It has been said that people don't care how much you know until they first know how much you care. This type of caring and spiritual love comes from the heart, not from the mouth. It results from one's relationship with God. Therefore, the goal of cultural competence is not to offer politically correct comments (from the mouth), but rather comments that reflect true spiritual caring (from the heart).[35]

Pray continually. Pray first, last, and always. Ask God for wisdom, for understanding, for discernment. Pray that the Holy Spirit will work through you to make God's truth and love real in the situation. Pray for an opening to talk about Jesus Christ.

AN EXAMPLE OF CROSSCULTURAL NURSING

Sonia, a friend of ours who works in India, exemplifies the best in crosscultural nursing. One of her patients was an elderly Sikh gentleman who was dying. She went out of her way to give him excellent care and in so doing endeared herself to his family. When the man died, the family asked her to take part in the funeral services. She agreed—and prayed for wisdom as to how she should participate in the ceremonies. After arriving she asked the Sikh priest if she would be permitted to sing a Christian hymn. He agreed, and when the time came, she stood and sang. While singing, she noticed tears in the eyes of the priest.

I (Arlene) asked her what she would do if a dying Hindu patient wanted her to chant prayers to Shiva, a common Hindu practice with dying patients. She replied that she could not do that, but she often asked for permission to pray to her God until the Hindu priest arrived. Patients rarely refused. She would send for the patient's religious leader if she was requested to do so. She prays for wisdom in her nursing interventions, guided by knowledge of Scripture and trusting the Holy Spirit to lead her. She models the meaning of Christian crosscultural nursing.

---

[35]Campinha-Bacote, "Spiritual Key to Cultural Competence," 20-22.

FOR FURTHER THINKING

1. Would it be ethical for a Christian nurse to encourage a patient from another religion to convert to Christianity? Why or why not?

2. To what extent would it be appropriate for a nurse to share personal faith convictions?

3. How would you answer a patient who wanted you to participate in a cultural tradition that you know would be harmful to the patient?

THEOLOGICAL REFLECTION

Read Psalm 67:1-7, Matthew 28:18-20, Acts 1:8, Romans 12:1-21, and Galatians 2:11-14.

1. According to Psalm 67, Matthew 28:18-20, and Acts 1:8, how does God view other cultures?

2. What principles does Romans 12:1-21 give in regard to crosscultural communication? What skills should we be developing?

3. The incident in Galatians 2 revolves around cultural practices. What was the problem here? Can you think of a nursing situation where you needed to participate in cultural practices in order to relate well with those in your care?

4. Where would you draw the line in participating in crosscultural practices? What guidelines would you use in deciding? (See Rom 2:1-16; 14:13-23; 1 Cor 10:23-33; Phil 4:8-9.)

Case Study: A Prayer for Sarah

Kimberle is a registered nurse and a grief counselor in a women's health unit of a community hospital. The surrounding neighborhood has a large Arabic population. Most of her Arabic patients are Muslim women, modestly dressed from head to toe. Their hair and neck are draped in a *hijab*. Sarah was one of these patients.

As Kimberle entered Sarah's room, Sarah lay in bed, curled up in a fetal position holding her abdomen. She was alone and crying quietly. Her head was still covered with her hijab, and only her tear-stained brown eyes were visible. She was approximately fourteen weeks pregnant and had been admitted for a threatened/inevitable abortion.

Kimberle quietly sat down next to her and touched her arm softly. She attempted to assess her physical condition as well as her ability to communicate. The previous shift had reported, "She doesn't speak English." She pointed to her abdomen and said the Arabic word for pain with a questioning tone in her voice. Eventually Kimberle discovered that Sarah did speak some English. She later expressed how touched she was at Kimberle's desire to talk to her in Arabic. She said, "It made me feel like you cared about me, like you wanted to be my friend."

After making Sarah as comfortable as possible, Kimberle silently prayed for wisdom and guidance for how to help her spiritually as well as she moved on to check on her other patients.

However, she was suddenly called back to Sarah's room to find her panicked in the bathroom. She was sitting on the toilet shaking and crying with a look of fear in her eyes. She was holding her breath, moaning and beginning to bear down. Kimberle grabbed two gloves and reached underneath Sarah to grab the fetus. She cradled the fetus, still attached to Sarah, in her hand as she helped her back to the bed. She gently placed the fetus on a clean white pillowcase. The baby had ten little fingers and ten tiny toes. Everything looked appropriate to size and shape for a thirteen- to fourteen-week fetus.

Sarah cried silently and held her child in her hands. Kimberle softly asked Sarah, "Would you like me to say a *Du' a*?" This is a word in Arabic for a prayer for blessing and comfort.

Kimberle held Sarah's hand and prayed, as they both held the baby, "Lord God, I come before you in time of need. You know the needs of Sarah's heart. Please be with her, Lord; strengthen her and speak with her; comfort her. Draw close to her, and help her to see how much you love her. God, grant her peace." They embraced and cried together.

Sarah had delivered the placenta by the time the physician arrived to examine Sarah. Kimberle took the fetus and laid it on a small pillow, gathered a tiny pair of booties, a baby identification band, and a memory quilt for Sarah. Volunteers provided these tokens for remembrance to comfort families who had to leave the hospital with empty arms.

The doctor stayed only about five minutes, but she encouraged Sarah to donate the fetus to a nearby university hospital that does genetic testing. Sarah readily signed the forms.

For many couples, genetic testing and investigation can help them learn what caused the miscarriage, but Kimberle realized that Sarah needed to know that the fetus would not be cremated and that burial options would be available to the parents. Cremation of a fetus that has reached a point of human recognition violates the Muslim faith.

Kimberle privately approached the doctor who had witnessed the consent signing and expressed her concern. The doctor shrugged her shoulders and told Kimberle not to make a fuss.

Kimberle asked Sarah if she understood what would happen to the remains after the testing and asked her what her faith taught in regard to this situation. Sarah said she was unsure but would talk with the *imam* (the spiritual leader in the mosque). In the meantime, Kimberle held the release papers, knowing that once the process was put in motion, she would be unable to stop it.

After Sarah talked with her *imam*, she and her husband decided to bury their child. Kimberle helped make arrangements in the time period required by her religion. Ceremonial washing was performed at the hospital, and her child was buried the next morning.

The morning after the burial, Kimberle decided to tell Sarah about the Old Testament story of David and his child that died (2 Sam 12). Muslims use the Qur'an for their scriptures, but they respect Jesus as a prophet and will usually be open to the Bible, especially the Old Testament. Kimberle explained that although David was unable to bring the child back to life, he knew that he would one day go to be with the child (v. 23). She further explained that God had provided a way for her to see her child again through knowing Jesus as Savior.

Many weeks after Sarah was discharged, Kimberle received a note from her. She wrote, "I can't stop thinking about you and how you spoke with me. Something very different—I cry and smile both together. Thank you. Love, Sarah."[36]

---

[36]Adapted from Kimberle S. Deller, "A Prayer for Sarah," *Journal of Christian Nursing* (2003): 18-19.

DISCUSSION QUESTIONS

1. In what ways did Kimberle demonstrate excellence in cultural care?

2. How does she maintain the integrity of her own Christian faith while meeting the spiritual needs of a Muslim patient?

3. Is it ethical for a Christian nurse to clearly present the gospel to a Muslim patient? Why or why not? (For further help on this question, see Julia Emblen and Perry Peverall, "Spiritual Care: Lingering Questions," *Journal of Christian Nursing* [2002]: 16.)

4. To what extent would it be appropriate for a nurse to share personal faith convictions?

5. If you were Sarah's visiting nurse, making a visit after her discharge from the hospital or seeing her in a well-baby clinic, how would you apply cultural humility in following up on Kimberle's spiritual care?

PART THREE

THE ENVIRONMENT

CONTEXT FOR CARE

7

THE SEEN ENVIRONMENT

Purpose: To explore the effects of the physical environment on faith and health

Objectives: After reading this chapter and completing the exercises, you should be able to:

1. Describe the nursing environment
2. Compare a biblical understanding of the natural environment with popular views of *nature/natural*
3. Define *energy* according to modern and postmodern worldviews
4. Describe the positive and negative effects of the natural environment on health

Keywords: environment, cosmology, natural, nature, energy field, *chi*, *prana*, vital energy, life force

AFTER YEARS OF HOSPITAL NURSING, Liz started to work in a rural home-health agency covering eight counties. The tenuous living situation of many clients was nearly overwhelming at first. She prayed for guidance to know which of her clients needed special attention. One family—a mother and stepson—was particularly troublesome. The eighty-four-year-old woman was dependent upon her stepson for much of her care. The obese son was himself confined to a wheelchair. Even though the nursing care was simple enough, the dirty, foul-smelling house was repugnant. In spite of that, Liz discovered two likable people, discouraged about their situation but doing the best they could.

As Christmas approached, Liz decided that it was time to do something extra. She doubted that there would be any Christmas at this home. One afternoon, she went loaded with a small tree, decorations, Christmas cookies, and a few small gifts. The mother and son were overwhelmed! Tears flowed.

Liz learned much that afternoon about the past life of this woman who had survived some very difficult times. She began to pray earnestly for them and wondered how to tell them of God's love for them.

Some time later, Liz and a friend spent an afternoon there helping with cleaning and laundry. Much trash was bagged and taken away. Because there was no washer in the home, Liz took several loads of laundry with her. As she lay in bed that evening, she thought about this family, so needy and yet trying to maintain some dignity. She thought of others in her caseload, many of them angry, frightened, or lonely people. "God," she prayed, "you have put these people in my life. You love them and know their needs. Let me be your hands for them."

The Environment in Nursing

Modern public health nursing was born in the optimistic glow of late-nineteenth and early twentieth-century science. Florence Nightingale's promotion of district nursing, distinct from sick nursing, was her vision for improving the general health of the British population.[1] Her *Notes on Nursing*, written for every woman who had charge of the health of others, focused on the immediate environment of the ill person. Nightingale believed that controlling the environment "put the patient in the best possible condition" for nature to do its healing. Discovering the laws of nature would enable us to do this.[2] District nursing brought this knowledge to the homes of the average person. Early American public health nursing was directed toward teaching people how to live in a healthy way. In many ways these efforts were successful: parents had their infants vaccinated, schoolchildren learned about healthy diets, pregnant women attended prenatal clinics, and people learned first aid to care for injuries and wounds.

Yet a committee appointed by the National Institute for Medicine reported in 1995 that nurses need better preparation to deal with stubborn environmental

---

[1] Diane Garey and Lawrence R. Hott, *Sentimental Women Need Not Apply: A History of the American Nurse* (Florentine Films, L. Hott and D. Garey, 1988).

[2] "In watching diseases, both in private homes and in public hospitals, the thing which strikes the experienced observer most forcibly is this, that the symptoms or the sufferings generally considered to be inevitable and incident to the disease are very often not symptoms of the disease at all, but of something quite different—of the want of fresh air, or of light, or of warmth, or of quiet, or of cleanliness, or of punctuality and care in the administration of diet, or each or all of these." Florence Nightingale, *Notes on Nursing: What It Is and What It Is Not* (1860; repr., New York: Appleton, Dover, 1969), 8.

health issues.[3] The committee defined *environmental health* as "freedom from illness or injury related to exposure to toxic agents and other environmental conditions that are potentially detrimental to human health." The environmental hazards addressed by the committee fell into four classes: chemical, physical, biological and psychosocial.[4] There was general agreement about addressing the health problems in these areas. Yet the committee noted that there is "heated debate over others that exist between health and social problems," such as interpersonal violence.[5] A great number of the problems public health nurses encounter fall into this contested area of social causes of disease. We will consider it in the next chapter.

Some health care workers, in reaction to failures of modern medicine, have turned to another solution. *Life* magazine once carried a photo of Andrew Weil, a physician advocate of natural holistic healing therapies, covered with mud and sporting a green herb.[6] The picture symbolizes those who see the hope for health in a return to the unspoiled world of nature. Decrying the failures of aggressive scientific medicine and technology, they offer a bewildering menu of therapies ranging from herbs to energy manipulation to shamanistic rituals to mystical channeling of spirit beings. In contrast to those in the public health movement who promote controlling the physical and social environment through public policy, these advocates of "natural healing" by and large eschew government regulation in health issues. They advocate instead a kind of do-it-yourself approach. Rather than controlling the environment, their philosophy is one of merging with or finding harmony with it.

Much current nursing literature on the environment has similar themes. One nurse educator describes her understanding of the environment as "alive, whole and interacting," reflected in the Gaia hypothesis, which states that the world is "a system made up of all living things and their environment. There is no clear distinction, only graded intensities, between living and nonliving

---

[3]Committee on Enhancing Environmental Health Content in Nursing Practice. The committee was established by the Institute of Medicine and published its report: Andrew M. Pope, Meta A. Snyder, and Lillian H. Mood, eds., *Nursing, Health, and the Environment: Strengthening the Relationship to Improve the Public's Health* (Washington, DC: National Academy, 1995).

[4]Dorothy Kleffel, "The Environment: Alive, Whole and Interacting," in *Exploring Our Environmental Connections*, ed. Eleanor A. Schuster and Carolyn Brown (New York: National League for Nursing, 1994), 14-15.

[5]Kleffel, "Environment," 14-15.

[6]George Howe Colt, "See Me, Feel Me, Touch Me, Heal Me," *Life*, August 1996, 34-50.

matter."[7] She looked to the ideas of the ancient Greeks and Romans and traditional Native Americans, as well as Eastern philosophy, for her understanding of the environment. She eventually concluded that the entire planet is our nursing client.[8]

For some nurses this language of merging takes on religious overtones:

> We must rejoin ourselves, individually and collectively, with a caring consciousness, a living cosmology that unites and attunes scientific forces with the myth, mystery, and metaphor of the mythic and mystical forces that reside on the other side of the universe that is continually turning over.
>
> The last step is crossing over the internal bridge of our consciousness and entering into this *living caring cosmology for our Lost Mother.*[9]

Both the public health approach and the merging with nature approach are based on certain assumptions about the world around us, about the environment, and about the larger reality in which we live. The public health approach reflects the modern paradigm of science and reason in which the goal is to control the environment, including people if need be, in order to eradicate disease. The second approach of merging and harmony with the environment is characteristic of the postmodern paradigm, to which many thinkers in nursing are turning.

The seen environment is the physical environment that can be felt, weighed, measured, seen, heard, tasted, and smelled. Technology and instruments extend human ability to investigate both the microcosm and the macrocosm. The natural sciences of physics, chemistry, biology, microbiology, astronomy, and so on study the seen environment. Energy fields in the seen environment are aspects of physical energy. God gave humans the responsibility to care for and develop the seen environment. God's power and wisdom are shown in the seen environment.

The seen environment is not spiritual or mystical. Mystical energy fields are mental constructs only. There is no evidence for their existence.

---

[7]Kleffel, "Environment," 7.
[8]Kleffel, "Environment," 12.
[9]Jean Watson, "A Frog, a Rock, a Ritual: Myth, Mystery, and Metaphors for an Ecocaring Cosmology in a Universe That Is Turning Over," in Schuster and Brown, *Exploring Our Environmental Connections*, 35.

Early nursing theories were primarily concerned with the patient's imme-diate physical environment or, in the case of community health, the larger environment including housing, transportation, food, water, and so on. Today many include the social environment as well. Some include the whole earth and even the universe. Martha Rogers removed time boundaries past and present in the environment.[10]

What does the Christian worldview tell us about our human dwelling? In the remainder of this chapter we will consider the seen environment, the natural world. In the next chapter we will turn to the unseen spiritual envi-ronment and its influence on our social relationships.

THE MEANING OF NATURAL

What do we mean when we refer to the natural environment? It is important to be clear about this because the term *natural* has taken on many connota-tions today. We are referring to the world of physical (material) things, those aspects of creation studied by natural science: biology, chemistry, physics, and all their various branches. The natural world is the carbon-based dimension in which we live.

Natural has become a code word today representing opposition to ex-cessive use of technology, a "back to nature" approach similar to the "merging with nature" view discussed earlier. Natural foods are raised without com-mercial fertilizers. Natural childbirth is delivery without use of anesthetics, most often by midwives. Herbal medicine is preferred over synthetic, manu-factured drugs. Naturopathic medicine, a movement of the early 1900s, is reemerging. Naturopathy asserts "the healing power of nature" and focuses on nutrition, lifestyle, and environment.[11]

When Florence Nightingale spelled *nature* with a capital *N*, she was close to, if not totally, endorsing this view. From a Christian perspective there may

---

[10]Martha E. Rogers, *An Introduction to the Theoretical Basis of Nursing* (Philadelphia: F. A. Davis, 1970), 118. Martha Rogers first opened the door for nursing to think more expansively of the human environment. She asks, "Can human field boundaries be identified within the space-time dimensions?" While Rogers stresses the mutual interaction and modification of persons and the environment, she is also optimistic about the positive direction of evolutionary change in both. Conscious human interventions for changing both themselves and the environment merely assist in this positive movement.

[11]Joseph E. Pissorno Jr., "Naturopathic Medicine," in *Fundamentals of Complementary and Alterna-tive Medicine*, ed. Marc S. Micozzi (New York: Churchill Livingstone, 1955), 170-73.

be much that is right about some of these approaches. On the other hand, embedded in the explanations there are often assumptions about nature that are not supported by Scripture.

Does nature have the power to heal? Yes and no. If we mean by this that God has built into our bodies processes that destroy invading organisms and restore damaged tissues, the answer is yes. The immune system and processes of tissue regeneration belong to the natural world. They are not wise and benevolent in themselves; such attributes belong only to the Creator.[12] Natural processes are simply working as their Creator designed them. Nursing interventions support these natural processes: dressing changes to remove drainage, exercises for cardiovascular and muscular strengthening, rest to conserve energy, nutrition to sustain the immune system and tissue repair, bathing and turning to prevent skin breakdown, and teaching healthy lifestyles. As we do these things, we are fulfilling God's intention that we care for and develop the natural world.

Does nature have power to heal? If by that we mean that the body has consciousness and intention in itself for healing and should be left to itself, then the answer is no—nature does not heal. Nature is not a wise and benevolent physician. It has no conscious intentions of its own. Only God, who created the natural world, is wise and has good intentions for creation.[13] As we saw above, God has given humankind the responsibility to carry out his intentions. Nursing is one way of doing so.

---

[12]Edward B. Davis and Michael Hunter write the following about the scientific revolution of the seventeenth century: "Perhaps most fundamental, however, was the adoption at this time of a new world view, involving a complete change in the way in which nature was conceived. . . . The mechanical philosophers of the seventeenth century challenged prevailing Aristotelian and Galenic notions, which typically depicted nature as a wise and benevolent being. Associated with such views were phrases like 'Nature does nothing in vain,' 'Nature abhors a vacuum' and 'Nature is the wisest physician.' By contrast, thinkers such as René Descartes (1596–1650), Pierre Gassendi (1592–1655) and Robert Boyle (1627–1691) held that the world was a vast, impersonal machine, incapable of acting consciously." Robert Boyle, quoted in *A Free Enquiry into the Vulgarly Received Notion of Nature*, ed. Edward B. Davis and Michael Hunter (Cambridge: Cambridge University Press, 1966), ix.

[13]Robert Boyle (of Boyle's Laws) was a Christian believer as well as a scientist. "For Boyle it was inappropriate both scientifically and theologically to speak of 'Nature' doing anything at all. . . . By denying 'Nature' any wisdom of its own, the mechanical conception of nature located purpose where Boyle believed it belonged: over and behind nature, in the mind of a personal God, rather than an impersonal semi-deity, immanent within the world." Davis and Hunter, eds., *Free Inquiry*, x.

> **Natural Discernment**
>
> Recent studies show that using so-called natural herbs is often useless and sometimes actually harmful. For example, ephedra, found in herbs and used for weight loss, has been linked to some deaths. Some herbs used in Chinese medicine to boost energy contain ephedra. See Dr. Stephen Barrett's website for reliable information regarding natural medicine and herbs. Even though Dr. Barrett is a religious skeptic, his scientific research is reliable (www.quackwatch.org/).

ANOTHER QUESTION ABOUT NATURE

A question concerning many in nursing today, especially when confronted with claims of alternative therapies, is, "What is the ultimate 'stuff' of the natural world?" Nurses are acquainted with molecules and atoms. Most of us know something of the debate concerning light: does light consist of particles or waves, or both? We hear the terms *quantum physics, Heisenberg uncertainty principle,* and *field theory.* But we may fail to see the meaning of much of this for nursing. It seems sufficient to understand molecular functions in fluid and electrolyte balance and pharmacology, and radioactivity in radiation-based diagnosis and therapy. We are glad to benefit from research on viruses done with the electron microscope and from new treatments based on subatomic theories. Meanwhile, we give our attention to caring for people.

The concept of energy has long been familiar to nurses. We understand that metabolism releases energy for body functioning and work. We know that oxygen is required for metabolism and for the functioning of all body systems. We know about electrons in the electrical functions of the heart, brain, and muscles. We also know something about radioactivity—its use in diagnosis and treatment and its potential for harm. Some of us may know about field theories in physics. But what is the human energy field theory?

Martha Rogers introduced this concept of energy field to nursing. Using the language of physics, she described people and their environment as energy fields. It is important to note that in her view humans do not *have* or *generate* energy fields; they *are* energy fields. She meant something other than the electrical activity of muscles and nerves creating an energy field around a person; instead, being human equaled being an energy field. Failed early attempts to measure human energy fields at New York University, where Rogers was dean of the School of Nursing, were first explained by lack of sensitive instrumentation. Since then, explanations tend to focus on a unique energy not accessible to physical measurement.

Many nurses who followed Rogers's thinking abandoned the idea that physics itself supported what they meant by *human energy field*. They appropriated various ideas, many from the Eastern philosophies and religions.[14] Nurses began reading of *qi*, *chi*, *ki*, *prana*, and *vital* or *life force* as explanations for therapies based on human field theory. Translated as "energy," these terms all convey the notion that there is a life-giving energy flowing through the universe, through the earth, and through all living beings. Health results from balance and movement in this energy, and illness from blockage or depletion. Techniques to restore the balance and flow of energy vary from hand movements to directing of mental intentions toward individuals or situations. Food, exercise, and meditation are also used to restore the energy balance.

Because these energies, sometimes called *subtle energy*, cannot be measured directly, research has focused on their supposed effects: increased positive affect, decreased negative affect, pain relief, and sense of relaxation.

Still the modern reliance on physics dies hard, and many writers explain these effects by referring to quantum physics and electromagnetism. It is doubtful whether most of those relying on such explanations understand quantum theory. Yet this "quantum leap" in thinking is frequent in nursing literature. Using the language of science lends a sense of respectability to human energy-field theory and the interventions based upon it. Advocates go even further when they elevate energy field to the level of worldview.

Quantum mechanics does not apply to the world of people and things in which nurses work.[15] There is no evidence based on physics that "intention"

---

[14]Physicist Fritjof Capra popularized the parallels (in his view) between recent developments in physics and Eastern mysticism. In the preface to the first edition (1976) of his book *The Tao of Physics*, he explains how repeated mystical meditative experiences helped him to realize the consistency between modern physics and Eastern mysticism. By 1984 he would write in the revised edition that widespread reception of the book had confirmed his feeling that what he wrote would become common knowledge. He writes, "The philosophy of mystical traditions, also known as the 'perennial philosophy,' provide the most consistent philosophical background to our modern scientific theories." *The Tao of Physics*, rev. ed. (New York: Bantam, 1984), xviii.

[15]"'Mechanics' is the study of motion, and quantum mechanics refers to the study of the motion of entities that are small enough and move fast enough to have both observable wavelike and particle-like properties. When quantum mechanics is applied to large-scale, familiar phenomena, the effects are too small to be significant and we are left with the laws of classical mechanics intact.

alone, so central to energy-based theories, brings about changes either in the physiology of other persons or in the environment. Even if we limit the changes in our patients brought about by a nurse's intention to psychological or social changes, some communication, either verbal or nonverbal, must occur. Thoughts in the nurse's mind must be acted upon in order to bring about changes in another person.

The human brain is part of the seen world; the human mind belongs to the unseen world. The two are related and influence one another, yet they are distinct. Philosophers and scientists have debated the "mind-body" connection for years with no cause-and-effect explanation for how they do interact. But those who have elevated notions of nuclear physics to a worldview argue that brain and mind are fundamentally the same. Not willing to yield to a mechanical view of things, they see the environment as a giant conscious system encompassing all reality. (Others argue for some higher reality that is neither matter nor consciousness.)[16] All things—rocks, earth, cells—are seen as conscious, with innate powers of consciousness and healing. There is no mind-body separation in this view, for all is mind. Phenomena like *nonlocal* healing are explained by the ability of thought (alone) to influence far-distant events. Advocates claim to have reduced the amount of crime in a city when many people meditate at the same time.[17] Clearly, they have left the science of physics and have embarked on mystical philosophy.

Brilliant physicists continue to speculate about the fundamental nature of things. However, when matter is subdivided to its absolute smallest level, whether particles, waves, or energy, the next thing is nothing physical, and we *must* turn to either philosophy or theology. Eastern religions have elevated nothing to the *Nothing* or the *Void* as ultimate reality. In the Christian

Classical mechanics and quantum mechanics are in a sense at the opposite ends of the same continuum" (Therald Moeller et al., eds., *Chemistry with Inorganic Qualitative Analysis*, 2nd ed. [San Diego: Harcourt Brace Jovanovich, 1984], 208). The Heisenberg uncertainty principle states, "It is impossible to know simultaneously both the exact momentum and the exact position of an electron." This principle is significant only at the subatomic level. But some view this principle as an intrinsic property of nature, some as a statement of the limits of our knowledge, and others as a matter for philosophical thought.

[16]"He (Bohm) sees mind and matter as being interdependent and correlated, but not causally connected. They are mutually enfolding projections of a higher reality which is neither matter nor consciousness." Capra, *Tao of Physics*, 310.

[17]Hari M. Sharma, "Maharishi Ayruveda," in *Fundamentals of Complementary and Alternative Medicine*, 243-54.

worldview something does exist beyond the smallest possible division of matter—the personal God of the Bible. This is the God who creates out of nothing and who sustains all things by his word. God is the ultimate source of the life and energy sought by those using the human-energy theory. God is also the Creator of the whole continuum of motion, from quantum mechanics of the smallest particles to classical mechanics of the familiar world of things and people in which nurses work.

There are distinctions between kinds of created things in this world. The Genesis story of creation supports this idea. "Thus the heavens and the earth were finished, and all their multitude" (Gen 2:1). God had different kinds of things in mind when he created them. The concept of species is implied in the Hebrew word *min* that describes the reproduction of plants and animals in the Creation story. God made clear distinctions between the kinds of animals the Hebrews could eat (Gen 1:1-25; Lev 11:14-29). Even though God made many kinds of things from the same basic physical "stuff," their uniqueness and distinctiveness remains. Rather than turning to Nothing or the Void to find harmony and unity, we turn to God, the Creator.

We (Arlene and Judy) have had many conversations with believers in *chi*, both from cultures where this idea has a long tradition and from "new believers" in Western countries, about what this energy is. Could it reflect a longing for the tree of life from which Adam and Eve were banned after their sin? Could it be an attempt to gain life in a way that God has not made available to us, life that only he will restore when the time is right? It's an understanding that may help to explain why similar ideas are found in so many cultures and religions. The good news is that God will give us the eternal life for which we were created and for which we long. But the Bible makes it clear that he does that only through Jesus Christ.

THE NATURAL CREATION GIVES US CLUES ABOUT GOD

The first thing to say about our environment, then, is that it is the creation of a personal, loving Creator. All created things, living and nonliving, are dependent on God for their existence. At the same time, the created environment is distinct from God the Creator. This is quite different from saying, "Matter is all there is and all there ever was," as is assumed in the modern scientific worldview. It is also quite different from assuming the existence of an impersonal *chi* (breath or vital force) as the source of life.[18] Nor is this the same thing as viewing all reality as god or the earth as our mother. While creation is dependent upon God, God is not dependent for his being upon creation. In other words, the creation is not God.

However, while creation is not a manifestation of God, it does express much of what God is like, just as a work of art reveals much about the artist. The psalmist writes,

> The heavens are telling the glory of God;
> > and the firmament proclaims his handiwork.
> Day to day pours forth speech,
> > and night to night declares knowledge.
> There is no speech, nor are there words;
> > their voice is not heard;
> yet their voice goes out through all the earth,
> > and their words to the end of the world. (Ps 19:1-4)

Observing the natural world tells us that God is powerful, that he is wise, and that he provides for his creation. Psalm 104:27-30 gives us a picture of all creatures rejoicing in dependence on God's creative and gracious power:

> These all look to you
> > to give them their food in due season;
> when you give to them, they gather it up;
> > when you open your hand, they are filled with good things.
> When you hide your face, they are dismayed;
> > when you take away their breath, they die
> > and return to their dust.
> When you send forth your spirit, they are created;
> > and you renew the face of the ground.

THE NATURAL WORLD IS GOOD

"God saw everything that he had made, and indeed, it was very good" (Gen 1:31). Good, in Hebrew thinking, was not an ideal, but it was seen in concrete

---

[18]There has been a strong belief in the West that physics and chemistry alone could not explain life. Carl Sagan discusses the postulation of a *vital force*, an *entelechy*, a *tau* or a *mana* the animated life. Eighteenth-century chemist Joseph Priestly tried to find the *vital force* by weighing a mouse just before and just after it died. Of course it weighed the same. Sagan quips, "If there is soul-stuff, evidently it weighs nothing—that is it is not made of matter." *The Demon Haunted World: Science as a Candle in the Dark* (New York: Random House, 1995), 272.

experiences of God's actions. We experience God's goodness in the way he formed creation. Environmentalist Calvin DeWitt describes seven of the provisions God made for his creation: energy exchange, soil building, cycling (carbon cycle, hydrologic [water] cycle), water purification, creative fruitfulness, global circulation of water and air, and the human ability to learn from creation.[19]

What Scripture Tells Us About the Natural Creation

- It gives us clues about God.
- It was created good.
- It awaits release from bondage to decay and death when Christ returns to earth.
- It is to be cared for and developed by people.

Nurses experience nature's goodness all the time: when immune systems destroy invaders, when hearts pump effectively, when nervous systems conduct sensations and coordinate muscular movements, when eating healthful food causes children to grow and elders to work and play, when a loudly protesting infant is born healthy and with all her parts working. We rejoice in the goodness of nature when stress falls away in a mountain vacation. We depend on the goodness of nature to sustain us with water. Our very lives depend upon the goodness of the natural world.

It would be nice if we could stop at this point while thinking about the goodness of the natural world. But nurses also study pathophysiology. All is not well in the natural world, for in it we find sickness and death. Our environmental dwelling turns against us rather than supporting our lives. Those who advocate returning to nature because it is basically good are telling us some truth. The natural world is good because God created it that way. But they are not telling us the whole truth. Nature has no intentions toward us, benign or otherwise.

---

[19]"The biosphere is a symphony of symphonies. The creatures that inhabit earth's ecosystems maintain and sustain the living fabric of the biosphere—as they reproduce, they continue to bring forth life from death. Through all this process they cycle and recycle the basic stuff of creation, all powered by the sun. And over all this activity, God provides everything these creatures need to continue through the years and generations." Calvin B. DeWitt, *Earthwise* (Grand Rapids, MI: CRC Publications, 1994), 19.

When it sustains life, it is working the way God meant it to. Even then, human involvement is required. For example, newborns left on their own die; nature does not care for them. Beyond that, we all know that even with the best of human care, nature doesn't always sustain life. Our work as nurses revolves around illness and death. Babies are born deformed. Accidents happen. Why does this contradiction in the natural world exist?

THE NATURAL WORLD IS IN BONDAGE

So much of what happens seems meaningless and unnatural. A tornado suddenly rips through a community, leaving homes destroyed, hundreds of people admitted to emergency rooms, and dozens of people dead. A healthy young father falls into a grain bin as it is being filled; he suffocates and dies. A home-health nurse loses the struggle to prevent the amputation of the limb of a middle-aged man with diabetes. A beautiful baby girl is stillborn. A teenage boy dies after being hit by a drunk driver. A vibrant young teacher struggles daily with chronic pain. Families live in temporary shelters awaiting the receding of floodwaters that have destroyed their homes and farms. The stories go on and on.

The Bible tells us that things, including people, run down. It gives us some clues as to why there are sudden intrusions of death and suffering into our lives. Something is out of joint in the natural world. When the first humans rebelled against their dependence on God, the effects of that sin were devastating, not just for their relationship with God but for the natural world as well. God's original blessing of creation was reversed. He cursed the ground itself in judgment.[20]

Two effects of God's curse are the enslavement of nature and the entrance of death into the world. Animals, originally the joy and satisfaction of humans, now often became feared enemies. Work, which was to be creative and pleasurable, now became a struggle for survival. Childbirth, meant to be joyous, became a painful experience. Human bodies, instead of supporting the eternal longings of our souls, will be torn from us in death, returning to the dust from which they are made (Gen 3:15-19).

---

[20]"This is an expression of God's judgment, and indication of coming misfortune. The blessings are reversed. The joyous dance of creation becomes a dirge, as a shadow falls over things." David Atkinson, *The Message of Genesis 1-11* (Downers Grove, IL: InterVarsity Press, 1990), 93.

Paradoxically, God's curse on the natural world was made in hope. Paul depicts creation as groaning in labor pains, pains that promise new life ahead. "Creation itself will be set free from its bondage to decay and will obtain the freedom of the glory of the children of God. We know that the whole creation has been groaning in labor pains until now" (Rom 8:21-22). In some way the liberation of nature from God's curse is tied up with human liberation in God's new creation.

Those who see nature as benign are blind to the frustration and decay of nature. They lay the problems of the natural world solely at the feet of human beings, blaming them for mismanagement and deliberate spoiling of the earth and its natural resources. Again, they are telling us some truth. Much that is wrong with our environment is due to human shortsightedness and greed.

Many blame Christianity for the present environmental crisis. Christianity teaches that God wants humanity—the pinnacle of his creative activity—to subdue the earth and have dominion over all living things (Gen 1:28). It is important to note that God told this to the first humans before they had rebelled against their Creator. When God told Adam and Eve to have dominion, the implication was that humans were to be God's agents and to care for creation.[21] We are to rule and subdue the natural world by serving it, not by exploiting it. Blaming Christianity itself for our present ecological crisis misses the problem. The problem is that humanity (including Christ's followers) has not been faithful and obedient to its calling.

Some thinkers today are realizing that humans themselves are fundamentally flawed, greedy, and selfish. Rather than cooperatively caring for the natural environment, we hurry to take what we want and think little, if at all, of what others need. Eighteenth-century romantics like French philosopher Jean-Jacques Rousseau thought that human beings were intrinsically good until they were spoiled by civilization. Rousseau was an early advocate of the return to nature. Philosopher of science René Dubos counters such an optimistic view. He writes, "The fashionable view at present is that human nature was bad from the very beginning and civilization has only given wider ranges of expression to its fundamental bestiality."[22]

---

[21]Fred Van Dyke et al., *Redeeming Creation: The Biblical Basis for Environmental Stewardship* (Downers Grove, IL: InterVarsity Press, 1996), 91.

[22]Dyke et al., *Redeeming Creation*, 163-64.

Nurses see people who suffer from environmental problems in every work setting: schools, clinics, communities, physicians' offices, emergency rooms, inpatient units.[23] Classifications of environmental health hazards include living problems, work hazards, atmospheric quality, water quality, housing quality, food quality, waste control, radiation, and violence.[24] Nurses working among the poor know that they bear a disproportionate risk with exposure to such hazards.

WE ARE TO CARE FOR THE NATURAL WORLD

In the midst of the destruction of the natural world, God's word to us remains the same as it was to Adam and Eve: "Develop and care for creation." How can we obey this command in nursing? We begin by humbly recognizing our positions as God's stewards of creation. There are at least two ways for nurses to do this: (1) by holding a humble, biblically informed view of technology and (2) by exercising our influence for care of the environment.

Those who decry technology are right in claiming that it often increases rather than relieves suffering. One of the reasons given for the increasing acceptance of physician-assisted suicide is the fear of being kept alive too long by machines. Aggressive use of technology often reflects a refusal to admit our inability to cure every condition and to always defeat death. The suffering person is lost from view in the race to solve the physiological puzzle.[25]

At the same time, technology has given new ways to treat problems, enabled us to relieve pain, and helped amputees walk. Who would want to give up using life-saving drugs? Even our stethoscopes are technology. Instead of rejecting technology as such, we need to struggle with the hard questions of when and how to use it.

Technology is an extension of human ability to develop and care for the natural world. Developing new technologies can be fulfilling God's calling. But there are dangers. One of the pitfalls to be avoided is transferring trust

---

[23]See for example, Veronica Squires and Breanna Lathrop, *How Neighborhoods Make Us Sick* (Downers Grove, IL: InterVarsity Press, 2019).

[24]The classification was developed by P. Stevens and J. Hall in 1993. It was reprinted in Andrew M. Pope, Meta A. Snyder, and Lillian H. Mood, eds., *Nursing, Health, and the Environment* (Washington, DC: National Academy, 1995), 27-28.

[25]Sherwin Nuland writes about the fascination of physicians with solving the puzzle of an illness in his book *How We Die* (New York: Alfred A. Knopf, 1994).

from God to technology. Ultimately God owns and sustains life. Pride denies our dependence on God and places it on human abilities. There are limits to what we can do, even with the most sophisticated technology. There are also limits to what we should do. It is always tempting to try everything possible to extend life—or to create new life. We need to learn when to stop.

We need to continually ask questions. Does our technology really benefit our patients? Is it motivated by a concern for the patients' good? Are we fair in the way we use technology? Is it available to all who need it or only to those who can afford it? Do a few people benefit from costly technology, leaving few resources for basic health care of the poor? Consider that most discussions about advanced technology occur in rich countries of the world. The questions of when and how to use ventilators rarely arise in poor nations, where the concerns are for the basics of clean water and enough food.

The story of Margaret and her husband, Roy, demonstrates trust in God's guiding and sustaining grace—combined with willingness to use good medical care. They had lived in a developing country as missionaries. During their stay Margaret contracted an amoebic liver infection. By all indications she recovered fully, and later she and her husband returned home with their two small sons. Years later she developed cirrhosis of the liver, which could only be accounted for by the earlier amoebic infection. Over the years she had said that she did not want any extraordinary measures taken when she was dying, including transplants. Now came the test.

There was no hesitancy on her part. No, she would not consider transplantation. "I've had a good life, two fine sons, and I'm nearly seventy years old. I am not afraid to die. But then I might have ten years yet." However, she was willing to adjust her diet and to take medication to manage the ascites. She asked that the pastors and some of her close friends come to her home to anoint her with oil and pray for her. It was a moving time, full of love, tears, and faith.

How long will Margaret live? No one knows for certain. But meanwhile she and her husband have built a smaller retirement home near their children and grandchildren. She does not talk much about her situation, so that people will not think of her as an invalid. She plans to live fully while she is living. Margaret's life is in God's hands.

We are not against transplants. The ability to give life to another through donating organs is a wonderful thing. Neither would Margaret and Roy rule out transplants as such. Roy is a physician, and Margaret is a medical technologist. It is possible that they may even change their minds. But their story represents the kind of questioning we are suggesting.

Finally, we need to look and pray for creative ways to show concern for the natural environment. When we instruct patients how to dispose of needles and syringes properly, we are protecting the environment. When we press for changes in how institutions manage medical waste, we are preserving the environment. When we support community efforts to develop open spaces for parks and playgrounds, we are helping to sustain the vitality and beauty of the environment. When we participate in block cleanup programs, we are serving creation. When we suggest reusable coffee cups instead of Styrofoam cups at work and in our churches, we are helping the landfill problem. When we press for fair-housing laws so that poor people can live in safe, pollution-free homes, we are caring for the natural environment.

God, the Creator, alone is worthy of our loyalty and worship. He alone is the ultimate source of life and healing. Appropriately used, medications and technology can be God's gifts to us. But in the end, they cannot give us life and ultimate satisfaction.

> God is our refuge and strength,
> > a very present help in trouble.
> Therefore we will not fear, though the earth should change,
> > though the mountains shake in the heart of the sea. . . .
> "Be still, and know that I am God!" (Ps 46:1-2, 10)

For Further Thinking

1. How does the physical environment affect health?

2. In what ways does nature heal?

3. In what ways can nature harm?

4. To what extent do you exercise control of nature in your nursing practice?

Theological Reflection

Read Psalm 19, Romans 1:18-32, Matthew 5:13-16, 13:1-9 (18-23), and Genesis 3.

1. What can we learn about God from nature?

2. What can we learn about ourselves and our patients from nature?

3. Why is nature (and reason) alone insufficient for understanding God?

4. In what ways can nature alone mislead us in understanding human needs?

Case Study: Sam and Carolyn

Sam and Carolyn, both in their eighties and homebound, were founding members of their congregation. Their pastor became increasingly concerned about the couple's functioning capabilities and so asked Gretchen, the faith community nurse, to visit.

When Gretchen entered their home on a frigid winter day, she immediately noticed the lack of heat and a strong urine stench. Sam and Carolyn appeared neglected and unkempt. She realized that they needed much more than standard faith community nursing. They needed physical care.

Sam and Carolyn did not qualify for home care, but Gretchen could not leave them without help. She had eighteen years of experience in community health and hospice nursing. She believed that home visiting was consistent with the ministry of Jesus Christ, who ministered to the ill by going to them, not expecting the ill to come to a place of worship for healing.

Gretchen recognized that Sam and Carolyn needed both faith community nursing and home care in order to meet their immediate needs. Stubborn, gruff, and frugal, the couple would not allow strangers into their home. They refused to follow the physician's advice of relocating to a nursing home. They rejected Meals-On-Wheels. Sam and Carolyn had no children, and no relatives lived nearby. The couple considered the church as their family, so they allowed Gretchen to visit.

Gretchen drew on her home care skills to perform a physical assessment of Sam, as well as a functional assessment of the couple. She was able to get Sam the medical care he needed, as well as help him to die with dignity. Gretchen continued to support Carolyn in prayer as well as with her physical needs.[26]

---

[26]Adapted from Gretchen Quenstedt-Moe, "Parish Nursing and Home Care: A Blended Role?," *Journal of Christian Nursing* 20, no. 3 (2003): 26-30.

DISCUSSION QUESTIONS

1. How did the natural/physical environment affect Sam and Carolyn's health and access to health care?

2. What may have happened if Gretchen had not intervened?

3. If you had been a visiting nurse assigned to Sam and Carolyn and they refused to allow you to visit, how would you have followed up?

4. If you were visiting Sam and Carolyn as a faith community nurse, how would you have handled the situation?

5. What is our nursing responsibility in situations where those in our care decide to "let nature take its course" when we know it will be harmful?

6. What is the church's responsibility in regard to promoting and maintaining physical health?

8

THE UNSEEN ENVIRONMENT

Purpose: To explore the significance of the spiritual and psychosocial
environment in health care

Objectives: After reading this chapter and completing the exercises,
you should be able to:
1. Describe the unseen environment from a Christian
   perspective
2. Assess the effects of the unseen environment in your
   nursing practice
3. Explain the moral and ethical implications of the unseen
   environment in nursing
4. List practical guidelines for living wisely in the unseen
   environment

Keywords: revelation, unseen environment, two kingdoms, society,
moral certainty, ethics

RUTH WORKED THE AFTERNOON SHIFT ON MAIN 3, a telemetry unit in a small community hospital. Many of the patients were elderly, and most were seriously ill. She liked the challenge of making rapid and accurate assessment of changes in their conditions and then responding to help them. It was common for the same people to return again and again, so she knew many of the patients and their families well. When patients improved and returned home, she rejoiced. When they died, she grieved, but she enjoyed using the best of her nursing knowledge and skill. That was the good part.

But there was another side. The head nurse of the unit was an insecure and manipulative woman. She used her power to keep the staff on edge and suspicious of one another. Besides that, most of Ruth's colleagues had personal problems that kept them from concentrating on their work. Several were involved in tempestuous sexual affairs, some with one another. Others had all the characteristics of personality disorders. Gossip abounded—about each other, the administration, and patients. The climate on the unit was stressful and confused. More than that, it was evil.

After several months, Ruth's supervisor asked her to be the regular evening charge nurse. She accepted because she thought God had placed her in this situation for a reason. She saw her responsibility as mentoring the team leaders, some of whom had little idea of how to manage the nursing assistants and LPNs working on their teams. Soon everyone knew that Ruth had no time for prolonged gossiping in the utility room. Further, they knew that she would hold them accountable for their assignments. She was tough, but she was also fair. The word got back to Ruth that everyone liked working when she was in charge. There was still the problem with the head nurse. But eventually the head nurse was asked to resign. Life on Main 3 was far from perfect, but it was a lot better than when Ruth began.

What was going on in the environment on Main 3? In the modernist worldview, the problem would be defined as only lack of proper orientation of staff and inadequate leadership by the head nurse. A nurse working from more postmodern thinking might say that energy was unbalanced. Perhaps someone who knew *feng shui* would suggest rearranging the furniture in the nurses' station or painting the walls another color, maybe even rearranging the workstations. But the underlying problem was evil in the relationships of the staff. In the Christian view the environment on Main 3 went beyond psychological or social explanations. Ruth's leadership helped to eliminate unrighteous patterns and bring about order and productive working relationships. She brought God's shalom to Main 3.

Unknown to others on this unit, Ruth fervently prayed every day for them. She also prayed regularly with a trusted prayer partner and had a circle of close friends praying with her. Ruth correctly discerned that the problems on this unit were more than simply interpersonal conflict. There were evil forces at work—this was a spiritual battle.

My own (Arlene's) experience in home health care brought me face to face with the unseen in a different way. I went into homes where family life was so discordant that children were spoken to only in harsh language if they were addressed at all, where no one read stories to children, and where often the parents were still children themselves. They were so overwhelmed that they spent their days watching TV. Attempts to teach a better way seemed almost futile. Where should one begin? After watching well-intentioned government programs pour money into community-based programs for many years with little noticeable improvement in the lives of people, one comes to realize that the problems are much too large to be fixed by programs.[1]

Another story represents the positive side of the unseen environment. Over a period of several years I went with students in home health to see an elderly woman who was cared for by her daughter. A stroke had taken away the mother's ability to speak. She spent her days in bed completely helpless. The faithful care of her daughter was given at great cost of time and effort, but she would not have considered another way. I never asked her why she did it. I knew. Her Christian faith taught her responsibility for her mother and gave her strength to endure year after year. On some visits we talked of the Lord's sustaining grace.

Things in the unseen environment are seen by faith. They are realities not perceived by the five senses that serve us well in our space-time environment. Nurses have always known when observing birth, suffering, and death that there is something about people that goes beyond the physical body—something not explainable by physics. We see evidence of this in the courage and faith of the mother with multiple sclerosis whose husband has left her, out of frustration with her handicap. We see it in the mother of a boy killed in a gang fight when she forgives those who shot him.

In chapter seven we considered the natural environment, the seen world that can be weighed and measured. In this chapter we turn to the unseen environment, the world that can be perceived only indirectly. According to the modern worldview, we can know only the seen natural world, and human behavior can best be explained by the physical and social sciences. Many of those who adopt the postmodern position would agree with Christians that an unseen world exists. Recently a convention of ghost hunters was held not

---

[1] I (Arlene) was in a master's program in a school of public health from 1968 to 1970. During those years, federal money was pouring into programs developed in response to President Lyndon Johnson's 1964 "War on Poverty." Many of these programs were good ones, at least in theory, like Head Start programs and community-based mental health clinics. Many individuals benefited from them. But the hopeful goal of lifting entire social groups out of poverty was not accomplished. Today, we read much about the increasing disparity between the growing poor lower class in the United States and the increasingly wealthy upper class.

far from my (Arlene's) home. Members use instruments that detect electro-magnetic fields, cameras with special film, and other instruments to confirm their belief that ghosts inhabit certain locations. Historical buildings and sites are most likely to be haunted, they say. The Bible, however, gives us no reason to go looking for ghosts (spirits of departed persons). In fact, it strictly forbids us to do so (Deut 18:10-11).

If the unseen world is only indirectly perceived from the seen world, how can we learn about it? How do we interpret events that seem to relate to it? Is there a way to know truth about the unseen environment? Is one person's idea as good as another's? Some would say so. To answer these questions, we turn to Scripture.

GOD'S REVELATION OF THE UNSEEN ENVIRONMENT

The unseen environment is the spiritual aspect of creation. The unseen is where God dwells (Jn 1:18). It is also inhabited by personal beings, embodied and disembodied, human and nonhuman. It is the place where we find God's law, the foundation of morality. The unseen realm is where we find things that are eternal. Paul wrote, "What can be seen is temporary, but what cannot be seen is eternal" (2 Cor 4:18). We have a deep longing for the eternal even though our natural lives will end in death (Eccles 3:11).[2] These unseen realities are the most important aspects of our lives. Life without them is "vanity and a chasing after wind" (Eccles 4:16). But if we cannot see them, how can we know about them?

According to the modern worldview, there is no way to have certain knowledge of these things; we can only speculate about what they might be, if they exist at all. Since that is the case, we need to get on with practical re-alities that can be seen and known through science. We are given facts with no meaning, technical and political power with no morality, and human life with only practical value.

Those who fit into a more postmodern way of thinking tell us that each person must find her or his own spiritual truth. The way to do this is through

---

[2]Anthropologist Kristofer Schipper writes out of his own study of and involvement with Taoism. The highest goal of this ancient belief and practice is "Long Life." On the surface there appears to be little left of Taoism, but Schipper sees its presence in the revival of health and longevity practices of *qigong* and Chinese medicine. Kristofer Schipper, *The Taoist Body* (Berkeley: University of California Press, 1993), 9.

intuition or various mystical experiences. Examples include accounts of near-death experiences in which we are given descriptions of supernatural beings and their messages. This approach, however, leaves us totally unconnected to actual events in the seen world. We are left to each person's own imagination and experience, an unreliable way to learn the truth.

The search for spiritual understanding is ancient. Job asked, "Where then does wisdom come from? And where is the place of understanding?" (Job 28:20). Ezekiel condemned those who gave prophecies out of their own imagination (Ezek 13:2). Human minds can produce futile thinking, and wisdom can be turned to foolishness (Rom 1:21-22). Moral thinking becomes debased, leading to all manner of evil and debauchery (Rom 1:28-31). Paul warned sophisticated Greek pagans, "We ought not to think that the deity is like gold, or silver, or stone, an image formed by the art and imagination of mortals" (Acts 17:29). John counsels us to not believe every spiritual message (1 Jn 4:1). With Job we ask, "Where can wisdom be found?"

> *Where then does wisdom come from? And where is the place of understanding? It is hidden from the eyes of all living, and concealed from the birds of the air.*
>
> JOB 28:20-21

Wisdom dwells with God. Isaiah the prophet wrote, "Have you not known? Have you not heard? The LORD is the everlasting God, the Creator of the ends of the earth. He does not faint or grow weary; his understanding is unsearchable" (Is 40:28). The way to spiritual understanding begins with reverence and love for God and willingness to walk in his ways. "The fear of the LORD is the beginning of wisdom, and the knowledge of the Holy One is insight" (Prov 9:10).

Because God is personal and we too are personal, it is possible for God to communicate with us. When creation was new, God walked and talked with humans in an open and direct way. They walked together in the cool of the evening. But the disobedience of the man and woman broke that open relationship (Gen 3:1-24). Since then, God's communication with humans has come in different, more hidden ways. But he continues to speak.

How does God speak? He reveals his heart and mind to us in ways similar to the manner we tell each other about ourselves. The Bible tells us that God sometimes speaks directly to people in dreams and visions (Joel 2:28). God also reveals himself through his actions. When we become aware of the divine significance of actual events, we learn something of God. David and Karen Mains call watching for God in our daily lives "the God hunt" and seeing evidence of him "God sightings."[3]

Jesus Christ, however, is God's most complete revelation of himself. "No one has ever seen God. It is God the only Son, who is close to the Father's heart, who has made him known" (Jn 1:18). "All other revelations and illuminations are simply clarifications and/or affirmations of this one incomparable revelation in human history."[4] Jesus told one of his disciples, Philip, who asked to see the Father, "Have I been with you all this time, Philip, and you still do not know me? Whoever has seen me has seen the Father. How can you say, 'Show us the Father'?" (Jn 14:9).

The Bible is the inspired witness of those who heard and experienced God's various revelations of himself. Its central theme is Jesus Christ. The Bible is the primary means God uses to break through our darkness and sin to bring us hope and light. It gives us a perspective for seeing the unseen in the everyday happenings of our lives. It helps us to know that things are not what they appear to be viewed from the seen world only. It gives us criteria for "testing the spirits," for judging the validity of the various spiritual experiences.[5]

The church hands down the interpretation of Scripture from one generation to another. However, "none of us can actually know the Word of God until God personally reveals himself to us. When God speaks, we will know it, for his word is 'living and active, sharper than any two-edged sword'" (Heb 4:12).[6]

"The Bible is a prism by which the light of God shines on us."[7] God's Spirit interprets the words of Scripture to us and awakens us to the significance of Jesus Christ for our lives. It is Jesus Christ who reveals God to us.

---

[3]David Mains and Karen Mains, *Tales of the Kingdom* (Elgin, IL: David C. Cook, 1983).

[4]Donald G. Bloesch, *Jesus Christ: Savior and Lord* (Downers Grove, IL: InterVarsity Press, 1997), 237.

[5]Paul tells us to test the spirits and not to accept all claims of spiritual insight as truth (1 Thess 5:19-21). The Bible warns repeatedly about false prophets and miracles (Mk 13:22; Deut 13: 1-5). We are told to judge all such claims *theologically*—how they agree with the rest of what we know about God as found in Scripture—and *morally*—how the lives of those claiming such insight and knowledge are evidence of godly living. The ultimate test is whether or not the person recognizes Jesus Christ as Savior and Lord.

[6]Donald G. Bloesch, *Holy Scripture: Revelation, Inspiration, and Interpretation* (Downers Grove, IL: InterVarsity Press, 1994), 53.

[7]Bloesch, *Jesus Christ*, 238.

God's self-communication to us is called *revelation*. Theologian Donald Bloesch describes revelation this way: "Revelation is indeed cognitive, but it is much more than this. It is an act of communication by which God confronts the whole person with his redeeming mercy and glorious presence. It therefore involves not only the mind but also the will and affections."[8]

When God speaks, he does not permit us to take a neutral position. We must choose to either accept his word and do what he tells us, or reject his word and rebel against him. It is an awesome thing to hear God speak. But when we receive his word with a humble and obedient heart, God teaches us wisdom. "He leads the humble in what is right, and teaches the humble his way" (Ps 25:9). When we receive God's revelation in faith, he opens our inner (spiritual) eyes to a transcendent dimension of reality, the unseen environment. The Scriptures refer often to eyes and ears of the heart. Paul prayed for a spiritual vision for believers in Ephesus:

> I pray that the God of our Lord Jesus Christ, the Father of glory, may give you a spirit of wisdom and revelation as you come to know him, so that, with the eyes of your heart enlightened, you may know what is the hope to which he has called you, what are the riches of his glorious inheritance among the saints, and what is the immeasurable greatness of his power for us who believe, according to the working of his great power. (Eph 1:17-19)

Paul was not interested in spiritual vision just out of curiosity or as a way to gain spiritual power. God mercifully shields us from much in the unseen world, showing us only those things necessary for our salvation. "The secret things belong to the LORD our God, but the revealed things belong to us and to our children forever, to observe all the words of this law" (Deut 29:29). God opens our spiritual eyes so that we can know him, his love, and his holiness. We also need to have our spiritual eyes opened to understand who we really are: created in God's image yet corrupted at the deepest level by sin. Spiritual vision helps to see our need for redemption and salvation, not just enlightenment, education, and social reform.

Knowing God's will must be expressed in the way we live. Paul prayed for the Christians at Colossae, "[May you] be filled with the knowledge of God's will in all spiritual wisdom and understanding, so that you may lead lives

---

[8]Bloesch, *Holy Scripture*, 48.

worthy of the Lord, fully pleasing to him, as you bear fruit in every good work and as you grow in the knowledge of God" (Col 1:9-10). Spiritual vision is given to help us understand more of God in order to please and honor him. As God's Spirit gives us both understanding and spiritual strength, our very character will be changed. We exhibit the fruit of the Spirit (Gal 5:22-23) and experience shalom personally and in our lives together (Is 32:17).

It is possible, however, to resist God's revelation, to close our eyes and ears, to harden our hearts. Paul quoted the prophet Isaiah when referring to those who refused to accept the message of Jesus that Paul preached.

'Go to this people and say,

You will indeed listen, but never understand,
    and you will indeed look, but never perceive.
For this people's heart has grown dull,
    and their ears are hard of hearing,
        and they have shut their eyes;
        so that they might not look with their eyes,
    and listen with their ears,
and understand with their heart and turn—
    and I would heal them.' (Acts 28:26-27)

To be without spiritual vision and hearing is spiritual death. Paul contrasted the lives of people who followed the Holy Spirit with those who followed what he called the *flesh*: "fornication, impurity, licentiousness, idolatry, sorcery, enmities, strife, jealousy, anger, quarrels, dissensions, factions, envy, drunkenness, carousing, and things like these. I am warning you, as I warned you before: those who do such things will not inherit the kingdom of God" (Gal 5:19-21). "Flesh" here does not mean our physical bodies but rather living only by what can be seen in the natural world and closing our hearts to God.

The experience of Ruth and her coworkers on Main 3 is an example of how the works of the flesh bring chaos to a nursing unit. It also shows us how the fruit of the Spirit in Ruth's life affected the climate of the whole unit. Main 3 reflected an ongoing, unseen spiritual struggle.

THE STRUGGLE IN THE UNSEEN ENVIRONMENT

What is going on in this unseen world? The Scriptures tell us of a struggle between two kingdoms. Each of them, the kingdom of this world and the kingdom of God, are competing for citizens. The outcome of this struggle is secure: the heavenly kingdom will prevail.[9] The decisive battle has been fought and won by the death and resurrection of Jesus Christ. But God, for his own reasons, has permitted follow-up battles to continue. The ruler of the "worldly kingdom,"[10] Satan, was once a powerful angel in God's presence. The Scriptures allude to a heavenly rebellion in which Satan lost his privileged position after trying to assume God's powers. Still powerful, he now rules over a large number of evil beings who plot with him against God's kingdom and its citizens.[11]

> *The god of this world has blinded the minds of the unbelievers, to keep them from seeing the light of the gospel of the glory of Christ, who is the image of God.*
>
> 2 CORINTHIANS 4:4

Satan's power, however, is deception, not truth. The devil and his hosts are not gods, but they pretend to be so. They are really feeble and bankrupt elemental spirits (Gal 4:9), and their power is that of the lie (Jn 8:44).[12] One of their primary tactics is working to deceive us about the truth of God (2 Cor 4:3-4).

The first story of human rebellion in the Garden of Eden recounts just such an act of treacherous deceit in which the serpent put doubts about God's love and goodness into the minds of Adam and Eve. He suggested that they should make their own decisions about good and evil rather than trust the Creator (Gen 3:1-5). He challenged them to reach for powers that were reserved for God alone. This is the core of the struggle that continues to this day in the unseen world. People, mere creatures, are trying to live as if they were not dependent upon a loving Creator. Human autonomy may seem good at first,

---

[9]Many religions see the struggle between good and evil as an eternal one; first one prevails and then the other. The Scriptures give us no such picture. Rather, the story of the Bible is how God works throughout history to bring those who so desire into his kingdom. Finally the two kingdoms will no longer exist together, and God's kingdom will prevail. See Revelation 11:15, 17.

[10]Paul identifies the devil, referred to as Satan in other places, as the ruler of this world. See Ephesians 2:1-2; 6:11-12.

[11]In Job 1:6-8 Satan is referred to as a heavenly being who both went about in the earth and was present in the Lord's heavenly court. Jesus referred to Satan as having fallen from heaven in Luke 10:18. Jesus did not dispute the idea that Satan was the ruler of demons in Matthew 12:24-27. The Scriptures are veiled as to the origin of these evil beings while they accept their reality. Many biblical scholars believe that when Satan fell from heaven, he took with him a large contingent of angels and that these fallen angels are demons. We think it wise to not say any more than what can be substantiated by Scripture.

[12]Bloesch, *Jesus Christ*, 44.

but it is a deception from the enemy, and eventually everything goes wrong. In truth, unless we give our loyalty to God and his kingdom we remain as prisoners in what Scripture calls "the power of darkness" (Col 1:13).[13] The Bible calls rebellion against God sin.

The effects of sin and rebellion are everywhere around us—violence, confusion in sexuality, alienation in families and communities, oppressive social structures. A great number of the social causes of disease identified by the NIH Committee referred to in chapter seven are spiritually rooted. How much can nursing, or even the whole health care system, do about family violence and sexual abuse? Nursing deals with the symptoms and has some success. But the root problems lie elsewhere, somewhere outside a world controlled by science.

EFFECTS OF THE UNSEEN IN SOCIETY

In the Genesis story of humanity's first rebellion against their loving Creator, we find the seeds of all the destruction caused by sin: fear of God rather than trust; shame with nakedness; alienation between men and women; fear between humans and animals; pain in childbirth; frustration in work; and death (Gen 3:8-24). Soon we learn of the first murder, Cain killing his brother Abel, and later we read of the continued effects of human revenge (Gen 4). This is the human story, and it occurs over and over again throughout history.

James Boice identifies the social effects of trying to build human society apart from dependence upon the loving Creator God: (1) a loss of roots and a restlessness; (2) closeness without community; (3) idolatrous worship of physical beauty; (4) pride in power and violent strength.[14] Boice refers to Simone Weil's conclusion that "the only cure for uprootedness is a rediscovery of the human being as God's creature and of God himself as the source of those basic elements without which a proper civilization cannot function: order, liberty, obedience, responsibility, equality, the right to express one's

---

[13]Scripture is clear that we are born prisoners of Satan and that only through Christ can we be rescued from this dark kingdom. When people declare their autonomy, they are only fooling themselves. We are actually slaves of sin. "But thanks be to God that you, having once been slaves of sin, have become obedient from the heart to the form of teaching to which you were entrusted" (Rom 6:17).

[14]James Montgomery Boice, *Two Cities, Two Loves* (Downers Grove, IL: InterVarsity Press, 1996), 73-75.

opinion, security, private property, truth and others." "She was exactly right," says Boice. "Our only true roots are in God."[15] Like that of our biblical ancestors, our culture today is increasingly hard, arrogant, self-seeking, and violent.

Nurses recognize the results of living independently from God in their work. The busyness and restless activity characterizing our lives are often attempts to camouflage the terror of rootlessness. How many of the stress-related diseases nurses both experience and treat have their roots in such restlessness? Stress-management practices that fail to deal with the root problem are like feeble attempts to staunch massive bleeding with Band-Aids.

People live in close proximity in today's urban culture. Yet they are lonely. We see the symptoms of loneliness in people who turn to drugs and alcohol for escape. Others call hotlines late at night to hear the voice of someone telling them why they should not commit suicide.

Fueled by social media, our culture idolizes those having perfect bodies and sexual charm. Even though some women protest against it, beauty is marketed in pageants, and goods are sold by sexually explicit advertising. "But [women] will continue to be exploited in the worst way and will even willingly submit to that exploitation until they discover that they are creatures made in the image of God, not of the latest rock star or movie idol."[16] The thousands of young people struggling with anorexia and bulimia are slaves to this lie.

Finally, our culture is increasingly marked by worship of raw power, with a resulting increase in violence and crime. Nurses working in emergency rooms, both rural and urban, can attest to this. We see the struggle for power in the politics of health care, both at the unit and agency level and in the larger arena of professional and economic maneuvering for control. Author Cheryl Forbes writes that the point of power is to be visible.[17] How much energy is spent today on image building and "power dressing"? It is present even in nursing. We are certainly not opposed to looking smart and dressing well. But when service and substance get lost in the drive for power, then power is wielding us.

---

[15]Boice, *Two Cities, Two Loves*, 74.

[16]Boice, *Two Cities, Two Loves*, 76.

[17]"More than one manager has told me that he loved office politics—the intrigue, the maneuvering —and that he was good at it. These managers manipulated others, tried to divide and conquer staff members, hinted that certain people were not as good at their jobs as others thought, whispered promises they never intended to keep." Cheryl Forbes, *The Religion of Power* (Grand Rapids, MI: Zondervan, 1983), 20.

We do not like to think of life in this way. Modern people have long thought that human progress on all fronts was inevitable, that we merely had to cooperate with the inevitable by gaining more knowledge and providing better education. Even today, when the myth of progress has been exposed as a lie and many people despair of the future of humanity, we still do not like to think about sin.[18]

We label human behavior sick rather than evil, except when the evidence is so overwhelming that it cannot be ignored, such as the massacre of thousands for "ethnic cleansing."[19] Then the problem is usually in "those people," often in other countries. We do not like to think of ourselves as sinful, as persons capable of morally twisted behavior and selfishness.[20] But morally twisted behavior is the end result of living apart from God and thus as slaves to sin (Rom 8:15-17).

MORAL CERTAINTIES IN THE UNSEEN ENVIRONMENT

Previously, we have considered the way the unseen is expressed in social behavior. Our relationships and interactions have moral implications. Understanding another aspect of the unseen, the moral dimension, is critical. Nursing today is searching for a moral anchor, but like the culture around us there is no acceptable agreement as to what that is. The lack of moral clarity to guide decision making in the clinical setting can place added stress on nurses. Legal, social, traditional, and professional criteria are variously put forth as the place to begin to sort out the boundaries of right and wrong, however, these reference points are often inadequate for the gravity of the moral uncertainties faced by nurses today. Social behaviors that were once categorized as illegal or immoral have now been legitimized through law in many states (assisted suicide and marijuana use as examples). Hobus and

---

[18]Historian Christopher Lasch, in his extensive writing, exposed the development and collapse of the idea of progress. One example is *The True and Only Heaven* (New York: W. W. Norton, 1991).

[19]The Scripture does characterize sin as disease in some places, but it is a disease brought on by rebellion (Is 1:4-6).

[20]Eugene Peterson, "Teach Us to Care and Not to Care," in *The Crisis of Care*, ed. Susan S. Phillips and Patricia Benner (Washington, DC: Georgetown University Press, 1994), 70. Eugene Peterson reminds Christians that they of all people should not be naive or ignorant about sin. The Bible is both insistent and convincing on the subject. However, even unbelievers should not have difficulty acknowledging the reality of sin. "It is, as Chesterton once pointed out, the only major Christian doctrine that can be verified empirically."

Schreiber describe the ramifications of legal drug use that have followed what they call a "prevailing mindset" that "if use of drugs is legal, they must be harmless."[21] Thus, the law does not protect against or prevent moral implications. Some nurse ethicists, wanting a more enduring foundation, argue for natural law ethics.[22] Others are turning to an ethic of care. All these ethics begin in the seen world and are based on human experience or reason. Nursing, now considered a secular profession, cannot accept a religious foundation for its ethics. Would recovery of our spiritual vision help us? We believe that it would.

Philosophers and even unsophisticated people in all ages and places recognize a moral reality (Rom 1:19-23). As we expressed in an earlier book,

> Because we live in a moral universe created by God, it is not strange that wise people throughout history have discovered universal-moral principles like justice, benevolence and truth. How often have you cried out in the midst of a frustrating situation, "That's not fair!" There wasn't time for deep theological reflection. The feeling just came from your gut. Aristotle observed that we know what justice is when we feel the wounds of injustice.[23]

The moral aspect of creation is not only "out there," it is within us as well. God created us in his likeness, and our moral calling is to express God's character. "The law of God for our behavior corresponds with the way we are made and with the world in which he asks us to be moral agents." Those who advocate a natural law ethic are right when they argue for a moral creation. Paul writes about those who do instinctively what God's law requires because it is written on their hearts (Rom 2:14-15).

Reflecting on our general sense of morality, however, leaves us perplexed. What does natural law tell us? What does it mean to be kind and just? Those who advocate assisted suicide, for example, sprinkle their arguments with the word *compassion*. Justice means different things to people. Furthermore, we

---

[21]Steven Hubus and John Schreiber, "Integration of a Biblical Worldview and Substance Abuse," in *Nursing as Ministry*, ed. Kristen Mauk and Mary Hobus (Burlington, MA: Jones and Bartlett, 2019), 283-303.

[22]Natural law is "a body of unchanging moral principles regarded as a basis for all human conduct." Lexico.com (Oxford: Oxford University Press, 2020), s.v. "natural law," www.lexico.com/definition/natural_law.

[23]Judith Allen Shelly and Arlene B. Miller, *Values in Conflict* (Downers Grove, IL: InterVarsity Press, 1991), 81

do not do even the good we know to do; our wills are bound (Rom 1:15-16). We are then not only perplexed; we are guilt-ridden as well. We need more than a moral creation to guide us. We need to know our moral Creator.

Christians believe that morality is rooted in the character of God. God is a God of justice and righteousness, love, and mercy. "Righteousness and justice are the foundation of your throne; steadfast love and faithfulness go before you" (Ps 89:14). God's law meets our need for moral understanding. "The law of the LORD is perfect, reviving the soul; the decrees of the LORD are sure, making wise the simple" (Ps 19:7). God's law does not change (Ps 33:11; 119:152). God's law is true. "The sum of your word is truth; and every one of your righteous ordinances endures forever" (Ps 119:160). God's word teaches us the distinction between good and evil (Heb 5:14; Rom 12:2). Finally, God's law observed results in a life of shalom. "Great peace have those who love your law; nothing can make them stumble" (Ps 119:165).

Ethicist John Kilner describes a biblical ethic for health care that brings together the best of other ethical theories. He identifies his approach as God-centered, reality-bounded, and love-impelled.

First, a God-centered ethic begins with God, what his purposes for us are and what his image in people looks like. Because our reasoning is both limited and sinful, we need more than ethical principles—we need a guide, the Holy Spirit, to help us discern the complex issues we face, and we need moral strength to do what is right.

Second, a reality-bounded ethic defines good and evil for us and give us moral guidance for the various aspects of our lives. Here Kilner includes such things as contributing to the needs of others and viewing people as holy ones to be treated with special care. Kilner identifies four ethical guides as especially pertinent for health care: (1) promoting life, (2) acting justly, (3) respecting freedom, and (4) telling the truth. There are times when we are not sure what should be done in specific situations. Then we need to discern how to apply these guides. Our guide, the Holy Spirit, helps us.

Finally, a biblical ethic is love-impelled, building others up and helping them to experience as much good as possible. Neighbor love is expressed in community and takes into account how our actions will affect others.[24]

---

[24]John F. Kilner, *Life on the Line: Ethics, Aging, Ending Patients' Lives, and Allocating Vital Resources* (Grand Rapids, MI: Eerdmans, 1992).

Nurses struggling with the moral implications of a health care system driven by economic profit are reflecting God's moral concern for justice. When we cry out against injustice in the care of the poor, we are expressing God's moral indignation. When coping with ethical issues relating to arrogant use of technology, we need to remember that we are accountable to God. Patients and caregivers wanting total control over the beginning and end of life are grasping for an autonomy that God did not give to us. In the morally uncertain climate today, nursing needs to recover its spiritual vision. We need a God-centered ethic.

NURSES AND THE UNSEEN ENVIRONMENT

The unseen environment has vast implications for nursing. In the above discussion we have touched on the social and moral implications. Now we conclude by identifying several practical ways that we can live wisely in this environment as nurses.

First of all, we can actively seek biblical wisdom. Derek Kidner coined the phrase *godliness in working clothes*.[25] Scripture gives us much practical wisdom for relating to patients and coworkers, for conducting ourselves with those in authority and for doing our work in an ethical way. Biblical wisdom leads to spiritual discernment that guides our actions as Christian nurses. God's word promises us that "His divine power has given us everything needed for life and godliness, through the knowledge of him who called us by his own glory and goodness" (2 Peter 1:3).

Second, we need to remember that we are in a spiritual battle with evil. When relationships in our work are devious and confused, we need to be aware that we are not fighting against certain people so much as against unseen spiritual beings. We are given spiritual weapons for this battle: truth, righteousness, peace, faith, salvation, Scripture, and prayer (Eph 6:10-18).

We also have good news to bring to our patients and coworkers, news that we can learn only from God's revelation of himself in Jesus Christ. It is good news that pushes back the kingdom of darkness and fear that holds many of our patients and coworkers in its grip. In a later chapter we will consider how to give spiritual care—how to share this good news.

---

[25]Derek Kidner, quoted by David Atkinson, *The Message of Genesis 1–11* (Downers Grove, IL: InterVarsity Press, 1990), 170.

Another practical consideration concerns the truth that things are not always what they seem. Knowing this has significance for nursing research. Nursing is moving more and more to qualitative research methods to capture narrative data to describe the personal nature of caring and the lived experience of illness. The frameworks through which we perceive and interpret nursing phenomena are derived from particular understandings of the unseen. Christian nurses will want to make such frameworks explicit and then evaluate them based on biblical and theological knowledge. For example, most nursing research assumes an understanding about the person. We want to ask, How does this view compare to what the Bible teaches us about people? This is not to say that we cannot learn some truth from theories not explicitly Christian, but it does mean that we need to be clear about the limitations of the interpretive frameworks we use. We need to discard those that give us a totally wrong understanding.

> *May you be made strong with all the strength that comes from his glorious power, and may you be prepared to endure everything with patience, while joyfully giving thanks to the Father, who has enabled you to share in the inheritance of the saints in the light.*
>
> COLOSSIANS 1:11-12

KEEPING OUR FOCUS

Finally, a word of hope. Our environment abounds with evidence of sin and evil. But there is good news. As socially devastating as sin is, it is not the most important side of the struggle in the unseen environment. The universe is still God's creation. We pointed out at the beginning of this section that the decisive battle in the unseen struggle has already been won by Jesus Christ. The evidence is an empty cross and an empty tomb on the first Easter. God is still present and acting. Eugene Peterson writes, "We live on holy ground. We inhabit sacred space. This holy ground is subject to incredible violations. This sacred space suffers constant sacrilege. No matter—the holiness is there, the sacredness is there. If our lives, and in this case our caring, are shaped in response to the violations, to the sacrilege, and not out of the holy, they are shaped wrongly."[26]

In this light Peterson counsels us to be restrained in our acts of caring because "responding to a person in need . . . takes place in an environment

---

[26]Peterson, "Teach Us to Care," 74-75.

already surging with life, prodigal with energy, vitality, beauty."[27] He calls us to worship, to stop our activity of caring long enough to discover what God is doing. Those of us who care for others should look for God in every situation.

Consider that in his wisdom and providence, God has placed each of us right where he wants us. Each day we need to ask God to open our eyes to see him acting, our ears to hear him speaking to us—through our patients, through those with whom we work, through the often confused or evil situations in which we find ourselves. We do this by taking time to let God first speak to us in his Word so that our vision is clearer and our hearing more acute. We do this through private and corporate worship. We do it through hearing the counsel of other nurses who also walk with God. These are all ways to heed Paul's words to keep our focus on what God is doing in our environment (Col 3:2). We can then enter each day knowing that we are not alone, for God is with us.

FOR FURTHER THINKING

1. In what ways does the spiritual and psychosocial environment affect health?

2. How would you describe your work environment?

3. Think of a time when you were put into the role of patient (either in a hospital or as an outpatient). What impressed you, positively and negatively, in the health care environment?

THEOLOGICAL REFLECTION

Read each of the following "beatitudes" and Scripture references, and then consider what difference each would make in your nursing environment. How could you begin to change your environment to make it a better place to work?

1. Blessed are nurses who treat others with dignity and respect, seeing them as the image of God. They humbly learn from others, even the lowly, and willingly teach others. They will grow in understanding and knowledge (Phil 2:3).

2. Blessed are nurses who do not mourn the lack of time, but make the most of time with their patients. Their gentle words comfort those who suffer. They, too, shall be comforted (Eph 5:15-16).

---

[27]Peterson, "Teach Us to Care," 73.

3. Blessed are nurses who consider new ideas for better patient care. As they advocate for their patients, they shall obtain mercy (Is 43:19).

4. Blessed are nurses who consistently strive for excellence despite the challenges they face. They will be satisfied with their profession (Phil 4:8-9).

5. Blessed are those who support and forgive one another, helping one another to learn from mistakes. They too will be forgiven (Mt 6:14).

6. Blessed are nurses who maintain personal integrity, resisting temptations to take shortcuts that would endanger patients. As they seek consistency in all that they do, they shall receive the respect and trust of their patients and colleagues (1 Pet 3:8-12).

7. Blessed are nurses who help one another and work as a team. They resolve conflicts quickly and fairly. They listen to each other and value each other's contributions to the team. They shall be called servants of God (Mt 25:40).

8. Blessed are you when you take courage, persisting in quality care even when you are misunderstood or undervalued by others. Many were persecuted before you. Rejoice and be glad, for great is your reward in heaven (Mt 5:11).[28]

Case Study: A Nurse Reflects

It is 10:00 p.m. on Thursday evening. In four months, I will be a first-time mother. Presently, I am in my first year as manager of a thirty-four-bed oncology unit in a community hospital. Eighty percent of my staff nurses are new to hospital nursing. Tonight, I will work with the night shift. My goals are to open communication, stand in solidarity with this shift, and to educate, encourage, and observe.

Currently we are experiencing a nursing shortage. Just two years ago, hospitals were merging and laying off nurses. In that tight market many new graduate nurses accepted positions in long-term care. I recently hired several of them—each one eager to get some acute care experience. Now they want relief from high demands and shrinking resources.

Managers try to rethink the nursing care model, inject pride in the profession, and promote high nursing standards while staying afloat fiscally. As an

---

[28]Adapted from Diane Stegmeir, "Beatitudes for Nurses," *Journal of Christian Nursing* (2004): 38.

idealist who likes promoting ideals, I am frustrated. Many of our nurses feel battered. Mandatory overtime and a high census take their toll. We struggle to deliver competitive customer service to an informed and increasingly sick consumer who demands more information, more expertise, and more caring.

I'm beginning to appreciate the influence of business on health care. To remain fiscally solvent, I have advocated shorter lengths of stay, disciplined staff for using excessive sick time, and waited long months to replace necessary equipment. I have reduced hiring, struggled to maintain safe staffing, and then increased hiring again. We have lost many nurses to the other local hospital that offers higher wages, weekend incentives, and access to gym facilities. I have listened to nurses explain that they simply need more money, more flexibility, and greater benefits for what they do.

Newly graduated nurses come with less clinical experience and seem to place little value on sacrificial service. At first glance, today's nurses seem to be an unmotivated, undedicated, selfish workforce—unconcerned with professional standards, unwilling to participate in unit-based improvements, and unwilling to be inconvenienced. In reality, they are tired.

I start my time on the night shift explaining why I am there and what the staff can expect from me. Before long I am trying to mediate a conflict between the charge nurse and her staff. She doesn't expect the problem to be resolved. She tells me that it is unfair for her to have a complex assignment, plus the additional responsibilities of charge nurse. She fears losing her license if she makes a mistake. She reminds me that in other places charge nurses receive additional compensation.

I start to feel defensive but want to be available for just such concerns. Why hadn't she expressed her concerns before? Why is she so adamantly refusing to accept what I see as professional responsibility that is well within her expertise? She is one of my better nurses. I start to feel discouraged.

I wish that I had more management training and knew how to handle this situation. Instead of listening, I defensively lecture her on the role of the professional nurse. I explain that compensation is being discussed, that I am working on solutions for night-shift staffing and remind her that any solution I have proposed has been put down by the night shift. Then I invite her to continue telling me her concerns and to participate in finding solutions. She doesn't seem to take me seriously.

The night routine begins. I restart an IV, review charts, answer call lights, and get a cup of tea for an anxious patient with a grave prognosis. I answer the phone and accept an admission. After reporting the admission to the reluctant charge nurse, I help her to decide which of the two nurses will take the patient. She shrugs her shoulders, saying she will just take the patient. She doesn't want any conflict. I encourage her to appropriately assign the patient to the nurse who has the less complex assignment but one more patient than the other nurse. We talk briefly about equity being greater than equivalent numbers.

I talk with the night supervisor, assist a nurse with rhythm interpretation, help to admit the new patient, and then spend a few minutes with the nursing assistant. I want her to receive some additional training so I can justify her not floating when I hire a second full-time aide. She has worked on this unit for over ten years. I would like to reward her longevity. She agrees that a second aide would be a great help. I am relieved.

At the end of the shift, I leave with my mind still whirring and wonder if I will be able to sleep. I am worried about straining my pregnant body and wonder how I will balance nursing with motherhood. Most of my friends tell me there is nothing more important than this new life I am nurturing. They assure me I will be transformed, concerned for nothing else than the new baby. I am not sure.

I passionately see nursing as a vocational calling to professional service. I want to instill this vision in others. I want to see nursing restored to a valued public service with intelligence, compassion, dignity, and reasonable compensation. I know that I am making a difference.

I wonder how to develop leaders in an age of self-service. I ponder what is fair and reasonable. I consider what I can do next week to help the night shift. I question whether we can continue to recruit nurses in the face of such difficult demands. I worry how nursing will navigate the waters of business and health care and remain compassionate.

Two thoughts help me day to day. First, I think of how God put Queen Esther in a difficult position "for such a time as this" (Esther 4:14). Second, Jesus said that we are salt and light in the world (Mt 5:13-14). Salt slows down the rotting process. Light reveals problem areas and effects change. I want to be salt and light in nursing. I care deeply about nurses and supporting positive structures where nurses practice. In doing so, I hope that I can faithfully represent Christ in the world.[29]

---

[29]Adapted from Jill McCullough, "Can I Really Be the Ideal Nurse?," *Journal of Christian Nursing* 17, no. 3 (2000): 20.

Discussion Questions

1. What issues does Jill describe that contribute to today's nursing environment?

2. What unseen forces seem to be at work in this situation?

3. How have you experienced similar pressures in your own work situation?

4. Using Jill's example of Queen Esther (Esther 4:14), how could a Christian nurse work with management to make a difference in nursing practice?

5. What would it mean for you to be "salt and light" (Mt 5:13-14) in your work situation?

6. What difference could prayer make in your work environment? Discuss some ways that you could intentionally pray for your colleagues.

9

A STORIED ENVIRONMENT

Purpose:	To identify the relationship between God's story and nursing practice
Objectives:	After reading this chapter and completing the exercises, you should be able to:
	1. Define hope
	2. Describe sources of hope
	3. Describe the effects of the *myth of progress* in health care
	4. Explain the role of *God's story* in giving meaning to human stories
Keywords:	story, hope, myth of progress, metanarrative

ELAINE STRUGGLED WITH AN INNER PROMPTING that she thought was God's voice: *Go talk to the patient in room 321.* She was not at all eager to enter the room. The patient, Mary Ann, had been admitted to the surgical unit after a suicide attempt. Elaine had little experience with suicidal patients and feared saying or doing the wrong thing. Finally, she had a short break in her work and went to 321. Elaine felt that God gave her a special boldness as she asked Mary Ann what precipitated this attempt to take her own life. "My husband said he doesn't love me anymore, and he wants a divorce," Mary Ann muttered quietly.

At that moment Elaine knew why God had urged her to go into this room. "Five months before, my husband had said the same words to me. I knew the pain of hearing those words, and I could identify with her desperation." When it seemed clear that Mary Ann did not want to say more, Elaine shared her own story, all the while feeling odd telling a stranger her problem. But she could tell that Mary Ann seemed eager to hear more. "Did you get a divorce?" she asked.

"No, we didn't," Elaine said. "He decided that he was confused when he said it, and he wants to try again. I have prayed that God will help me forgive him,

and we are depending on God to heal our marriage." She then identified
herself as a Christian believer.

"I'm a Christian too," said Mary Ann. "But my husband moved out."

Elaine wished that she could assure Mary Ann that her husband would
come back, that everything would be fine, that God would heal their marriage, and they would live happily ever after. "All I could do was remind
her what a powerful God we have, and that although her husband had left
her, God hadn't."

Then Elaine had to leave because a patient had returned to the unit from
surgery. "I'll be praying for you," she said to Mary Ann and gently squeezed
her hand.

Elaine wrote this story for the *Journal of Christian Nursing* seventeen years
later, after celebrating her nineteenth wedding anniversary. She concluded
with the following paragraph:

> I didn't know much about caring for suicidal patients, but I discovered that day
> that God does. Sometimes in nursing, he calls us to listen to his voice and obey,
> because he knows everything about our patients. He knows their deep needs
> better than we do. He knew that Mary Ann needed to know she was not alone,
> that even other Christians were suffering the same pain she was. She needed
> someone to remind her that God will bring us through every crisis life has to
> offer. I felt grateful and privileged that he used me to pass on his hope to her.[1]

The hope Elaine offered to Mary Ann was not a bland optimism that things
always work out. Her own pain prevented her from doing that. The hope she
offered was in the God of hope, the God who works to achieve his purposes
in our lives, often in ways unseen.

Nurses have always been bearers of hope by their words and by their acts
of caring. As we saw earlier, nursing was taken around the world by
Christian missionaries who often worked with few resources. Nurse historian Linda Sabin cites the example of Mrs. Charles Lewis, a missionary
nurse in China. Mrs. Lewis put the following notice in a 1915 *American
Journal of Nursing*: "We are looking for two or three more good, conscientious nurses who are anxious to be useful in laying the foundations for re-
liable nursing in the future China. Thirty-two hundred patients were seen

---

[1]Elaine Creasman, "The Patient in Room 321," *Journal of Christian Nursing* (1994): 22-23.

at our clinics in Pautingfu last year, and 823 operations were done, and yet, we must beg for nurses to go and help with this work."[2]

Christian missionaries obey the words Christ spoke before ascending to heaven: "Go therefore and make disciples of all nations, baptizing them in the name of the Father, and of the Son and of the Holy Spirit, and teaching them to obey everything that I have commanded you. And remember, I am with you always, to the end of the age" (Mt 28:19-20). Along with their preaching, missionaries have offered practical actions to make life better for those they were serving.[3] Christ's command and the promise of his presence have enabled them to continue their work as bearers of hope.

DEFINING HOPE

Mary Thompson, whose research focused on nurturing hope in patients, defines hope in this way: "Hope is the expectation of attaining a goal, the knowledge and feeling that there is a way out of difficulty. It is a perspective on life that results in action. Hope enables a person facing a potentially despairing situation not to give up."[4] Hope expects new things to happen in the future. Life isn't just the same old thing over and over. Growth and progress are possible.

Hope has always been a vital aspect of nursing, for both nurses and their patients. The hopeful nurse finds strength to continue working in the face of great odds. Common nursing wisdom tells us that more often than not patients who have hope improve physically and emotionally to a greater degree than those without hope. Nurses were among the first to do research on how hope affects the healing process.[5] We have hope that, even though it may take

---

[2]Linda E. Sabin, "Claiming Our Heritage: Bridge to a Lasting Future," *Journal of Christian Nursing* (1997): 5.

[3]See chapter one in this book. "Since late antiquity, when Eastern Orthodox Christians established the first hospitals, religious organizations have frequently led the way in providing for the institutional care of the sick." Ronald L. Numbers and Darrel W. Amundsen, eds., *Caring and Curing: Health and Medicine in the Western Religious Traditions* (New York: Macmillan, 1986), 2.

[4]Mary Thompson, "Nurturing Hope: A Vital Ingredient in Nursing," *Journal of Christian Nursing* (1994): 10-17.

[5]In their investigation of past research, Carol J. Farran, Kaye A. Herth, and Judith M. Popovich conclude, "Although other outcomes may be identified in future qualitative and quantitative studies, there is sufficient evidence to support the biological and psychosocial effects of hope and hopelessness on individuals and families." *Hope and Hopelessness: Critical Clinical Constructs* (Thousand Oaks, CA: Sage, 1995), 191.

some time, treatments will be effective. We urge our patients to hope that medications will work, that surgery will be beneficial, that exercise will improve muscle strength. We encourage them to trust the skill of their caregivers. We help them find hope, in the face of crippling disease, for some improvement or for slowing their decline. Just being alive is reason for hope. Death is the end of hope, at least for this life.

WHISTLING IN THE DARK?

Nurses write much about the benefits of hope. But what if we can no longer offer hope that improvement is possible or that our nursing interventions will help? For example, how could Elaine offer hope to Mary Ann concerning her marriage when there seemed to be no hope for it? Often it seems we are urged to "hope in hope." The positive psychological benefits of hope are stressed. But why should anyone hope for a better future when all evidence belies the possibility? Are we merely "whistling in the dark"?

Two theorists who have influenced nursing, one a nurse and the other a developmental psychologist, are examples of unfounded optimism. Martha Rogers was one of the first to explicitly include the time dimension in nursing theory. Time, the fourth dimension, adds a sense of movement and liveliness to her nursing theory.[6] By including this fourth dimension of time, Rogers opened new ways of thinking about nursing. From her perspective, increasing complexity, diversity, and rhythmicity of the life process were inevitable and good.[7] Her ideas appealed to many when she first proposed them, and they still do. Rogers's theory is optimistic. It assumes that people and societies always move over time in a positive direction.[8]

---

[6]Barbara Sarter, in her study of Martha Rogers's theory, emphasizes that the concept of four-dimensionality (all reality for Rogers) is not space and time. "Reality is nonlinear, nontemporal, nonspatial. . . . Nontemporal refers to the relativity of time and to the 'relative present' for a given individual. Paranormal phenomena, such as precognition, telepathy, reincarnation, and meditative modalities, which indicate an awareness 'beyond waking' can be explained by the postulate of four-dimensionality." Perhaps the term *timeful* might better express Rogers's meaning. While she rejected the idea of linear time as a constraint for people, her ideas of wave phenomena and rhythmicity have no meaning apart from time. Barbara Sarter, *The Stream of Becoming* (New York: National League for Nursing, 1988), 62.
[7]Martha Rogers, *An Introduction to the Theoretical Basis of Nursing* (Philadelphia: F. A. Davis, 1970), 115-16.
[8]Rogers, *Introduction to the Theoretical Basis of Nursing*, 55. Rogers had a positive view of evolutionary progress. "The theory of progressive evolution finds expression in man's sequential development. The life process is a becoming. The evolution of life exhibits an invariant one-way trend."

Erik Erikson's *Childhood and Society*, published in 1950, was the impetus for nursing's interest in the life cycle, first taken up in psychiatric and pediatric texts and eventually spreading throughout the entire curriculum. Erikson proposed his theory at a time when psychology and sociology were eagerly accepted as means to create a new humanity capable of living in harmony rather than always being at war. Erikson's optimistic interpretation of Darwinian theory shapes his psychosocial theory.

Both Martha Rogers and Erik Erikson were basically hopeful about the future. Erikson, born in 1902 in Europe, and Rogers, born in 1914 in the American South, lived in the years when the "myth of progress" was beginning to weaken in intellectual circles. Yet the dying of a cultural assumption is prolonged, and both of them, along with many others in academia, continued to express this optimism. Historian Roy Swanstrom characterizes the "cult of progress" this way:

> The experts were not thoroughly agreed about what progress meant, but the general feeling was that year by year, century by century, mankind was moving toward the day when material well-being would replace poverty and deprivation; rationality would replace myth and superstition; liberty and democracy would replace despotism and tyranny; a world-wide human brotherhood would replace hatred and war; and humanity would be the ruler rather than the victim of the forces of nature. Note the implication that while the conditions of life are constantly improving in quality, the human race itself is growing in both virtue and wisdom.[9]

French psychologist and pharmacist Emile Coué (1857–1926) even coined a slogan for this movement: "Every day in every way, I'm getting better and better." He noted that patients recovered faster when he praised the effectiveness of the medicines he prescribed and believed that optimistic affirmations fostered the recovery process.[10]

Lillian Wald is an example from nursing history of one who practiced this belief in human progress. Along with Mary Brewster, she founded the Henry Street Settlement House in 1893 on New York City's lower east side. She was

---

[9]Roy Swanstrom, *History in the Making: An Introduction to the Study of the Past* (Downers Grove, IL: InterVarsity Press, 1978), 61.

[10]See "Everyday in Every Way I'm Getting Better and Better," *Present Outlook*, accessed September 25, 2020, http://presentoutlook.com/day-by-day-in-every-way-im-getting-better-and-better.

a strong believer that public health nursing would assist human progress by applying scientific knowledge. Forty years after founding Henry Street she could write the following: "Increasing emphasis is laid on detecting and overcoming defects in children—cardiac, dental, visual, aural, and others. In this effort it may be repeated that the nurse is the indispensable interpreter of the aims and methods of modern medical science."[11]

Wald was an enthusiastic supporter of the newly developing field of "mental hygiene" and taught the Henry Street nurses to secure treatment for mentally ill members of the families in their care. She also believed that "in the nurse's approach to her cases, she needs to know the fundamentals of modern psychology so that her own relationship with them may be sound and productive."[12] Wald's passion was progress in human relations in the broadest sense, and she saw education, supported by government policy, as the means for social engineering. She did not expect miracles but "something better—the opportunity to work out for ourselves a planned and controlled way of life."[13] The ideals of public health nursing today still reflect Wald's century-old vision.[14]

Wald's passion was progress in human relations in the broadest sense, and she saw education, supported by government policy, as the means for social engineering.

Others shared this hope for the benefits of public health. A 1949 textbook of hygiene and public health even promotes "the control of racial health through the application of a knowledge of heredity and through sex hygiene."[15] Such an optimistic view of eugenics in 1949 is frightening. Where was the writer when the work of Nazi physicians in concentration camps was revealed to the world in 1945? Was he naive, or did he approve?

---

[11]Lillian D. Wald, *Windows on Henry Street* (Boston: Little, Brown, 1934), 85.

[12]Wald, *Windows on Henry Street*, 107.

[13]Wald, *Windows on Henry Street*, 336.

[14]We have noted several times that Florence Nightingale's thinking was reflective of this view. Swanstrom observes, "The epitome of the new optimistic spirit was the first world's fair, held in London in 1851, whose huge Crystal Palace attracted thirteen thousand exhibitors and six million visitors and gave dramatic visual demonstrations of human ingenuity and prowess. Without question it left the clear impression that human progress was indeed the key to all history" (*History in the Making*, 63). Florence Nightingale would have been thirty years old at this time. The Crimean War, during which she instituted reforms in the care of wounded British soldiers, was fought from 1853 to 1856. She published *Notes on Nursing*, a book that reflects this positive attitude, in 1860.

[15]Earl B. Erskine, *Hygiene and Public Health* (New York: Prentice-Hall, 1949), 4.

THE DECLINE OF THE MYTH OF PROGRESS

Why was the idea of progress so prevalent? Scholars attribute this attitude to the Enlightenment and the secularization of a biblical understanding of human history. According to theologian Robert Jenson, Westerners have understood human life as realistic narrative. We think that the sequence of events in our life should make a certain kind of "dramatic sense" because they fit within a real *universal* story.

Today many have lost faith in the idea that our lives should make sense within a larger story. The reason is that "modernity was defined by the attempt to live in a universal story without a universal storyteller." Jenson explains: "The entire project of the Enlightenment was to maintain realist faith while declaring disallegiance from the God who was that faith's object. The story the Bible tells is asserted to be the story of God with His creatures; that is, it is both assumed and explicitly asserted that there is a true story about the universe because there is a universal novelist/historian."[16]

We see the effects of "disallegiance from God" in society. God, no longer taken seriously in public life, is relegated to private life. We explain the natural world and human life without reference to God. Modern science has *desacralized* the environment—pushed gods and demons out of the human dwelling. By contrast, in many cultures past and present, the environment itself is considered *sacred*. Everything has religious significance, and "every human experience is capable of being transfigured, lived on a different, a transhuman plane."[17] In the modern worldview, people must create significance for their own lives.

But living without God as the "universal storyteller" is a project doomed to fail. Two world wars, continuing revolutions and military actions, and "cleansings" of various sorts—ethnic, social, and political—have shattered utopian dreams of progress. Rising crime rates, government scandals, family breakdown, and the widening gap between rich and poor undermine optimism for the future. Our accumulation of material comforts and our technological advances have not been accompanied by the expected moral improvement. As a result, many today see human history as meaningless,

---

[16]Robert W. Jenson, "How the World Lost Its Story," *First Things* 36 (1993): 21.

[17]Mircea Eliade, *The Sacred and the Profane: The Nature of Religion* (New York: Harcourt Brace Jovanovich, 1959), 171.

without story. "If there is no God, or indeed if there is some other God than the God of the Bible, there is no narratable world," writes Jenson.[18]

This loss of a sense of meaningful history affects not only humanity as a whole; many today have lost hope that their personal lives have any significance. For a time we can live *as if* things will indeed work out for the better. But then reality hits. Erikson's theory provides a stark example. His work locates personal identity within human culture and society. But he gives us no larger story and no universal storyteller. After the final stage of development comes death and the end of one's identity.[19]

Nurses see this loss of story in patients who are self-destructive, who live with no hope and no goals, who are indeed afraid to hope. They see it in patients whose personal identity is confused. They see it in fellow nurses whose frantic attempts to find meaning in life are self-demeaning and destructive: multiple sexual affairs, partying, debt-accumulating shopping sprees. They see it in patients (and themselves) suffering from stress-related health problems because they are "seeking immortality through work."[20] They see it in the growing demand for legal access to assisted suicide when loss and illness threaten patients' identity as competent and capable individuals in control of their lives. Living without a story is a terrifying thing.

RETURNING TO GOD'S STORY

Would returning to the biblical story help nursing to find a source of hope? We believe so! Is such a return a regression to the past? We believe it is a return to reality! The Bible tells a grand and true story, God's story of redeeming his creation and rescuing humanity from captivity to sin and its effects. Rather than human progress, the Bible tells us of a perfect creation from which humanity fell. But God is rewriting the story of human rebellion and sin with a new conclusion. He is creating a new humanity, a new kingdom.

---

[18]Jenson, "How the World Lost Its Story," 21.

[19]I (Arlene) addressed Erikson's theory in my doctoral dissertation, "Becoming Good." Erikson's well-known chart of developmental stages of the individual ends with the stage of maturity. Some nurse writers refer to death as "the final stage of development," but this seems at best a euphemism. While survivors might be said to "develop" as a result of the death, what about the one who died? The standard response is that answers to this question belong to religion, not nursing. But this is just the point. There is no larger story within which to place our own stories of facing and responding to suffering and death.

[20]"I will be among the few who cheat death of its victory by gaining a reputation that outlives them." David P. Gushee, "How Immortality Almost Killed Me," *Christianity Today*, March 3, 1997, 43.

> ### Views of Human History
>
> - The *biblical* story is linear—it has a beginning and an end with purpose and direction.
> - *Chaos*—the human story has no purpose, pattern, or significance.
> - *Circular* or *cyclical*—life is an endless repetition of cycles.
> - *Mechanical*—humans are products of nature with no freedom for change.
> - *Progressive* or *developmental*—human institutions and thought emerge naturally from simple to complex over time.

The biblical idea that human history is linear—has a beginning and an end, purpose and direction—contrasts starkly with other views both ancient and modern: (1) chaotic views in which the human story has no purpose, pattern or significance; (2) circular or cyclical views in which life is merely an endless repetition of cycles, sometimes called the eternal return; (3) mechanical views in which humans are merely products of nature with no freedom or possibility of change; and (4) progressive or developmental views in which human institutions and thought emerge naturally from the simple to the complex over the course of time. In the biblical worldview, human history has a course and moves toward a goal *not inherent* in the nature of things. The goal is outside of history, in God's own purposes. God's superintending of human history, as well as sustaining the natural world, is called *providence:* "God's faithful and effective care and guidance of everything which He has made toward the end which He has chosen."[21]

What are God's plans and purposes for humanity? First we must understand that they are beyond our ability to discover through reason or experience alone. God is unlimited and holy in his understanding and ways. We are limited and sinful. Our minds are simply incapable of fully comprehending God's mind and of interpreting our lives. If we are to know God's purposes, God must reveal them to us (Is 55:8-9). In fact, he wants us to ask him about his ways, so that he may help us understand his grand story.[22]

---

[21]"History," *Holman Bible Dictionary* (Hiawatha, IA: Parsons, 1994).

[22]Scripture tells us that we can seek to know God's ways. Moses, the leader of the Hebrew exodus from Egypt, prayed, "Show me your ways, so that I may know you and find favor in your sight" (Ex 33:13)—a prayer often repeated by God's people since then. This does not mean that God shows us the future; rather, he shows us how to live in such a way that we enter into and cooperate with his plans for us. Because we are made in God's image, our actions have significance because they contribute to the meaning of the whole.

In chapters seven and eight we said that there is trouble in God's creation. God's story is not one of bland optimism in which evil is ignored or discounted. But—in contrast to the best of human plans—God's unchanging plans and purposes will be fulfilled in spite of his rebellious creatures.[23]

> For I am God, and there is no other;
>   I am God, and there is no one like me,
> declaring the end from the beginning
>   and from ancient times things not yet done,
> saying, "My purpose shall stand,
>   and I will fulfill my intention. . . ."
> I have spoken, and I will bring it to pass;
>   I have planned, and I will do it. (Is 46:9-11)

What is the story God tells us? In the Bible we read of God's creating a new humanity, those who live under his reign. He is creating a new kingdom in which his laws are not imposed from the outside but come from the hearts of its citizens (Ezek 36:27). Further, God himself will live among his people (Rev 21:3), and God himself will banish hostility and violence. No abusive spouses will rip families apart. No rabid dogs will bite children, and no deadly viruses will sap life (Is 11:6-9).

Jesus of Nazareth is the central figure in God's new story. With the birth of Jesus in Bethlehem two thousand years ago, God opened the possibility of a new relationship between God and people. Jesus, conceived by the Holy Spirit, carried in the womb of Mary and born in a stable, was the long-awaited Messiah, God's anointed one, coming to save his creation. God entered human history, becoming fully human and at the same time fully God. God, living everyday life with ordinary people—fishermen, tax collectors, mothers and children, even prostitutes—is the amazing center of this story. Historian of religion Mircea Eliade says, "Since God was *incarnated*, that is, since he took on a *historically conditioned human existence*, history acquires the possibility of being sanctified. . . . For God's interventions in history, and above all his incarnation in the historical person of Jesus Christ, have a transhistorical

---

[23]We are not puppets; we can choose to reject God's purposes (Eph 2:2; Is 65:2).

purpose—*the salvation* of man."[24] God was working within the ordinary events of life to fulfill his purposes.

Jesus lived about thirty-three years. During his public ministry, only three years long, he gathered about him a small group of followers, preparing them to continue his ministry after he left. During those three years Jesus inaugurated the coming of the kingdom of heaven to earth, promising that it would grow from a tiny seed into a large tree (Mt 13:31-32). His kingdom does not exist in a geographical location; it is within those who have come under God's rule. Jesus taught that we enter God's kingdom by spiritual birth, not physical birth (Jn 3:1-16). He claimed to be the only means of entry: "I am the way, and the truth, and the life. No one comes to the Father except through me" (Jn 14:6). But the invitation for citizenship is extended to all people (Mt 28:18).

Most new nations come to birth through war and public declarations. But the heavenly kingdom came through weakness and death, not through an army of angels. It was Christ's death on the cross, a shameful Roman execution, which rescued us from our sins. He was vindicated when he "was raised on the third day" (1 Cor 15:4). Unlike gods in other religions who live in a mythical realm, Christ died a physical death and was raised bodily from the tomb. Forty days after his death and resurrection he returned to heaven. Now he rules over all things—the past, the present, and the future. One day he will return with the armies of heaven to rule as the all-powerful king (Eph 1:20-23).

Living in the Extended "Third Chapter" of God's Story

We can think of the biblical story as being told in four chapters: (1) creation, (2) rebellion and sin, (3) redemption, and (4) new creation. Actually chapters two and three overlap, and chapters three and four run parallel for a while. But eventually chapter four, the new creation, will be the full resolution of this age-long story. The rebellion and sin of the second chapter will be over, and the redemption of chapter three will be completed. It is to this third chapter—where sin and rebellion, redemption and the beginnings of the new creation, are all being played out together—that we now turn.

---

[24]Eliade, *Sacred and the Profane*, 111-12.

Chapters in the Biblical Story

- Creation
- Rebellion and sin
- Redemption
- New creation

The church as Christ's body on earth keeps and tells the story. Those who respond to Christ's call are his disciples. He told his followers, "You did not choose me but I chose you. And I appointed you to go and bear fruit, fruit that will last" (Jn 15:16). Practical actions of care are "bearing fruit." They are signs of our faith in the end of the story. John, the writer of the book of Revelation, heard these words from heaven: "Death will be no more; mourning and crying and pain will be no more" (Rev 21:4). The sure hope that one day God himself will heal creation has inspired Christians through the ages to work in hope. Christian nurses are participants in God's story.

Today, as nurses take up our roles in God's story, Jesus is still with us (Mt 28:20). After his ascension he poured out his Spirit, enabling his followers to bear witness to him by word and deed. Peter explained to an amazed crowd at the first Pentecost, "This Jesus God raised up, and of that all of us are witnesses. Being therefore exalted at the right hand of God, and having received from the Father the promise of the Holy Spirit, he has poured out this that you both see and hear" (Acts 2:32-33). After healing a crippled man a few days later, Peter explained to puzzled religious leaders that it was the name of Jesus that had healed the man (Acts 3:15-16).

The presence of Jesus enables Christian nurses to persevere in hope in very difficult circumstances. His Spirit guides us as we respond to him. It was the Spirit of Jesus who urged Elaine to talk to Mary Ann in the opening story. Elaine could not assure Mary Ann that her husband would return. She was not even certain how her own marriage would work out. Elaine offered the hope of God's presence instead.

We might ask, "So what good is believing God's story if we may not get what we desperately need or want?" People sometimes answer this question by glibly saying that everything works out for the best in the end. But these words are not true. Awful things usually lead to awful results. For example, abused children often become abusers themselves.

What then is a better response? The apostle Paul wrote to Christians suffering for their faith, "We know that all things work together for good for those who love God, who are called according to his purpose" (Rom 8:28). These words, often spoken as bland and useless assurance, are addressed to lovers of God, members of his kingdom. The promised good is God's long-term purpose and not necessarily our immediate desires. The goal of God's story is creating a new humanity, new people who love him. God is working in his people, making them like Jesus Christ (Rom 8:29). So the good that God brings out of bad things comes when he uses them to make us like Jesus. That may take a long time. Jesus said our first goal in life should be to seek the kingdom of God and his righteousness (Mt 6:33). What we should fear most is losing our souls, not our lives (Mt 10:28).

But God is not concerned only with his long-term goal for us. He suffers with those who suffer chronic pain. He grieves with the mother whose child is dying. He designs the wonderful processes that heal our bodies so they function. Jesus said, "Are not two sparrows sold for a penny? Yet not one of them will fall to the ground apart from your Father. And even the hairs of your head are all counted. So do not be afraid; you are of more value than many sparrows" (Mt 10:29-30).

What Elaine can promise Mary Ann is that nothing can separate her from the love of God, not even the breakup of her marriage. Nothing that happens must cause us to lose our souls. Nothing can make Jesus turn away from us. His loving presence is constant (Rom 8:39).

Christians have found hope in this assurance through the centuries. This is the hope that will sustain nurses in the changing health care system. This is the hope that we can offer our patients when all other hopes are lost.

HOPEFUL LIVING IN HARD TIMES

When Jesus' disciples asked him about the future, he told them that the dates and times of future events were not for them to know. They were to simply get on with the tasks at hand, trusting God for direction and empowerment. They were to be witnesses for Jesus wherever they lived and worked (Acts 1:6-8). Jesus himself modeled this almost casual attitude toward life. He did not schedule his activities as modern people do. He went from place to place seemingly without preplanning. He was open to the interruptions of individuals along the way—people like blind beggars, untouchable lepers, mothers wanting their children to be blessed.

Yet there was a consistency to his life that reflected his mission. He left one place after healing many when still more were gathering to see him. "Let us go on to the neighboring towns, so that I may proclaim the message there also; for that is what I came out to do" (Mk 1:38). He did speak often of going to Jerusalem and predicted that he would be captured, executed, and then vindicated. Jesus possessed an inner coordination and purpose that directed his life. He was not driven to achieve a goal, yet he moved steadfastly toward what he knew the Father had in store for him. The unity of his life sprang from his understanding of the way in which God carries out his purposes.

Living in God's true story, learning how he works out his purposes, trusting when we can't see him working: these all enable nurses to live in hope. We want to bear this hope to patients and colleagues (Eph 1:20-23). We do not need to merely "hope in hope." We know the God of hope who fills us with peace and joy in believing, so that we may abound in hope by the power of the Holy Spirit (Rom 15:13).

Phyllis Karns is one such bearer of hope. She tells the story of Joanne, a thirty-five-year-old woman with a terminal illness. Joanne's greatest concern was for the care of her children after her death.

Phyllis showed her two instances in the Bible where mothers gave their children over to the care of others in less than ideal situations. One was Hannah, mother of the prophet Samuel, who allowed him to be raised in the household of a corrupted priesthood (1 Sam 1:24-28). The other was Moses' mother, Jocebed, who relinquished her son to be raised by a heathen princess in a climate of wealth, power, and pagan religion (Ex 2). Each of the mothers was willing to trust God to be faithful in overseeing the growth and development of her child and to accept that God truly loved and would take care of the child.

Phyllis prayed with the dying mother, who was able to trust Jesus as Lord of the future for her children as well as for her own life after her death.[25]

---

[25]Phyllis S. Karns, "Building a Foundation for Spiritual Care," *Journal of Christian Nursing* (1991): 13.

STORY AS A WAY OF KNOWING

We have focused thus far on living in God's story as the only way to find the hope so important in nursing. But story is also a way of knowing, a way of discovering truth. Nurse educator Patricia Benner writes of the power of story for nursing as ethical practice.[26] Theologian Stanley Hauerwas argues that narrative is central to explain the truth of Christian life both for learning our identity and for learning moral truth.[27]

Stories give content to moral words like love and justice, courage and temperance. But how do we know when stories are true stories, not necessarily true in the sense that they actually happened but true in the sense that they tell us right things? For example, if we tell a story about "good" nursing care where a nurse refused a patient's request that would lead to her or his death, how can we know that it is truly good? Perhaps another nurse telling the story would label it bad care, saying that the patient's wishes should have been followed.

It is God's story that shows us the way. We continually test the smaller stories of our lives against his story. How do they fit within it? Do they continue to tell God's story, or do they belong to another story of sin and rebellion? The amazing thing is that God actually invites us to help tell his story by our lives.

God's story also teaches us who we are: historical beings dependent on God and others. We often introduce ourselves by telling the story of our lives. However, it is not only others who learn to know us by our stories; we learn to know ourselves. Many fearful nursing students have been amazed to discover that they actually knew more than they thought about patient care. Likewise, patients who trembled at the prospect of a painful treatment have come through amazed at their own strength. This is why telling stories to children and adults can be a powerful source of encouragement.

Because God is telling his story in our environment, we can have hope, we can know ourselves, and we can know moral truth. The key for nurses is to live within his story and to tell it to ourselves and each other over and over. To learn it well.

---

[26]Susan S. Phillips and Patricia Benner, eds., *The Crisis of Care* (Washington, DC: Georgetown University Press, 1994).

[27]Stanley Hauerwas, *The Peaceable Kingdom* (Notre Dame: University of Notre Dame Press, 1983), 28.

For Further Thinking

1. What gives you hope?

2. As you review your personal life story, what events became turning points that continue to influence the way you think and act today?

3. In what ways does knowing God's story in the Bible affect your nursing practice?

Theological Reflection

Read Luke 10:1-12. This story of the "good Samaritan" was instrumental in the development of nursing as a ministry of the church.

1. What main point was Jesus making by telling this story?

2. How do the details expand on the concept of Christian caring?

3. Based on this story in Luke 10, what should characterize our nursing care today?

Case Study: Jesus Healed the Woman

Martha Heimbach, age eighty-three, had been a resident in an extended-care facility for about six weeks. Although she was recovering well from a fractured hip, she seemed increasingly confused and disoriented. Then her pastor visited with a copy of an old photograph of Martha's confirmation class of 1938. He asked her to identify the people in the photograph.

When Martha's nurse, Jennifer, brought Martha's afternoon medications, she asked about the photograph. Martha suddenly brightened and began to tell Jennifer about the people in her confirmation class and some of her early experiences singing in the choir and helping with church suppers.

Jennifer then asked Martha how her faith was helping her as she recovered from her broken hip. "I know God is with me. I pray a lot and I read my Bible."

"What's your favorite Bible story?" Martha probed.

"Oh, I always liked the story of how Jesus healed the woman who touched the hem of his garment," Martha replied. "You know, I never had any children. I prayed and prayed, but God never gave me any babies. But he also showed me that he had other things for me to do. I took care of my mother-in-law for twenty-three years after she had her stroke, and she was really good to me. And I played the piano every week at the old folks' home. They enjoyed that so much! My favorite hymn is 'Beneath the Cross of Jesus.'"

"So in a way, Jesus did heal you like he did the woman in the Bible story, because he gave you other ways to invest yourself in the people you loved— and they loved you in return," Jennifer suggested.

"Oh yes! It would have been nice to have babies, but I'm just as happy without them."

DISCUSSION QUESTIONS

1. How did having the opportunity to reminisce and tell her own story help Martha to connect with God's story?

2. In what ways did the Bible story help her to make sense of her own story?

3. If you had been the nurse in this situation, how would you continue the conversation?

4. What would you hope to accomplish? What outcomes would you expect?

5. Briefly describe a time when you were able to connect with a patient by either telling your own story, or listening to the patient's story.

6. How did faith intersect with your story or your patient's story?

PART FOUR

HEALTH

OUTCOMES OF CARE

10

WORKING TOWARD SHALOM

Purpose: To establish a biblical understanding of health as shalom

Objectives: After reading this chapter and completing the exercises, you should be able to:
1. Compare definitions of *health* in the nursing literature with the biblical concept of shalom
2. Describe the cultural influences on a person's understanding of health
3. List five dimensions of health
4. Explain the implications of your definition of health on your nursing practice

Keywords: health, healing, culture, shalom, wholeness, relationship

SUSAN STOOD ON MY (JUDY'S) DOORSTEP, a glowing picture of health. Her eyes flashed with enthusiasm for life, and a deep sense of joy radiated from her face, but the large mass on her neck betrayed another force at work in her body. Susan was on her way home from radiation therapy for a rapidly growing thyroid cancer, but she had never felt more alive.

She wanted to tell me how much her relationship with God and the friendships she had developed within the church congregation meant to her, and how that gave her a different perspective on her illness. She knew she was dying, but she felt at peace. She was ready to meet God, and she knew that her husband, Joe, would not be left alone—people in the church would continue to care for him.

Susan's view of the church had not always been this positive. As a young woman, Susan and Joe were active church members in a neighboring congregation. She raised her family in a Christian home and taught Sunday school for several years. However, after her daughters were confirmed they gradually drifted away from the church. When her oldest daughter became engaged, she called the pastor asking him to officiate at her wedding. The pastor refused, stating that since she was no longer an active member, it was against his policy to perform the ceremony for her. The incident hurt Susan deeply. She grew angry and bitter toward God and the church. She and Joe withdrew from the congregation and did not participate in any church activities for about twenty years.

During those years away from their church, Joe passed our church building every Sunday morning on his way to the golf course. Each time, he felt something drawing him into the building. Finally he began attending worship, then joined a Sunday school class, where he once again began to grow in his faith and delighted in the fellowship with people in the church. For years the Sunday school class prayed with him that Susan would release her bitterness and return to church with him. She slipped in occasionally but kept her distance. Then tragedies began to strike. First a son-in-law died in an automobile accident. Then Susan's brother died of thyroid cancer. Within months Susan faced the same diagnosis.

Throughout all the crises, the church ministered to Susan through notes, visits, flowers, and prayers. Finally, her resistance broke down. She came back into a vital faith and began to enjoy the fellowship of the community of God's people.

As Susan's illness progressed and she became homebound, I visited her as a faith community nurse. We discussed the importance of taking her pain medication and why she didn't have to worry about becoming addicted. We developed a strategy to deal with the side effects of her medication. Our primary focus, though, was on her relationships: with her husband, her family, the church community, and God. We prayed together, wept, and hugged. Susan died just before Christmas. Her funeral was a celebration of life and faith—a testimony to the health God offers us in his shalom.

What Is Health?

The popular media portray health as youthful appearance, hard muscles, sleek bodies, clear skin, and cavity-free teeth. Nursing literature is increasingly moving to the other extreme. Health is "expanding consciousness," according to nursing theorist Margaret Newman.[1] It is "essentially synonymous with

---

[1]DeAnn M. Hensley, Kimberly A. Kilgore, Jill Vass Langfitt, and LaPhyllis Peterson, "Margaret A. Newman: Model of Health," in *Nursing Theorists and Their Work*, ed. Ann Marriner (St. Louis: Mosby, 1986), 371.

becoming, which is an open, rhythmically co-constituting process of the human-universe interrelationship," according to theorist Rosemarie Parse.[2]

One nursing text compiled the current definitions of health found in nursing literature and listed these:

- a dynamic process
- determined subjectively and objectively
- a goal
- being able to take care of yourself
- optimal functioning in body, mind, and spirit
- integrity of self
- a sense of wholeness
- coping adaptively
- a subjective experience
- growing and becoming
- a broad concept[3]

According to current nursing literature, health is indeed a broad concept; so broad, in fact, that it ceases to be an adequate goal for nursing. Margaret Newman even states, "Health encompasses conditions that heretofore were described as illness, or in medical terms, pathology."[4] For the most part, contemporary nursing definitions of health focus primarily on a state of mind. Older definitions and conventional wisdom (as represented by television commercials) focus on the body. The World Health Organization (WHO) idealistically defined health in 1946 as "a state of complete physical, mental, and social well-being and not merely the absence of disease or infirmity." It was a definition that medical ethicist Daniel Callahan says set the stage for a conception of health that literally encompasses every element of human happiness.[5]

Earlier I said that Susan radiated health despite her tumor. She obviously did not meet the WHO standard of health. On what basis could I say that Susan

---

[2]Rosemarie Risso Parse, "Human Becoming: Parse's Theory of Nursing," *Nursing Science Quarterly* 5 (1992): 13.

[3]Janice B. Lindberg, Mary Love Hunter, and Ann Z. Kruszewski, *Introduction to Nursing: Concepts, Issues and Opportunities* (Philadelphia: Lippincott, 1994), 198-99.

[4]Hensley et al., "Margaret A. Newman," 371.

[5]Daniel Callahan, "The WHO Definition of 'Health,'" *Hastings Center Studies* 1, no. 3 (1973): 77-87.

was "healthy"? What is the difference between that understanding of health and Margaret Newman's? Susan demonstrated health in her attitudes and relationships, but the tumor itself was not encompassed in her health—it remained a very serious pathology. However, if we view the person as an integrated whole, created to live in harmony with God, self, others, and the environment,[6] then health means being able to function as God created us to be. It involves reconciliation with God and others, forgiving and accepting forgiveness, loving and being loved, finding meaning and purpose in life leading to a sense of joy and hope, as well as freedom from physical ailments.

Health is a state of complete physical, mental, and social well-being and not merely the absence of disease or infirmity.

WORLD HEALTH ORGANIZATION

HEALTH IS CULTURALLY DEFINED

To some extent, health is culturally understood. Nursing theorist Madeleine Leininger explained, "Our rapidly growing multicultural world makes it imperative that nurses understand different cultures to work and function effectively with people having different values, beliefs, and ideas about nursing, health, caring, wellness, illness, death, and disabilities."[7] She saw human caring as the heart of nursing and as a universal phenomenon. "*Health* refers to a state of well-being that is culturally defined, valued, and practiced, and which reflects the ability of individuals (or groups) to perform their daily role activities in culturally expressed, beneficial, and patterned lifeways."[8] Hence nurses must draw their goals for nursing from the persons or groups in their care.

Biblical anthropologists Bruce Malina and Richard Rohrbaugh attempt to uncover the cultural understanding of health found in the time of Jesus.[9] They stress that in ancient Mediterranean culture a person's state of being was more important than the ability to act or function. "Illness is not so much a biomedical

---

[6]Adapted from Judith Allen Shelly and Sharon Fish, *Spiritual Care: The Nurse's Role* (Downers Grove, IL: InterVarsity Press, 1988), 33.

[7]Madeleine M. Leininger, ed., *Culture Care Diversity and Universality: A Theory of Nursing* (New York: National League for Nursing, 1991), 6.

[8]Leininger, *Culture Care*, 48.

[9]Bruce J. Malina and Richard L. Rohrbaugh, *Social-Science Commentary on the Synoptic Gospels* (Minneapolis: Fortress, 1992), 70-72.

matter as it is a social one. It is attributed to social causes, not physical ones. Because sin is a breach of interpersonal relationship, sin and sickness go together. Illness is not so much a medical matter as a matter of deviance from the cultural norms and values."[10] Malina and Rohrbaugh view Jesus' healings primarily as restoring the person to the worshiping community. Healing is directly related to the cultural belief system.

Missionary physician Tony Atkins describes the African view of health in a similar way, as a function of community. He explains, "It is an indigenous concept that acceptance within, and harmony with family and society are important elements in healing and preserving the health of people."[11] He compares the African view to the biblical understanding of health and concludes, "For the Jew, as for many people in tribal societies today, health was essentially a positive quality that derived from the fact that people existed in total harmony with the world and in harmony with God."[12]

A BIBLICAL UNDERSTANDING OF HEALTH

The biblical understanding of health is closely related to the concept of shalom. Often translated as "peace," shalom actually incorporates all the elements that go into making a God-centered community—peace, prosperity, rest, safety, security, justice, happiness, health, welfare, wholeness. Christian philosopher Nicholas Wolterstorff defines shalom as "the human being dwelling at peace in all his or her relationships: with God, with self, with fellows, with nature."[13] The future new Jerusalem described in Revelation 21:2-4 illustrates the meaning of shalom:

> *Shalom is the human being dwelling at peace in all his or her relationships: with God, with self, with fellows, with nature.*
>
> NICHOLAS WOLTERSTORFF

> And I saw the holy city, the new Jerusalem, coming down out of heaven from God, prepared as a bride adorned for her husband. And I heard a loud voice from the throne saying, "See, the home of God is among mortals. He will dwell

---

[10]Malina and Rohrbaugh, *Social-Science Commentary*, 71.

[11]Tony Atkins, "What Is Health?" *Health and Development* (1984): 5.

[12]Atkins, "What Is Health?" 6.

[13]Nicholas Wolterstorff, "For Justice in Shalom," in *From Christ to the World: Introductory Readings in Christian Ethics*, ed. Wayne G. Boulton, Thomas D. Kennedy, and Allen Verhey (Grand Rapids, MI: Eerdmans, 1994), 251.

with them; they will be his peoples, and God himself will be with them; he will wipe every tear from their eyes. Death will be no more; mourning and crying and pain will be no more, for the first things have passed away."

Like the WHO definition, the concept of *shalom* is too broad to be the goal of nursing, but it provides a perspective through which we can frame our understanding of health. Linked to the biblical understanding of the person, shalom points us to how the healthy person functions. It includes the physical, psychosocial, and spiritual dimensions of the person.

Biblical scholar Walter Brueggemann explains this perspective of health as shalom.

> *Health* refers to stability enough to share in the costs and joys, the blessings and burdens of the community. To be healthy means to be functioning fully in terms of the norms, values, and expectations of the community.
>
> *Healing* refers to the restoration and rehabilitation of persons to their full power and vitality in the life of the community. Sickness, then, does not refer primarily to physical pain as much as to the inability to be fully, honorably, and seriously engaged in the community in all its decisions and celebrations.[14]

Hence, we should not be surprised when a terminally ill patient rallies long enough to attend a daughter's wedding or celebrate Christmas with a son returning from an overseas military assignment. Research that demonstrates the value of support groups, prayer, and worship attendance in maintaining physical health illustrates this perspective.

The spiritual dimension is not just one part of the person, it encompasses the whole being. The late theologian Paul Tillich illuminated the idea of *dimensions* by saying that the person should not be considered "as a composite of several levels, such as body, soul, spirit, but as a multidimensional unity." The dimensions do not "lie alongside, but within each other."[15] He then describes six dimensions: mechanical, chemical, biological, psychological, spiritual, and historical. He proposes that health cannot be defined apart from its opposite—disease—and disease affects all dimensions of the person. True healing takes place only when all six dimensions are healthy; however, in this

---

[14]Walter Brueggemann, *Peace* (St. Louis: Chalice, 2001), 199.

[15]Paul Tillich, "The Meaning of Health," in *On Moral Medicine: Theological Perspectives in Medical Ethics*, ed. Stephen E. Lammers and Allen Verhey (Grand Rapids, MI: Eerdmans, 1987), 162.

life we must usually be content with limited healing. Ultimate healing comes through Jesus Christ, who is the *sōtēr*—a Greek term that means both "savior" and "healer."

The interrelationship between health and salvation in the New Testament is striking. When a group of men brought their paralyzed friend to Jesus, they were surprised to hear Jesus say to him, "Your sins are forgiven" (Mk 2:5; Lk 5:20). He then went on to heal him physically. There seems to have been a relationship between the man's need for forgiveness and his illness. When a woman with chronic vaginal bleeding touched the hem of Jesus' garment, he replied to her, "Your faith has made you well," implying a relationship between faith and healing (Mt 9:22).

The Greek word *sōzō*, used here and elsewhere for "healing" (see Mk 5:23; 6:56; 10:52; Lk 8:48-50; 17:19; 18:42; Acts 4:9; 14:9; Jas 5:15), is translated in other passages as "salvation" (see, for example, Mt 1:21; 10:22; 19:25; 24:22; Mk 16:16; Lk 13:23-24; Jn 3:17; 10:9; Acts 2:21; 4:12; 11:14; Rom 10:9). When Jesus cleansed the ten lepers (Lk 17:11-19), only one returned to thank him. Jesus told that man, "Your faith has made you well [*sōzō*]." All ten were cleansed of leprosy, but only the one who returned found complete healing—and it was intimately wrapped up in his ability to praise God.

The whole point of Jesus' healing people was to restore them to a fuller, richer relationship with God and the faith community. Theologian Jürgen Moltmann explains, "Healing consists of the restoration of disrupted community, and the sharing and communication of life. Jesus heals the sick by restoring their fellowship with God."[16] Theologian Thomas Droege expands this idea:

> Since wholeness is more than physical well-being, the healings of Jesus also effected changes in the meanings and values of those whom he encountered. Jesus consistently called people to repentance. He invited people to turn away from those things that brought division and disintegration into their lives and to become responsible for their own health as well as the health of others.[17]

---

[16]Jürgen Moltmann, *The Spirit of Life: A Universal Affirmation* (Minneapolis: Fortress, 1992), 191.
[17]Thomas A. Droege, "The Healing Ministry of Jesus as an Example of Wholistic Health Care," in *Theological Roots of Wholistic Health Care*, ed. Granger Westberg (Hinsdale, IL: Wholistic Health Centers, 1979), 19.

Such a definition goes far beyond the scope of nursing, but it also reveals something of our relationship to other members of the health care team and to the Christian community. Because people are multidimensional beings in need of holistic healing, we are also a multidimensional healing community. Nursing encompasses only one dimension of health care. However, the role of the nurse does not necessarily "lie alongside" medicine and pastoral care; in many ways it is "within" both. It involves recognition that both the nurse and the person receiving care are members of a community and dependent upon God. Healing requires us to function harmoniously within those communities and in partnership with God.

IMPLICATIONS FOR NURSING PRACTICE

Functioning under such definitions leads to some fuzzy distinctions, but it acknowledges what we already know and reduces the spirit of competition. There will be times when nursing stretches to include practicing medicine. Nurses in developing countries with scarce resources and few physicians have always gone far beyond the limits of traditional nursing—diagnosing, treating, prescribing, and even performing surgery.[18] Today's advanced practice roles also push hard into the once ironclad bounds of medicine.[19] In a similar way, nursing borders on entering into the role of clergy—even to the point of organizing through religious orders or working as faith community nurses and deacon nurses on churches' ministerial staffs. Rather than fight turf battles, we need to recognize that the pursuit of health must remain multidimensional and interprofessional. Just when we think we have the lines drawn properly, they will shift again.

What then are the implications of this multidimensional understanding of health for nursing? Florence Nightingale understood nursing to be taking "personal charge of the health of others."[20] If we are to take charge of it, we must know what it is!

---

[18]See, for example, J. Birney Dibble, *Outlaw for God: The Story of Esther Bacon* (Hanover, MA: Christopher, 1992). An LCA missionary nurse in Liberia, Esther Bacon often taught the missionary doctors how to perform surgery and deliver babies in culturally appropriate ways.

[19]Betty Souther, "Congregational Nurse Practitioner: An Idea Whose Time Has Come," *Journal of Christian Nursing* (1997): 32-34. Souther, the director of the Center for Health Studies at Houston Baptist University, has developed a new Master's of Science in Nursing program to prepare parish nurses to perform in a role once reserved for physicians.

[20]Florence Nightingale, *Notes on Nursing: What It Is and What It Is Not* (New York: Appleton, 1860), 3.

Nurse educator Ruth Stoll defines health as having five dimensions:

Wholeness. Health is wholeness, the harmonious unity of the person within himself and outwardly with God and his environment.

Transformation. Health is a dynamic process of internal transformations progressively reflected in the person's outward behavior.

Relationship. Health is the experiencing of loving, just and forgiving relationships with God, self and others that provide meaning and purpose in life.

Coping and adaptation. Health is a reality-oriented perspective that allows the person to adapt and cope with internal and external change and stress.

Human paradox. Health is creative living with the human paradox of being and becoming, of living with sin, redemption and restoration.[21]

Theologian Karl Barth defined health simply as "the power to be as man exercised in the powers of the vital functions of soul and body."[22] In other words, it is to be all that God created us to be. Missionary physician Daniel Fountain cautions: "Health cannot be defined. It is not simply an object for analysis. To render it such is to think secularly about health. Health is life, a gift we receive, an endowment we are to develop, and a journey we are to pursue. We can observe and analyze much along the way. We can manipulate and improve certain aspects of health and life. But we can never comprehend the whole."[23]

Stoll's Dimensions of Health

- Wholeness
- Transformation
- Relationship
- Coping and adaptation
- Human paradox

While it may be true that we can never fully grasp the concept of health (hence, the wide range of definitions), most people instinctively know what it means to be healthy. Perhaps Tillich's insistence that health can be defined only in contrast to its opposite—disease—can help direct our understanding.

---

[21]Ruth I. Stoll, *Concepts in Nursing—A Christian Perspective* (Madison, WI: Nurses Christian Fellowship, 1990), 158.
[22]Karl Barth, "Sickness and Illusion," in *On Moral Medicine: Theological Perspectives in Medical Ethics,* ed. Stephen E. Lammers and Allen Verhey (Grand Rapids, MI: Eerdmans, 1987), 155.
[23]Daniel Fountain, *Health, the Bible and the Church* (Wheaton, IL: Billy Graham Center, 1989), 52.

People all over the world, in every culture, seek health care when pain or disability prevents them from attending to the activities of daily living. What are they hoping to find? At first they are looking for relief from pain, ability to function, and restoration to their social environment. This level is primarily physical. Beyond that, people may seek to eliminate the underlying causes of the immediate problem. At this level the psychosocial and spiritual dimensions enter into the health care spectrum.

When our operational definition of health neglects the physical dimension, nurses can justify avoiding the hard—and often unpleasant—work of caring for the body. We also eliminate the primary motivation most people have for seeking health care. Pain, nausea, fever, and conditions that limit our ability to work and play drive us to seek help.

God created us with bodies. The physical is real. It is not an illusion. Regardless of how strongly certain nursing theorists may argue that the biological functions are illusory and can be controlled by the mind, our bodies are still subject to injury and illness. We have only to stub a toe to be convinced. While the mind certainly has a great deal to do with wellness and healing, disease is real. Bacteria and viruses can invade even the strongest immune system. Cancer and heart disease afflict the most ardent health enthusiast.

The physical dimension certainly dominates most people's thinking about health. Bioethicist Daniel Callahan suggests that the best definition for health might be "a state of physical well-being."[24] But that definition will not satisfy today's nursing theorists—or the biblical concept of shalom.

Our definition of health must also include the psychosocial and spiritual dimensions. It is here that the postmodern nursing theories stepped into the gap left by our overdependence upon the scientific "medical model" of health care. Holistic health care, according to these theories, strikes a chord in people who have been conditioned by our modernist culture to expect that every physical problem can be "fixed." They turn to alternative therapies when scientific medicine does not work completely, results in unpleasant side effects, or proves exorbitantly expensive. One of the primary drawing points of these alternative therapies is the emphasis they place on personal control, as well as their appeal to ancient spiritual wisdom.

---

[24]Callahan, "The WHO Definition of 'Health,'" 172.

In the early 1960s physician Halbert Dunn began talking about "high level wellness,"[25] which set the stage for viewing health as an individual achievement that can be controlled by the mind. There is a great deal of truth to this concept. Every nurse can relate stories of people who overcame great odds to recover rapidly because of sheer willpower, or others who died when they lost hope. But the mortality rate remains 100 percent. In fact, if one compares life expectancy in populations where alternative therapies are commonly practiced (such as in China or India) with others where allopathic medicine prevails, the numbers are tilted greatly in favor of Western medicine.

A Christian view of health must also incorporate a realistic understanding of human suffering and mortality and the hope of eternal life. There are forces at work in the world that we cannot fully control, even with science or mind control—microorganisms, genetics, environmental pollutants, violence, accidents, spiritual influences. We are not God. We will eventually get sick and die. To view health as shalom means to stand with those who are sick and dying and to encompass them in the fellowship of the Christian community and the presence of God.

PUTTING HEALTH IN A LARGER CONTEXT

The Christian, then, places health within a larger context. It can be a radiant health in the midst of terrible physical disability. Conversely, health can be absent in a person with a well-toned body. Health usually shows itself as "a state of physical well-being,"[26] but ultimately it is shalom, a God-centered wholeness that enables the person to live in harmony with self, God, others, and the environment.

Medical ethicists Stephen Lammers and Allen Verhey assert, "Definitions of health turn out to be important because in doing the defining, we must explore the relationship of health to other human goods; the relationship of health and responsibility, both of individuals and of the medical [or nursing] profession; and the relationship of health and those conventional modes of treating and coping with illness."[27] So how does health shape our goals for nursing?

---

[25]Halbert L. Dunn, *High Level Wellness* (Arlington, VA: R. W. Beatty, 1961).
[26]Callahan, "The WHO Definition of 'Health,'" 172.
[27]Stephen E. Lammers and Allen Verhey, eds., *On Moral Medicine: Theological Perspectives in Medical Ethics* (Grand Rapids, MI: Eerdmans, 1987), 150.

Let's go back to Susan, my radiantly healthy dying friend. As a nurse I acknowledged the value of expert scientific medical care and dealt with her physical condition. At the same time, as a faith community nurse I represented the caring Christian community and worked toward a different kind of health. During those months before she died, Susan was surrounded by family, friends, and a Christian community that included her visiting nurses. Together we had worked toward shalom.

Health is essentially living according to God's purposes, even in the face of suffering and death. It includes the physical dimension; therefore, we work toward maintaining optimal physical function and providing comfort measures. However, complete health also means living in harmonious relationship with God and our neighbors; therefore, nursing also includes assisting patients in establishing and maintaining a relationship with God through Jesus Christ, as well as facilitating healing relationships among people.

> *Health is essentially living according to God's purposes, even in the face of suffering and death.*

A final example illustrates this kind of health. Several years ago my (Judy's) phone rang. A weak voice mumbled slowly, "I . . . can't . . . take it! I'm . . . I'm . . . going to . . . commit . . . suicide."

George was an old friend. I recognized his voice immediately. Mouth and tongue cancer had been slowly robbing him of life over the past ten years. His wife, Anna, had died a year before. He lived alone now. A month earlier he had been admitted to the hospital five times for various complications, then transferred to a nursing home, where he refused to stay.

"Have you taken anything you shouldn't?" I asked, fearing the worst.

"No, I'm too scared. But you said to call if I ever felt this way, and I do."

I dropped everything and drove to his house. Knowing George was a hunter, with guns in the house as well as pills, I feared what I might find. When I arrived, George was sitting in a recliner looking dejected, surrounded by boxes of gastrostomy feedings, bottles of pills, and medical equipment. He grabbed my hands and poured out his feelings of agony. I listened, then prayed for him, taking his concerns to the Lord. Then he rose out of his chair, fell on his face sobbing and pleaded with the Lord himself. A short time later, with George back in his recliner, his brother arrived while we were talking.

Table 10.1. Healing in the New Testament

Encounter	Assessed Needs	Intervention	Outcome
Leper—Mt 8:2-3; Mk 1:40-41; Lk 5:12-13	To "be made clean"	Jesus stretched out hand and touched him, saying "Be made clean!" Sent to priest and directed to offer prescribed gift	Leprosy cleansed Restored to worshiping community Told others about Jesus (against Jesus' orders)
Centurion's servant—Mt 8:5-13; Lk 7:1-10	Paralysis and terrible distress Close to death	Jesus spoke (from distance)	Physical healing Faith of centurion affirmed
Peter's mother-in-law—Mt 8:14-15; Mk 1:30-31; Lk 4:38-39	High fever	Jesus touched (took) her hand and lifted her up	Fever left Able to function in her social role
Demoniac(s)—Mt 8:28-32; Mk 5:1-13; Lk 8:26-33	Danger to society (attempts to restrain him were unsuccessful), bizarre behavior (howling, nakedness), self-mutilation, demon possession	Jesus confronted demons and cast them into swine	"Clothed and in his right mind" Desire to follow Jesus Patient and swineherds became evangelists in surrounding country Community asked Jesus to leave
Paralytic—Mt 9:2-7; Mk 2:3-12; Lk 5:18-25	Forgiveness Physical healing	Jesus forgave sins, then healed the paralysis	Able to get up, carry his mat and walk home Glorified God
Jairus's twelve-year-old daughter—Mt 9:18-26; Mk 5:22-42; Lk 8:43-48	Resuscitation (patient appeared dead or close to death), healing	Jesus took parents and Peter, James and John into the girl's room, took her by the hand and told her to get up Jesus told father, "Do not fear, only believe"	Patient got up out of bed, walked around and was able to eat Her spirit returned to her Skeptical crowd amazed
Woman with hemorrhage—Mt 9:20-22; Mk 5:25-29; Lk 8:43-48	Chronic vaginal bleeding (12 yrs) Long history of unsuccessful medical treatments Financially exhausted	Touched Jesus' clothing (self-care) Jesus insisted that she identify herself	Bleeding stopped immediately Felt in her body that she was healed of the disease Made well through her faith Shalom ("Go in peace")
Two blind men—Mt 9:27-31	Cure for blindness Mercy	Jesus inquired about their faith, touched their eyes and told them they would be healed according to their faith	Eyes opened Spread the news about Jesus throughout that district
Mute demoniac—Mt 9:32-33	Demon possession	Cast out demon	Patient spoke; crowd amazed, but Pharisees skeptical
Blind, mute demoniac—Mt 12:22; Lk 11:14	Demon possession	Cured him	Patient could speak and see; crowd amazed, but Pharisees skeptical
Boy with epilepsy—Mt 17:14-18; Mk 9:17-27; Lk 9:37-42	Safety issues Demon possession	Disciples unable to heal because "lack of faith" Jesus cured him	Demon came out Boy cured instantly
Demoniac—Mk 1:23-26; Lk 4:33-35	Inappropriate behavior, seizures, demon possession	Jesus cast out demon	Demons came out of patient Jesus' fame spread

Table 10.1. *(continued)*

Encounter	Assessed Needs	Intervention	Outcome
Deaf mute man—Mk 7:31-37	Deafness, speech impediment	Jesus provided privacy, put his fingers in patient's ears, spat and touched patient's tongue, saying "Be opened"	Patient could hear and speak clearly Crowd spread the word about Jesus
Blind man—Mk 8:22-26	Vision impairment	Jesus provided privacy and healed in two stages by applying saliva to the patient's eyes, laying on his hands	Vision gradually restored, sent home
Widow's son—Lk 7:11-15	Apparent death	Jesus touched the bier and told patient to arise	Patient sat up and began to speak Crowd fearful, praised God
Infirm woman—Lk 13:11-13	Evil spirit–imposed disability for 18 years; bent over; unable to stand up straight	Jesus called to her that she was healed, then laid his hands on her	Patient immediately stood up straight and began praising God
Man with dropsy—Lk 14:1-4	"Dropsy"	Jesus "took him and healed him"	Apparent object lesson for Pharisees Man healed
Ten lepers—Lk 17:11-19	All had leprosy and were forced to keep their distance from healthy people	Jesus cleansed all 10 of leprosy and told to go show themselves to the priests (return to community)	One patient returned to thank Jesus, was commended for his faith and sent on his way
Man with severed ear—Lk 22:47-51	Right ear severed by sword	Jesus touched the ear and healed it	Physically healed
Official's son—Jn 4:46-54	Lay ill, near death	Jesus said, "Go; your son will live"	Son healed, father and entire household believed
Disabled man—Jn 5:1-9	Ill and disabled for 38 years, lying by pool at Bethesda Apparent feelings of aloneness and helplessness	Jesus asked him if he wanted to get well, but ignored his excuses and told him to stand up, take up his mat and walk Later, Jesus confronted him and told him not to sin anymore or worse things could happen to him	Healed, up and walking, going to the temple and apparently reformed
Blind man—Jn 9:1-7	Born blind, financially destitute	Jesus put mud made with his saliva on patient's eyes, then told him to go and wash in the pool of Siloam	Physically healed (able to see), believed, witnessed to family and others in community
Lazarus—Jn 11:1-44	Ill, apparently dead	Waited until patient was dead four days, wept and went to tomb, asked the stone be removed, prayed, "Lazarus come out"	Lazarus came out, still wrapped in strips of cloth Jesus told crowd that it all happened so that they would believe
Paralyzed man— Acts 3:1-26	Congenital deformities of feet and ankles, unable to walk, carried by friends so he could beg	Peter told him to stand up and walk in the name of Jesus Took him by the hand and raised him up	Feet and ankles made strong, jumped up and began walking and leaping and praising God Crowd filled with wonder and amazement

Table 10.1. *(continued)*

Encounter	Assessed Needs	Intervention	Outcome
Sick people—Acts 5:12-16	Assorted sick and demon-possessed people brought by friends and relatives	People carried the sick out into the street so that Peter's shadow would fall on them as he passed by	All cured Apostles held in high esteem by people, but persecuted by Jewish authorities
Unclean spirits—Acts 8:6-8	Large numbers of sick people—paralyzed, lame, demon possessed	Philip proclaimed the Messiah to them and performed signs (healing)	Many cured Great joy in the city
Saul's blindness—Acts 9:17-19; 22:12-13	Saul struck blind during a vision of Jesus	Ananias instructed in a vision to go to the home where Saul was staying; Saul prayed; Ananias laid his hands on Saul and told him he'd been sent so he could be healed and filled with the Holy Spirit	Scales fell off Saul's eyes, vision restored, was baptized, ate and regained his strength
Aeneas—Acts 9:33-34	Bedridden for 8 years, paralyzed	Peter told him, "Jesus Christ heals you; get up and make your bed"	Immediately got up All the residents of Lydda and Sharon saw him and turned to Lord
Tabitha—Acts 9:36-41	Became ill, died	Peter prayed at bedside, then told patient to get up; after opening her eyes, she sat up and Peter took her hand and helped her up	Peter showed her friends that she was alive Many believed in the Lord
Disabled man—Acts 14:8-10	Could not use feet, crippled from birth	Paul looked at him intently, saw he had faith and loudly told him, "Stand upright on your feet"	Man sprang up and began to walk Crowd thought Paul and Barnabas were gods, wanted to offer sacrifices Paul preached Jews persecuted them
Slave girl—Acts 16:16-18	Possessed spirit of divination, earned a great deal of money for her owners by fortune telling	Paul got annoyed and ordered the spirit to come out of her	Spirit came out immediately, so girl was no longer useful to owner; Paul and Silas arrested on trumped up charges
Eutychus—Acts 20:9-12	Overcome with sleep during Paul's long sermon and fell out the third floor window, died	Paul bent over him, took him in his arms and said, "Do not be alarmed, for his life is in him"	Boy taken away alive, friends and family comforted, Paul went back to preaching
Publius's father—Acts 28:8-9	Sick in bed with fever and dysentery	Paul visited him and cured him by putting his hands on him	Cured, then other sick people on the island came and were also cured Paul received many honors and islanders took care of his physical needs

Jake asked George how he was doing. George looked at me and said, "You tell him." We talked about his suicidal feelings and discussed options. Jake settled into the other chair. Assured that George was in good hands for the time being, I left.

George is a broken man. However, the brokenness has come not so much from his cancer as from his loneliness. As long as Anna was with him, he faced the repeated surgeries and painful procedures with a sense of optimism and strength. Even after Anna died, George seemed to do pretty well as long as he could come out to the healing services at church. But now he was alone, isolated in his home despite occasional visits from friends, family, and the visiting nurse. He felt as if God had left him as well. Although talk of individualism, self-care, and autonomy falls easily from our tongues today, God made us for community. Healing—wholeness—comes only in community, not in self-actualization or radical autonomy. Wholeness is not an achievement, something we can accomplish. It is a gift from God and a way of living in community.

How can we bring *wholeness* to those in our care? First, we offer everything in our nursing knowledge and skill to bring comfort and healing. The visiting nurse came the next day to care for George's physical needs. She called his physician to get his pain and anxiety medications adjusted, and she revised his feeding schedule. But Christian nursing can't stop there. We give ourselves, as members of the body of Christ, to draw our patients into a community of caring. For George, that community went to work, planning follow-up visits, prayer calls, and other supportive measures. Ultimately, though, his wholeness will come through being reconciled to God.

By the next evening George was surrounded by friends and family. His sister called to say she would come and stay with him for two weeks. His pain and anxiety were under control. He no longer felt like committing suicide. In his words, "It was the difference between night and day."

What changed George's condition? The prayer? The physical interventions? The presence and support of a caring community? All of the above. George is still a very sick man—terminally ill—but he is experiencing health in a new way. He is living in shalom.

FOR FURTHER THINKING

1. What do you think most people are seeking when they consult health care professionals?

2. Based on television commercials and internet ads for medicines and nutritional supplements, how do you think our society defines health?

3. How would you define health?

THEOLOGICAL REFLECTION

Read Matthew 9:12-13, Luke 4:18-19, Luke 10:8-9, and John 10:10.

1. How do these passages describe Jesus' goals for ministry?

2. How can you apply Jesus' goals to your own ministry in nursing?

3. Select several New Testament healing accounts from table 10.1, read them from the Bible, and examine the outcomes. Look particularly for physical, spiritual, and psychosocial dimensions of healing. How does each of these encounters result in shalom?

Case Study: Seeking Shalom

Reflect on a person in your nursing experience who seemed to demonstrate shalom-type health. Briefly write your own case study, including all the details someone else would need to fully picture this person.

DISCUSSION QUESTIONS

1. In what ways did the person in your case study demonstrate shalom-type health?

2. How was this person's spiritual health expressed?

3. How did spiritual health affect the person's psychosocial health?

4. How did spiritual and psychosocial health affect the person's physical health?

5. What nursing interventions facilitated this health?

6. How was the need for these interventions assessed?

11

HOPE IN SUFFERING

Purpose: To investigate a biblical view of suffering

Objectives: After reading this chapter and completing the exercises, you should be able to:
1. Describe the biblical explanations of suffering
2. Explain the views of suffering in eight religious traditions
3. List four cautions when seeking relief from suffering through alternative therapies
4. Communicate realistic hope in the midst of suffering

Keywords: suffering, hope, mystery, religion, alternative therapies

IN A MOMENT OF DESPAIR, Joe Collins took a shotgun, placed it in his mouth, and pulled the trigger. He intended to blow his brains out. Instead he lost half his face. All that remained was one bulging eye, two holes where his nose should have been, and a mouth opening only big enough to hold the cigarette that constantly dangled from it. A heavy cloud of gloom hung over his head.

Joe Collins was my (Judy's) first patient. Our assignment was to "talk to patients." But Joe couldn't talk; he merely grunted occasionally. He was faced with extensive reconstructive surgery to give him back the life he didn't want to live. Joe's suffering overwhelmed me. I could not even look at him, much less carry on a conversation. I made his bed, scrubbed his bedside table until it shined, filled his water pitcher, and tried to ask a few questions he could answer with a grunt.

"How can a just and loving God allow people to suffer?" is the age-old question that confronts every nursing student as soon as clinical experience begins. Theologians call this question theodicy. Although Joe's physical suffering was self-inflicted, many other cases followed that were harder to understand—a twenty-three-year-old mother of a newborn, dying of ovarian cancer; a pediatric unit filled with hydrocephalic infants and toddlers dying of leukemia; an esteemed former professor paralyzed and brain-damaged from a stroke.

The questions loom larger when suffering comes closer to home—your mother is suddenly stricken with a myocardial infarction; a brother is killed in an automobile accident; your position at work is dissolved and you find yourself unemployed. You no longer just ask, Why? Now you implore, Why me?

Several years ago, as my father-in-law sat slumped in a wheelchair after years of struggling through the effects of a series of strokes, my husband asked him, "Pop, do you ever ask God, Why me?" My father-in-law, a retired pastor, had spent his life in dedicated service to God and other people. He deserved a better end than this.

Pop looked at his son and, with great effort, answered, "No, the proper question is, Why not me?"

Suffering is a great mystery. It doesn't make sense to us. Our culture concentrates time and attention on avoiding suffering. And when it becomes impossible to eliminate the suffering, many decide to remove the suffering person through euthanasia. Such action flies in the face of Christian hope.

Christians certainly don't have all the answers, but we can trust the God who does. The Bible and church history give us some helpful insights into suffering—insights that do not solve the dilemma but at least make it more bearable. Interestingly, the early Christians who suffered intense persecution and oppression did not ask the theodicy question.[1] That came later, as Christians had more leisure time to spend in reflection. Instead of asking why, the first-century church concentrated on supporting the sufferer (1 Pet 4:12-15; 2 Cor 8:1-2; Gal 6:2).

Our culture, on the other hand, has convinced us that we deserve what we get. If we eat wisely, exercise regularly, and avoid toxic environmental hazards, we'll live to a ripe old age. That philosophy is fine as long as we are healthy, affluent, and successful. But it rapidly fails when debilitating illness, unemployment, or failure strikes unexpectedly. Even Christians, who trust in God's grace, may subtly assume that a person must have done something wrong to deserve the problems that come—just as Hindus believe that suffering comes from bad karma. That is not a Christian perspective.

---

[1] Stanley Hauerwas, *Naming the Silences: God, Medicine and the Problem of Suffering* (Grand Rapids, MI: Eerdmans, 1990), 49.

THE MYSTERY OF SUFFERING

Suffering remains a mystery we cannot fully explain, but God has given us some hints about it, and we can summarize what we do know.

First, suffering came into the world through sin. Suffering was not part of God's original creation, but he gave us the freedom to disobey him, with suffering as a result of that disobedience (Gen 1–3). Therefore, all people, as well as all of creation, suffer (Rom 8:18-39). Although some suffering is the direct result of human behavior (for example, wounds from violence, sexually transmitted diseases from promiscuity, addiction from substance abuse), we cannot automatically blame an individual for his or her suffering (Jn 9:1-7; Job 1–2). Most suffering comes from factors over which we have no control. Satan causes some suffering (1 Pet 5:8-9; Rev 2:10), and involvement in Christian ministry often brings suffering (2 Cor 6:4-10; 2 Tim 1:8). Suffering is part of life. We can expect it. Rather than ask "Why me?" we should wonder, "Why not me?" (1 Pet 4:12-19).

Second, we can be assured that God is involved in our suffering. God lovingly walks with us in our suffering (Is 43:1-7). He suffers for us (Lk 22:1-71; 23:32-49; Heb 4:14-16). Through the death and resurrection of Jesus Christ, the power of sin was broken, so that one day suffering will cease entirely (Rev 21:1-4; Is 35:1-10; 53:1-12). In the meantime, God gives us the privilege of suffering for him (Phil 1:29). He uses suffering to refine, mature, and discipline us (Is 48:9-11; Heb 12:3-13; 1 Pet 1:6-9). He demonstrates his power and love in the midst of our suffering (2 Cor 12:7-10).

Third, we can respond to suffering in faith. Our own suffering equips us to help others who suffer (2 Cor 1:3-11; Rom 5:1-5). We join together with the body of Christ, the church, to care for those who suffer either physically, psychosocially, or spiritually (Mt 25:31-46; Lk 10:1-12, 25-37; 1 Cor 12:26).

Finally, we endure suffering with patience and hope, trusting in God's compassion and mercy (Jas 5:7-11). Although suicide or euthanasia may seem

---

A Biblical View of Suffering

- Suffering came into the world through sin.
- God is present with us in our suffering.
- We can respond to suffering in faith.
- We can trust God's compassion and mercy.

to be a way out of suffering, they are not acceptable to God (Ex 20:13; Num 11:15; Job 3:11-13; Jer 20:14-15; Phil 1:19-24). Suffering remains a mystery that cannot be fully understood or controlled (Job 1–2; 42); however, we can trust in God's unlimited love and compassion (Lam 3:22-24).

SUFFERING IN OTHER RELIGIONS AND BELIEF SYSTEMS

Other religions hold different views of suffering. As nurses care for people from different religious traditions, we should be aware of some of the major views. The descriptions below are general, and a nurse caring for persons of these religions will want to do more in-depth study, as well as learn from the patients themselves. Not only do these views of suffering apply to professed adherents of other religions and cultures, but many of these ideas have become common within our culture and even permeated the understanding of some Christians. Table 11.1 shows the belief systems in direct relation to one another.

Table 11.1. Suffering: A view from other religions

RELIGION	CAUSE OF SUFFERING	RESPONSE TO SUFFERING
Hinduism	Bad karma created in previous existence.	Resignation to fate in this life while trying to create good karma for the next life. Release from the cycle of life to nirvana with loss of individual identity as the goal.
Buddhism	Desire and attachment to people and/or things.	Acceptance of the Four Noble Truths and following the Eightfold Path to eliminate desire and finally to achieve enlightenment and loss of individual identity. Mahayana Buddhism values compassion.
Judaism	Suffering is a fact of life. Why an all-powerful and all-loving God allows suffering is a problem. Why the innocent suffer is a problem. Weakness is a cause of suffering for secular Jews.	Forsaking sins and developing character is sometimes the response. Remaining strong. Adherents work to prevent and relieve human suffering.
Christianity	Same concerns as Judaism. Evil entered human experience following the fall.	Knowing that God suffered for and with humanity in Jesus Christ. Jesus conquered death and suffering, he is with us in suffering, and he will return to rule in the New Earth. Adherents work to prevent and relieve human suffering.
Islam	Suffering is a fact of life. Allah is compassionate and all-powerful, and suffering is not outside his power.	Submission to the will of Allah. Voluntary suffering is sometimes meritorious. Alms-giving presents a social way to relieve suffering.
Animism (Spiritism)	Curses, magic, witchcraft, etc., lead evil spirits to cause sickness and other distress.	Placating or diverting the spirits by means of charms, amulets, potions, rituals, etc.
Naturalism	Entering the natural chain of cause and effect either through lack of knowledge or stupidity.	Knowledge gained through science is the way to gain control in the chain of natural cause and effect.
New Age Mysticism	Wrong thinking, including wrong commitments to others, causes suffering. Or it may result from imbalance of energy or life force.	Psychological or spiritual techniques to detach the self from wrong commitments and wrong thinking, e.g., meditation and yoga. Methods to manipulate energy achieve balance and relieve suffering.

Hinduism. In Hinduism, suffering is viewed as the result of bad *karma* or destiny created in a previous existence. In other words, the sufferer is paying for something done when he or she was another person or creature. According to the doctrine of *samsara* (transmigration), all life goes through an endless succession of rebirths. Hindus teach that the appropriate response to suffering is resignation to one's fate while, at the same time, trying to create good *karma* for one's next existence. Release and liberation from the wheel of life (*moksha* or *mukti*) comes when one realizes that his or her individual soul *(Atman)* is identical with the universal soul *(Brahman)*. The only way to finally escape suffering is to lose one's individual identity in the universal soul or the Absolute, a state of bliss called *Nirvana. Nirvana* is achieved by detachment from the finite self and attachment to reality as a whole.

The Hindu sees three basic approaches for achieving *Nirvana,* or salvation. (1) Salvation by knowledge *(Jnana Yoga)* is acquired by listening to the sages and the Hindu scriptures, practicing meditation by turning awareness inward, and realizing the *Atman-Brahman* identity. (2) Salvation can come by devotion *(Bhakti Yoga)* to a particular manifestation of God (Brahma the creator, Vishnu the preserver, and Shiva the destroyer and his wife Kali), and hope to break through to a union with God. (3) Salvation by correct works *(Karma Yoga)* is gained by performing ceremonies, sacrifices, pilgrimages, and other good actions without attachment of desire for their rewards. All of these methods may also include *Raja Yoga,* an involved technique of meditation that includes control over the body, breathing, and thoughts.[2]

Because Hindus view suffering as the result of *karma*, they may respond to illness or loss as something that they deserve. Hindu patients may suffer silently and seldom complain of pain.

Buddhism. The Buddhist sees suffering as the result of human desire and attachment to people and things. The goal of each Buddhist is to attain *Nirvana*, a release from suffering, desire, and the finite self. In *Nirvana* there is no enduring self, but a total awareness and total being leading to enlightenment. Buddhism is built on the Four Noble Truths: (1) Life is full of pain

---

[2]Kenneth Boa, *Cults, World Religions and the Occult* (Wheaton, IL: Victor, 1990), 19-20. Also see David Burnett, *The Spirit of Hinduism* (Tunbridge Wells, England: Monarch, 1992), 71-85, 190-204; and George W. Braswell Jr., *Understanding World Religions* (Nashville: Broadman & Holman, 1994), 31-34.

and suffering *(dukkha)*. This is especially evident in birth, sickness, decay, death, and the presence of hated things and separation from loved things. Even the forces that hold life together *(skandas)* are full of suffering. These include the body, senses, thoughts, feelings, and consciousness. (2) Suffering is caused by *tanha*, the desire or thirst for pleasure, existence, and prosperity. (3) Suffering can be overcome by eliminating these cravings. (4) This elimination occurs by following the Eightfold Path.

The Eightfold Path is a system of therapy designed to develop habits that will release people from the restrictions caused by ignorance and craving and lead to purification of consciousness or enlightenment. It consists of (1) right knowledge (the Four Noble Truths), (2) right aspirations (intentions), (3) right speech, (4) right conduct, (5) right livelihood (occupation), (6) right effort, (7) right mindfulness (self-analysis), and (8) right meditation.[3]

There are two main divisions of Buddhism: Greater Vehicle *(Mahayana)* Buddhism and Lesser Vehicle *(Theravada)* Buddhism, in which the ways of achieving *Nirvana* differ. Most Buddhists today follow Mahayana Buddhism, in which the ideal is to become a *bodhisattva*, one who concentrates on reducing the suffering of others. There is less emphasis on the withdrawal and meditation that characterizes Theravada Buddhism, and more on sacrificing oneself out of compassion for living beings. By meditating, though, the aspiring bodhisattva realizes that nothing we see has genuine reality and that the real nature of things is empty. Meditation is seen as the way to a mystical nondualistic experience of reality in which there are no distinctions and no self.[4]

Most cultural Buddhists simply believe that life is suffering, so it must be accepted without complaining. Buddhist patients may hesitate to report pain or express emotion. However, they appreciate a nurse who shows sympathy and persistently seeks to relieve their suffering.[5]

Judaism. Jews accept the reality of human suffering. The question raised in the Hebrew Bible (the Christian Old Testament) concerns the distribution of suffering: *Why do some people suffer and others not?* (Job 21:7-16; Ps 94:3-7). Why do the wicked not suffer when those who try to keep faith with God do?

---

[3]Boa, *Cults, World Religions*, 31-33; see also Braswell, *Understanding World Religions*, 52-58.
[4]Ninan Smart, *Worldviews: Crosscultural Explorations of Human Beliefs* (New York: Scribner's, 1983), 105-7. For nursing implications see "An Asian Patient: How Does Culture Affect Care?" *Journal of Christian Nursing* (1991): 4-9.
[5]Jeanette Yep, "An Asian Patient: How Does Culture Affect Care?—A Family Member Responds: Please Understand Us," *Journal of Christian Nursing* (1991): 6-8.

God is both compassionate and all-powerful, so why does this injustice occur? Suffering is sometimes explained as punishment for sin and other times as a means of testing character and faithfulness. But this does not explain all suffering. The Bible also speaks of a radical intervention by God in human affairs in which undeserved suffering will be made right by the coming of a messiah to set up God's kingdom.[6]

Many modern Jews hold a more secular view of suffering that emphasizes the need to survive it with courage and dignity. Because of the extreme suffering throughout Jewish history, many Jews today hold that they must be strong to defend themselves against further suffering. Some of them still look forward to a coming Messiah who will lead them to freedom and peace, while others maintain that only human efforts will reach these goals.[7]

Islam. For Muslims, suffering is to be expected as a part of living. God (Allah) is viewed as all-powerful and compassionate. Because Allah is all-powerful, everything that happens, including suffering, is under his control. The proper human response is to submit to the will of Allah in all things, including suffering. Suffering is sometimes viewed as punishment for evil, but more often as a means (instrument) of developing character. In some cases, voluntary suffering undertaken for God is seen as meritorious.[8] At the same time, there are social means for attacking suffering through alms-giving *(zakat).* There is a day of judgment in which each person's deeds will be weighed on a pair of balances to determine the person's destiny. Paradise is a place of sensuous delight and gratification.

The Five Pillars of Islam are the main religious practices. They are (1) reciting the *Shahadah,* "There is no God but Allah, and Mohammed is his prophet," aloud several times daily; (2) praying prescribed prayers *(salat)* five times a day; (3) alms-giving *(zakat);* (4) fasting during the month of Ramadan by not eating or drinking anything during the daylight hours; and (5) going on a pilgrimage to Mecca *(Hajj)* at least once in a lifetime. A Muslim must also be a good spokesperson for the faith.[9]

---

[6]John Bowker, *Suffering in the Religions of the World* (Cambridge: Cambridge University Press, 1970), 5-40.

[7]See, for example, Darrell J. Fasching, *Narrative Theology After Auschwitz: From Alienation to Ethics* (Minneapolis: Fortress, 1992).

[8]Bowker, *Suffering,* 99-136.

[9]Boa, *Cults, World Religions,* 71; Braswell, *Understanding World Religions,* 111-12.

It would be important for nurses to provide opportunity and privacy for Muslim patients to pray at the proper times and to observe fasting during Ramadan when medically permissible.

Animism. Many people in almost every culture believe that spirits animate, or live in, all things, both the living and the inert. This folk belief may be the primary religion of its adherents, but it underlies or coexists with many other religions as well. These spirits are associated with cures, magic, and witchcraft. The response to suffering is to find ways to placate the spirits or direct their attention away from the sufferer. Such techniques include charms (magic formulas), amulets, secret potions, rituals, and dances.[10]

Nurses may find that patients who think illness is caused by evil spirits will wear amulets or little sacks of herbs around their necks to ward off the spirit. These patients will not want to remove them. It would be important for the nurse to listen carefully to how an animist patient understands the cause of their suffering and take their concerns seriously. They may also attribute physical illness to spirits, and so believe that taking prescribed medication will not help.

Naturalism. For the naturalist, suffering is purely the result of natural causes. Humans suffer either because they do not yet know how to avoid the natural chain of cause and effect or because they step into the chain by their own poor choices. The response to suffering is to learn how to get control of the natural chain of events through science. When that is not possible, some advocate taking control of one's own death to eliminate suffering.[11]

Naturalists will seek medical care and usually follow the prescribed treatment. They may also seek assisted suicide when suffering seems overwhelming.

New Age. These spiritual approaches usually see suffering as the result of wrong thinking (imperfect consciousness) or unnecessary commitment to other people or material concerns. New Age philosophy draws from many traditions and religions, but especially from Westernized and romanticized

---

[10]David Burnett, *Clash of World: A Christian's Handbook on Cultures, World Religions and Evangelism* (Nashville: Thomas Nelson, 1992), 57-68. For nursing implications, see Hsin-chun Mao and Li-ling Yang, "Understanding the Spiritual Needs of Chinese Patients," *Journal of Christian Nursing* (1994): 39-41.

[11]This philosophy found its ultimate expression in the assisted suicide campaign outlined in Derek Humphrey, *Final Exit* (Secaucus, NY: Hemlock Society, 1991); Derek Humphrey and Jack Kevorkian, *Prescription Medicine: The Goodness of Planned Death* (Buffalo, NY: Prometheus, 1991).

Hinduism, Buddhism, Taoism, and Theosophy. *Monism* (the belief that all is one) usually surfaces as the most central belief. New Age philosophy decries dualistic thinking for separating all that exists, including humans, from the One, good from evil, the seen from the unseen, and matter from spirit. Self is viewed as the prime reality, so that as human beings expand their consciousness, they can transform themselves. Barbara Blattner, in her text *Holistic Nursing*, states, "People are responsible for their own bodies and minds. They can choose sickness or health. They have control over their lives and minds, their bodies, and their health."[12] Hence, people who suffer have chosen to do so.

New Age techniques for relieving suffering are drawn from energy manipulation and mind control, which are based on a monistic worldview. They may also use occult practices, attempting to control and manipulate the spiritual world. Many New Age thinkers appeal to Jungian psychology and quantum physics for explanations of the efficacy of their modalities.[13] Since they believe that dualistic thinking overburdens people with guilt and stress, various psychological techniques are used to relieve guilt feelings. However, because they often see no distinction between life and death, and pain and happiness, assisted suicide becomes an option for ending suffering.

SEARCHING FOR HEALING TECHNIQUES

What, then, can we do to relieve suffering? Are any alternative therapies "safe"? Can we incorporate practices based on other religions into our nursing care? Jesus admonished his disciples to be "wise as serpents and innocent as doves" (Mt 10:16). As Christians practicing in a pluralistic health care system, we need to heed his advice. Every new technique must be carefully evaluated, not only for its effectiveness but also for its philosophical underpinnings (see appendix for guidelines). At the same time, we can trust God to protect us from being unknowingly led astray.

---

[12]Barbara Blattner, *Holistic Nursing* (Englewood Cliffs, NJ: Prentice-Hall, 1981), 25.

[13]See, for example, Victoria E. Slater, "Toward an Understanding of Energetic Healing," parts one and two of *Journal of Holistic Nursing* (1995): 209-38, and Deirdre Davis Brigham, *Imagery for Getting Well: Clinical Applications of Behavioral Medicine* (San Francisco: Harper & Row, 1984). For a cogent critique of these modalities, see Elliot Miller, "The Christian, Energetic Medicine, 'New Age Paranoia,'" *Christian Research Institute*, June 9, 2009, www.equip.org/article/the-christian-energetic-medicine-new-age-paranoia/.

Some Christians believe that they can use certain alternative techniques by adapting them to a Christian understanding of their effectiveness. Others adamantly shun all practices that have any hint of Eastern philosophy or occult roots. At times we need to humbly agree to disagree when strong differences of opinion occur among Christians regarding holistic techniques. However, we are still responsible before God to be both wise and faithful. While some alternative therapies are just basic common sense—good nutrition, rest, relaxation, human touch—many of these therapies can lead those who practice them into idolatry.

Suffering often drives people to turn to alternative therapies out of desperation. They are willing to try anything, and sometimes the techniques *do* seem to bring temporary comfort. Christians may let down their guard when they see patients respond positively to various complementary approaches. Psychologist Elizabeth Hillstrom provides some helpful insights into why these therapies appear to work.[14]

First, they may be conferring actual physical benefits in ways that are not yet apparent to scientific inquiry. Research has shown real physical benefits of some herbal remedies, acupuncture, and acupressure. It has not been able to demonstrate *why* they work, but it does suggest, for example, that these therapies may cause the body to release endorphins. Some alternative therapies may also bring real physical improvements indirectly through reducing stress and giving hope, love, and a sense of meaning and empowerment.

In many cases, people attribute healing to alternative therapies when it is actually due to the body's ability to heal itself. Hillstrom quotes doctors as saying that 80 percent of physical ailments they treat would resolve themselves without treatment. Some benefits from holistic treatments can be attributed to the placebo effect. The placebo effect has an actual physiological basis.[15] It causes the body to produce endorphins, which reduce pain and worry, allowing the immune system to function more effectively. The beneficial effects of emotional support and the communication of caring and concern can also aid in healing.

---

[14]Barbara Hillstrom, *Testing the Spirits* (Downers Grove, IL: InterVarsity Press, 1995), 193.
[15]For example, see Shankar Vedantam, "Placebos May Be a Powerful Tool That Medicine Has Overlooked," *Morning Edition*, NPR, May 9, 2019, www.npr.org/2019/05/09/721685197/placebos-may -be-a-powerful-tool-that-medicine-has-overlooked.

If these were the only effects of alternative therapies, we could easily incorporate them into Christian nursing. However, there are problems involved. Some apparent healings are fraudulent and trick people into thinking they are healed. This can have devastating effects when the "healed" person stops taking essential medication or discontinues life-sustaining medical care. Furthermore, many holistic alternative therapies turn to occult spiritual beings for their power. Hillstrom warns that participating in these activities may well be flirting with the demonic, and we must keep in mind that God has strictly forbidden seeking help from the spirit realm.[16]

FINDING HOPE IN SUFFERING

Instead of looking to esoteric fads for healing techniques, we have a wealth of resources in our Christian heritage to bring comfort and healing to those who are suffering. Physicians Mary Greenwold Milano and David Larson cited numerous research studies to document that "not only can religious beliefs help patients to cope with their illness, but a patient's religious commitment has also been found to be associated with improved clinical status and outcomes."[17] In fact, regular church attendance turned out to be a significant factor in maintaining lower blood pressure rates in twenty studies conducted over thirty years.[18] Corporate worship, prayer, and Bible study have been shown to positively affect both physical and mental health.[19]

Sister Rosemary Donley outlines three distinct approaches to suffering within the Christian tradition. Interestingly, these approaches have been the heart of nursing from its beginning, and are second nature to most nurses.

> The first spiritual response is compassionate accompaniment. . . . The compassionate person need not offer meaning or alleviation. Rather the "other" offers a quiet sharing of the experience and helps the person to sustain the burden of the suffering. . . . They are motivated by the belief that, through their presence, the suffering person may experience the presence of the Lord from whom nothing can separate us. . . .

---

[16]Hillstrom, *Testing the Spirits*, 164-70.

[17]Mary A. Greenwold Milano and David B. Larson, "The Research Shows: Religion Is Healthy," *CMDS Healthwise*, fall 1995, 7.

[18]Susan S. and David B. Larson, "Warning: Research Shows Religion Is Good for Your Mental Health," *Christian Counseling Today*, October 1993, 28.

[19]David B. Larson and Susan S. Larson, "Clinical Religious Research," *Christian Medical and Dental Society Journal* (1992). Also see Mark Hartwig, "For Good Health, Go to Church," *Focus on the Family Citizen*, June 21, 1993, which has extensive endnotes of research cited.

To search for meaning of personal and communal suffering is a second type of spiritual response. . . . When suffering is endowed with the glorious role of bringing a person closer to God, the person experiences relief even when the suffering itself remains. . . .

The third, and perhaps most dramatic expression of a Christian response to suffering, is action to remove the suffering itself. . . . However, when a Christian response is reduced *exclusively* to action to remove suffering, there is a profound loss.[20]

The Christian tradition does not emphasize one approach to suffering over the others, so our task becomes determining the appropriate balance between technological intervention, meaning giving, and compassionate presence. Donley continues, "Perhaps the ordering that makes most sense in our highly technical environment is an integration of action to remove suffering and its causes with compassionate presence and meaning giving."[21] This results in nursing care that respects the person as reflecting the image of God. Physical healing is an integral dimension of the salvation offered to us through Jesus Christ.

The gospel gives us a clear mandate to provide excellent physical care, but we need not desperately seek a cure for every terminal illness or attempt to preserve biological function at any cost. Sometimes people experience healing in this life; sometimes they find it in the life to come. Christian faith gives us the perspective to realize that life is a gift from God—it is in his hands. This perspective also prevents that sense of hopelessness that sees assisted suicide as an option. However, there does come a time when chemotherapy can stop, when resuscitation efforts are futile, and invasive procedures no longer help.

At that point we still have something we can *do*. Christian nurses continue to offer hope in the face of suffering and death through compassionate presence and meaning giving. Such intervention is not an *imposing* of personal beliefs on a vulnerable patient, a concern expressed by many nurses. There is no sense of manipulative proselytizing, but simply sharing the good news of Jesus Christ.

Jesus sent his followers out not only to preach, but also to heal (Mt 10:8; Lk 10:9). Healing prayer, used appropriately with patients, is an effective nursing

---

[20]Rosemary Donley, "Spiritual Dimensions of Health Care: Nursing's Mission," *Nursing and Health Care*, April 1991, 179-80.
[21]Donley, "Spiritual Dimensions of Health Care," 182.

response to suffering. We will provide further guidelines for spiritual care in chapter fourteen.

For the Christian, a vital relationship with God gives strength not only to the suffering person but also to the nurse who provides that compassionate accompaniment and meaning giving. When we find ourselves looking for quick fixes for suffering, whether in technology, alternative therapies, or "assistance-in-dying," we need to pull back and examine our faith commitment. Sometimes we gain the faith and strength to care for others through our own experiences of God's faithfulness in suffering.

LEARNING FROM EXPERIENCE

It doesn't take long before we learn that the Lord does not allow us to profess understanding without giving us firsthand experience. The prophet Jeremiah spent time in a cistern; the apostle Paul ended up in prison; Jesus went to the cross. The truth of Romans 5:3-5 echoes throughout the pages of Scripture and into our own lives. "We . . . boast in our sufferings, knowing that suffering produces endurance, and endurance produces character, and character produces hope, and hope does not disappoint us, because God's love has been poured into our hearts through the Holy Spirit that has been given to us."

There are no shortcuts to hope. Several years ago I (Judy) experienced the confusing specter of the health care system from the other side. As I faced a series of painful procedures, major surgery, and the strong possibility of cancer, powerful emotions stormed my physical and spiritual being. And I, the strong and rational one who cares for others, fell apart.

Suddenly I found myself surrounded by the remarkably supportive community of the body of Christ. People began to pray. Friends called and prayed over the phone. Colleagues stepped in without hesitation to fulfill responsibilities I couldn't handle.

In the meantime I began to cry out to the Lord. I felt guilty that I was so scared. Where was my faith? Amazingly no one else asked that question. They just let me express my fears, listened, and cared. Each morning I would awake around four o'clock, tormented by the what-ifs. My devotional times stretched to two hours. I would begin reading the Bible, fixating in Psalm 16, pouring out my fears to the Lord; then I would promptly fall asleep. I would then awake feeling at peace. It was as if I were curling up in the lap of my heavenly Father, realizing that whatever happened, he would be with me and in control.

Gradually I began to see the good gifts of the Lord in the midst of my anxiety. Delays with tests and procedures, which at first seemed frustrating, provided time and opportunities to grow and experience the love and support of caring Christians. A visit from one friend, a Christian nurse, was a particular turning point. She asked me, "Are you afraid of dying? If so, we can talk about it." And as we talked, the fears began to lift. Suffering was beginning to produce endurance.

The object of my hope began to shift. No longer was I caught up in the immediate worries about the surgery and possible diagnosis, or even the practical concerns of whether I would live to see my children grow up, but a deep sense of the Lord's love enveloped me. When the fears began to well up again, the words of the hymn "God Will Take Care of You" began to drift through my head. Tears flowed as I realized the truth of those words. Even if I did have cancer, God would take care of me, my family, and all the pressing projects that made me feel indispensable. That realization began to free me from the bondage of fear, so I could begin to reach out again to other people in their needs and get on with the work at hand. Endurance began to produce character, making me more compassionate and understanding of others who suffer.

Throughout this process I began to see the reality of the hope we have in Jesus Christ—the hope that will not disappoint us. I experienced the power of God's love being poured out through the Holy Spirit through precious times of prayer, through a deepening love for God's Word, and through the overwhelming care and support of his people. I gained a new appreciation for the body of Christ and the important role that we have as Christian nurses to provide that compassionate presence and meaning in suffering.

Instilling hope is the heart of Christian nursing. Technical competence is extremely important, but to those who are suffering and afraid, the absolute fact of Jesus Christ's death and resurrection to restore us to relationship with God holds ultimate weight. That is not an abstract theological concept, but the practical reality that grounds our hope.

All people, as well as all of creation, suffer. Suffering came into the world through sin—the sin of Adam and Eve in the Garden of Eden (Gen 3). It is perpetuated by the sin evident in society, its structures, and ourselves. We all experience the effects of sin. The destructive forces of natural disasters, illness, and injury do not discriminate between the just and the unjust (Mt 5:45).

Although some problems are the direct result of a person's behavior—bitterness, pride, violence, sexual promiscuity, substance abuse, lifestyle choices—most suffering results from the general effects of evil in the world. We cannot blame an individual for his or her suffering. Suffering is simply part of life in a fallen world (1 Pet 4:12-19).

In the process, God uses suffering to teach and refine us. He lovingly walks with us through suffering (Is 43:1-7), assuring us that he will not allow anything more than we can bear (Heb 12:3-13). Our own suffering equips us to empathize with others in their suffering (Rom 5:1-5; 2 Cor 1:3-11). A nurse who has not suffered personally will find great difficulty providing emotional and spiritual support for others.

Nursing directly enters the suffering of this world, bringing the hope of comfort, strength, and healing. Our taproot draws its nourishment from the words of Jesus, who instructed his followers, "Truly I tell you, just as you did it to one of the least of these who are members of my family, you did it to me" (Mt 25:40).

> *Nursing directly enters the suffering of this world, bringing the hope of comfort, strength, and healing.*

We actually proclaim the kingdom of God when we care for suffering people (Lk 4:18-21). Through Jesus Christ, God not only announced the ultimate end of suffering, he himself took human form to suffer for our sake—making that hope possible. Right now, we live in a now-and-not-yet kingdom. Jesus' suffering and death on the cross definitively won the victory over sin in our world. Our hope for a new world order is certain. But the effects of sin still ripple through our lives. The reality of the kingdom will not fully appear until the parousia—the second coming of Christ. In the meantime, we endure suffering with patience and hope, trusting in God's mercy and compassion, but also reaching out in love to care for others who are suffering. Ultimately, we look forward to a time when illness, tears, and suffering will have been wiped away—when nurses won't be needed!

For Further Thinking

1. How would you answer a parent who asks, "Why does God allow my child to suffer? It seems so unfair!"

2. In what ways has God used suffering in your life? What did you learn from these experiences?

THEOLOGICAL REFLECTION

1. Read Romans 5:3-5. Note the progression in these verses. How have you seen this occur in either a person in your care or your own life?

2. Read John 9:1-7. Why had God allowed this man to suffer blindness? What implications does this account have in regard to our assumptions about the reason for a person's suffering? According to Jesus, how should we respond to suffering?

3. Read Romans 8:12-30. What further light does this passage shed on the reasons for suffering? What hope can we find in the midst of suffering?

Case Study: I'm Glad I Have AIDS!

Mary Ernst, RN, a divorced mother of three children, supported her family as a critical-care nurse. One day at work she accidentally stuck herself with a contaminated needle. A year later she went to donate blood for a friend who had been injured in a car accident. After her blood was tested, a physician informed her coldly that she was HIV-positive. She felt alone and hopeless. The physician offered no support.

When she told her pastor and his wife about the diagnosis, they seemed to assume that Mary had contracted the virus through sexual contact or by injecting illegal drugs. They, too, offered no support. People at church shunned her. Some asked her directly if she had been in a sexual relationship with someone with AIDS.

Feeling devastated, she joined the AIDS Coalition, a support group, where she met Tony, a man with AIDS who knew he had contracted the virus through his gay lifestyle. Tony encouraged Mary, telling her, "Hold on. There's still life to be lived." She also found friendship and comfort among other members of the AIDS Coalition.

Over the years, Mary supported Tony and others as they became ill and died. When Tony's lover died, Mary attended the funeral—one of only nine people in the congregation. Even his family abandoned him because of his lifestyle.

Mary also found hope and comfort through journaling and reading. One book, *Burden of a Secret* by Jimmy Allen, told the story of his family's struggle as his daughter-in-law and two grandchildren all died of AIDS as a result of an HIV-contaminated blood transfusion. In the process his son rejected God. The book helped Mary to see the dangers of keeping her own struggle secret. And she began to consider ways of reaching out to other people with Christ's love.

She had changed churches, so she went to her new pastor to share her vision and express her sense of calling to a ministry with hurting people. He prayed with her for direction. She also heard several ministry volunteers speak at the church, and opportunities for service began to unfold. She decided to begin an outreach ministry for people with catastrophic illnesses and to name it The Comfort Zone. She was recently honored as her church's Volunteer of the Year.

Even though Mary's work with The Comfort Zone increased, she did not abandon her friends at the AIDS Coalition. She knew the pain of rejection, and she refused to turn her back on them, even though most of them were in the gay lifestyle. She refused to condemn them. She chose to love them, even though she did not agree with their lifestyle.

Mary went out of her way to care for Tony, even buying him cigarettes when he wanted them. Tony could see that Mary loved him unconditionally. One day he began to ask questions, wondering why she treated him with kindness, when most straight people—especially Christians—condemned him.

Tony's questions increased. Finally he told her, "I want what you have."

She replied, "Are you ready to turn over what's left of your life to Christ?"

He was, so they prayed together as he committed his life to Christ. Before he died, Tony told Mary, "Get to the young people. Tell them to be careful. Sex is not a toy. I started experimenting as a youngster, and this is how I turned out. Now I regret it."

Tony eventually died peacefully and quietly.

Mary concludes, "Now when I put my arms around an HIV-positive person and say I love him and that Jesus died for him, I realize that my own diagnosis has meaning. I even have those days—not every day, of course—when I can say, 'I'm glad, Lord, that I have this disease, because it has opened doors for me to tell others about You.'"

Fourteen years later, Mary has retired from nursing. She is still alive and active in her ministry to people with catastrophic conditions.[22]

Today, with antiretroviral drugs, people do not die of AIDS as they did in the early years of the AIDS crisis, but the stigma remains. Mary serves as a model for nurses today as we care for those who suffer.

DISCUSSION QUESTIONS

1. How would you respond if you were diagnosed with a terminal condition?
    a. What would be your greatest fears?
    b. What would give you hope?
2. In what ways did Mary suffer after her HIV diagnosis?
3. How could her church community have been more supportive of her?
4. In what ways did God offer Mary hope?
5. Review the perspectives on suffering of other religions in this chapter. What hope could each of these religions offer Mary?
    a. Hinduism
    b. Buddhism
    c. Judaism
    d. Islam
    e. Animism
    f. Naturalism
    g. New Age

---

[22] Adapted from Carolyn Curtis, "I'm Glad I Have AIDS," *Journal of Christian Nursing* (2003): 16-17.

12

THE PARADOX OF DEATH

Purpose: To examine the Christian view of death and dying

Objectives: After reading this chapter and completing the exercises, you should be able to:
1. Identify reasons people fear death
2. Explain six paradoxes of death
3. List four things that Christians can take with them in death
4. Describe the differences between palliative care and hospice care
5. Describe practical nursing interventions for supporting a dying person

Keywords: death, dying, resurrection, spiritual body, heaven, hell, compassionate accompaniment, meaning, palliative care, hospice care

"I KNOW I SHOULDN'T LET DEATH BOTHER ME because I'm a Christian," a hospice nurse remarked, "but after seeing so many people die, I hate death! I've also become paranoid about every little symptom I see in myself or my family—I immediately assume that it is the beginning of a terminal illness. I live in constant fear of death."

Continuous exposure to death and dying brought this hospice nurse face to face with the nagging fears all of us harbor. Most of us can deny the inevitability of death most of the time. We can talk about the beauty of heaven and the hope of eternal life with objectivity and little emotional involvement. However, for those who experience the death of a loved one, the diagnosis of terminal illness, or constant exposure to dying patients, the coping measure of denial quickly fades. It is hard to deny what is so ominously real.

Christians are not immune to death and grief. Like other people, they suffer from the agony of death because life has meaning, relationships have depth and importance, and we are strongly aware of all the unfinished business in this life. Few of us are as confident as the apostle Paul, who could say, "For to me, living is Christ and dying is gain. If I am to live in the flesh, that means fruitful labor for me; and I do not know which I prefer. I am hard pressed between the two: my desire is to depart and be with Christ, for that is far better; but to remain in the flesh is more necessary for you" (Phil 1:21-24).

Regardless of how much we love and trust God, most of us fear death. We do not want to be separated from our friends and family, even if it means moving on to a better life. Most of us, if pressed, would say that as much as we want to meet Jesus face to face, we'd much rather stay right here with friends and family in our comfortable, familiar home.

Avoiding the Subject

Because Christians often believe that fearing death shows lack of faith, the bereaved and dying among us may suffer neglect as well as grief. We either avoid them entirely because we do not know what to say, or we offer pious platitudes that further isolate them. For instance, a widow may have difficulty attending church services because she feels betrayed by Christian friends who never came to visit during the six months her husband lay dying of cancer. A mother who lost her daughter in an automobile accident six months ago is still wracked by grief, but her pastor tells her that she should be happy because her daughter is with the Lord. Now she feels guilty as well as depressed. Perhaps we show our lack of faith most clearly when we refuse to acknowledge the horror of death.

Even those Christians who have grappled with their own fear of death and believe they have overcome it find that it is a continuing struggle, not a one-time victory. Nurses who see death daily find themselves becoming gradually drained of life and hope. Roberta Paige, a hospice nurse, relates the following anecdote:

> In a corner of the emergency department cubicle Ann sat with a chapel veil on her head praying the rosary. On the stretcher beside her lay Edward, her fiancé. Dark blood flowed through his nasogastric tube. He was also hemorrhaging from his rectum. Waxen and pale, Edward did not respond when I entered. He appeared to be asleep. Ann motioned me to her side and said that they were waiting for the Bishop to come, because Edward desperately wanted to be confirmed before he died.

The bishop came. Edward opened his eyes and smiled during the confirmation ritual. A short time later, he died.

The paradox of death seemed so evident in this place. The stench of blood and the sadness of a woman watching the man she loved ebb away countered the life that shined through Edward, more vividly perhaps because he was dying. As a Christian, I knew I should rejoice at this deathbed commitment to Christ. Instead, anger welled up inside me. I wanted to scream, "Death, I hate you!"[1]

Why does death threaten us so much? Why isn't the hope of eternal life with Christ sufficient to alleviate our fears? Doesn't the Bible say, "When this perishable body puts on imperishability, and this mortal body puts on immortality, then the saying that is written will be fulfilled: 'Death has been swallowed up in victory'" (1 Cor 15:54)? Perhaps we need to back up and look at what the Bible really does say about death.

The passage above from 1 Corinthians 15 is often quoted out of context. This sense of victory is not our present experience. The triumph is yet to come. We are not yet free from the sting of death. In the meantime, we are at war with an enemy. Earlier, in 1 Corinthians 15:22-26 we are told,

> For as all die in Adam, so all will be made alive in Christ. But each in his own order: Christ the first fruits, then at his coming those who belong to Christ. Then comes the end, when he hands over the kingdom to God the Father, after he has destroyed every ruler and every authority and power. For he must reign until he has put all his enemies under his feet. The last enemy to be destroyed is death.

We need not feel guilty about fearing death. Death is the last enemy of God. It would be strange not to fear such an enemy.

Even Jesus struggled with death. He mourned at the tomb of his friend Lazarus, even though he knew he would raise him from the dead. The Gospel of John says Jesus was "greatly disturbed in spirit and deeply moved" (Jn 11:33). The Greek terms imply a deep, agonized groaning. The death of a friend pained Jesus to the depths of his being.

Although Jesus went to his own death willingly, he did not go without extreme anguish. He wrestled in prayer, saying, "My Father, if it is possible, let this cup pass from me; yet not what I want but what you want" (Mt 26:39).

---

[1]Roberta Lyder Paige, letter to Judith Allen Shelly. Reprinted by permission.

Seeking support from his friends, he told his disciples, "I am deeply grieved, even to death; remain here, and stay awake with me" (Mt 26:38). Even Jesus needed comfort at the time of death.

THE INCONVENIENCE OF DEATH

The disciples were not shining examples of supportive care. They fell asleep. Three times Jesus had to wake them and remind them of the seriousness of the situation and his need for them. But Jesus recognized their problem, saying, "The spirit indeed is willing, but the flesh is weak" (Mt 26:41). We can remember the disciples' weakness when our own care for dying patients falls short of the ideal. Jesus understands our failures too.

One incident in my (Judy's) experience continues to haunt me, reminding me that I would have done no better than the disciples in watching with Jesus. I was working three to eleven, the only RN on a hectic surgical unit with a reduced staff. Five patients returned from the recovery room on my shift. Nine others had intravenous drips and still needed frequent vital-sign checks. We had an emergency admission who needed extra attention. And in the room at the end of the hall was a woman in isolation, dying of hepatitis with her sixteen-year-old daughter at her side.

I didn't have time for a patient in isolation or for a distraught teenager. The patient didn't belong on our floor anyway; she was a medical patient. She was hemorrhaging copiously from esophageal varices and aspirating blood despite a nasogastric tube. Her IV infiltrated. Her blood pressure was fading.

The daughter frantically began to shout, "Somebody do something!"

I paged the medical resident, who responded, "The woman is dying. Why should I come?"

In desperation I hustled the daughter out of the room and tried to clean up the patient and get her tubes in working order. As she left the room, the daughter told me, "If Mama's dying I want to be here!"

I closed the door and set to work, inwardly angry because I did not have time for this. As I removed the tape from the infiltrated IV catheter, the patient winced and said, "You don't have to be so mean." I felt a stab of guilt as I realized my anger was showing. Within minutes the woman died, her daughter waiting outside the door. Suddenly I felt consumed with guilt. Not only had I prevented the girl from spending those final moments with her mother, she was now alone with no one to comfort her. I had been "asleep" to the needs of the patient and her daughter because of my own inability to cope, just as Jesus' disciples slept while he suffered the agonies of death alone.

Death is almost always inconvenient. It defies our need for control and predictability. I could at least call the supervisor to help me, but families whose lives are interrupted by the death of a loved one face a more drastic disruption. They may be left without a home or income. They may owe thousands of dollars in medical expenses. The loss of companionship and radical change in lifestyle may precipitate deep depression. Regardless of how carefully a family plans for death with wills, insurance policies, appointment of guardians and alternative housing, death is always a rude interruption. Even when death brings relief from pain and suffering, it is seldom easy for the survivors.

TERROR AND HOPE

For the Christian, death is a paradox. It is both the hope of eternal life and the fear of the unknown. It is relief from pain and physical limitations—and the agony of separation. It is the joyous expectation of seeing God—and the fear of his wrath. It is universal (everyone must die), but each of us must die alone. It is the final release from all that binds us, and yet it is the ultimate enemy that came into the world through sin.

> *Death is the final release from all that binds us, and yet it is the ultimate enemy that came into the world through sin.*

In the Scriptures, death is both physical and spiritual. The greatest fear of the Old Testament writers was not physical death, but the anticipated separation from God. The psalmist cried out, "Is your steadfast love declared in the grave, or your faithfulness in Abaddon? Are your wonders known in the darkness, or your saving help in the land of forgetfulness?" (Ps 88:11-12).

The Old Testament writers believed that death meant separation from God.[2] An understanding of this concept gives a fuller appreciation for the agony Jesus felt as he went to the cross, for his loss was total. His cry of "Eli,

---

[2]Hans Walter Wolff, *Anthropology of the Old Testament* (Philadelphia: Fortress, 1974), 106-7.

Eli, la'ma sabach-thani?" ("My God, my God, why have you forsaken me?") in Matthew 27:46 was his expression of terror at being separated from the Father even briefly. It is from that excruciating horror that we are freed by the death and resurrection of Jesus. But physical death remains, even for the Christian.

Herein we face another paradox. If the final victory over death is not yet realized, what happens to those who die in the interim? Jesus could tell the thief on the cross, "Today you will be with me in Paradise" (Lk 23:43), and Paul assures us that "neither death, nor life . . . nor anything else in all creation, will be able to separate us from the love of God in Christ Jesus our Lord" (Rom 8:38-39). But what happens between physical death and the second coming of Christ? One answer lies in 1 Thessalonians 4:13-18:

> But we do not want you to be uninformed, brothers and sisters, about those who have died, so that you may not grieve as others do who have no hope. For since we believe that Jesus died and rose again, even so, through Jesus, God will bring with him those who have died. For this we declare to you by the word of the Lord, that we who are alive, who are left until the coming of the Lord, will by no means precede those who have died. For the Lord himself, with a cry of command, with the archangel's call and with the sound of God's trumpet, will descend from heaven, and the dead in Christ will rise first. Then we who are alive, who are left, will be caught up in the clouds together with them to meet the Lord in the air; and so we will be with the Lord forever. Therefore encourage one another with these words.

Perhaps the key to understanding this passage lies in the Greek word *koimōmenōn*, which most Bible translations render as "sleeping," but the NRSV translates as "died." Sleep may be the closest experience we presently have for the concept of eternity. We go to sleep and awake with little or no sense of the time elapsed. The dead in Christ enter into eternity. They are freed from the constraints of time, so that "one day is like a thousand years, and a thousand years is like one day" (2 Pet 3:8). So Jesus could say to the thief on the cross, "*Today* you will be with me in Paradise" (Lk 23:43, italics ours). In eternity the kingdom of God has already come, because there is no time, but on earth we still await its coming.

Another paradox is that the Bible portrays death as both a natural event and an enemy. Genesis 25:8 reports, "Abraham breathed his last and died in a good old age, an old man and full of years, and was gathered to his people." Nothing could seem more natural and appropriate. Job 5:26 says, "You shall come to your grave in ripe old age, as a shock of grain comes up to the threshing floor in its season." Here death seems to almost fulfill the purpose for life.

Death presents us with a paradox of terror and hope. For many people the fear of God's judgment overshadows the hope of eternal life in Christ. Matthew 25:31-46 makes it clear that we will be judged for our actions (or inaction). Matthew 7:21 warns us that outward profession of faith is not sufficient for entrance into heaven. Jesus expects us to do "the will of my Father in heaven." The question of faith versus works can be confusing when reading such passages. According to James, though, works are the evidence of our faith (Jas 2:17). Those who truly belong to Christ will show the fruit of the Spirit in their attitudes and behavior (Gal 5:22-24). However, our salvation—our entrance into eternal life in Christ—is by grace alone. No record of good works is going to get us into heaven (Eph 2:8-9). Believers may endure discipline and even punishment from God for their own good (Heb 12:5-6), but they can rest assured of God's grace. Jesus assures us, "Anyone who comes to me I will never drive away" (Jn 6:37).

ENDING AND NEW BEGINNING

Another biblical paradox about death is that it is both the end and a continuation of our life on earth. The relationship with God initiated on earth continues and grows in heaven. We also have the sure hope of being reunited with other believers after death. Looking to the future, death is merely a transition for the Christian. But looking backward, death is absolute and final. We cannot call back anyone from the dead. The Bible gives strong warnings that we are not to tamper with the realm of the dead (see, for example, Deut 18:10-12; Is 8:19; Lk 16:19-31).

Consulting the dead through séances, mediums, spirit guides, out-of-body experiences—or whatever the current fad may be—is off limits for Christians (Lev 19:31; Deut 18:9-14; Gal 5:19-21). In the first place, in doing so we merely deceive ourselves, for (except for Jesus and those he raised) the dead cannot return and communicate with us. But, more important, attempts to obtain hidden information from the dead show a blatant lack of faith in God. It is closely akin to Adam and Eve's act of disobedience in the Garden of Eden where they were enticed by the serpent to gain forbidden knowledge so they could be "like God" (Gen 3:5). The Lord has revealed all that we need to know about death in order to live fully. We do not need to seek further insights from forbidden sources.

The paradox of death both frightens and intrigues us. It is perhaps at the thought of death that we are forced most clearly to consider the meaning of life. To a person who feels life has no meaning or purpose, death may seem a welcome release. On the other hand, a person with close relationships and a strong sense of purpose may hang on to life in the face of overwhelming obstacles.

Because death is universal; it is often called the "great equalizer." On the surface the statement appears to be true. Both rich and poor, famous and unknown, good and bad people die. The cliché "you can't take it with you" grew out of the realization that all of the things we accumulate on earth—wealth, possessions, power, status—are left behind at death. But for the Christian neither statement is entirely true, for we look beyond this earth to eternal life. There are a number of things we can take with us.

First of all, we take our relationship with God with us. In fact, Jesus is coming back to personally escort us into the presence of the Father (Jn 14:1-3). Although from this side of death we appear to die alone, in actuality the familiar words of the Twenty-Third Psalm, "Even though I walk through the darkest valley, I fear no evil; for you are with me," tell us that this is merely a perception problem. We are not alone.

We can also take with us the expectation of reunion with Christians who have died before (and after) us (1 Thess 4:17). In eternity we will all be together; there will be no separation. We will have all the joys of human fellowship without the pain and suffering caused by sin in our earthly lives.

Finally, we can take our bodies with us. Not our aching, imperfect physical bodies, but "spiritual bodies," which will be recognizable, just as Jesus was when he returned from the grave (1 Cor 15:35-50). Death is not to become one with the universe or enter into a cycle of reincarnation. Neither is it the final stage of development. It is personally entering into the presence of the living God to worship and enjoy him forever (Rev 21:1-22:5). We maintain our personal identity.

HEAVEN AND HELL

But what about those who die without Christ? As much as we would like to ignore this issue, judgment is the other side of the gospel message. There can be no "good news" until we first acknowledge the "bad news." John 3 tells us, "For God so loved the world that he gave his only Son, so that everyone who believes in him may not perish but may have eternal life" (v. 16). John goes on to explain, "Those who believe in him are not condemned; but those who do not believe are condemned already, because they have not believed in the name of the only Son of God" (v. 18).

The issue of judgment for the unbeliever puts the Christian nurse into a quandary. Nursing teaches us to be nonjudgmental, yet we cannot sit idly by and watch a dying unbeliever slip into eternal condemnation. Christian nurses vary in their responses. Some fly into a panic, becoming insensitive and obnoxious in their deathbed evangelism. Others say nothing but carry a growing burden of guilt over their failure to witness. Most of us fall somewhere in the middle of the spectrum of responses. Occasionally we may experience the joy of leading someone to Christ. For the most part, we offer gentle physical and spiritual care, perhaps seeing a glimmer of faith sparked in our patients, but seldom see a deathbed conversion. Sometimes we feel guilty because we should have done more; other times we feel guilty because we were overbearing, straining the relationship with a patient.

Believer and unbeliever alike frequently ask the question, "How can a loving God send a person to hell?" There are no easy answers. Hell is a terrible end. Although the biblical picture of hell is varied and metaphorical, the one constant is that it is eternal separation from God (see, for example, Deut 32:22; Mt 5:22; 8:12; 10:28; 18:9; 22:13; 24:51; 25:30, 41; Lk 16:24; 2 Pet 2:4). We know from the Scriptures that God does not want anyone to go to hell (2 Pet 3:9). The whole purpose of Jesus Christ's birth, death, and resurrection was to save us from eternal condemnation (Jn 3:16-17, 1 Tim 1:15). It is only those who choose to live apart from God who are condemned to hell (Jn 12:47-50), but at the point of death that choice seems final and awful (Lk 13:23-30).

Stephen Travis puts the biblical concepts of heaven and hell into focus by defining them in the context of our relationship with God:

> If this be so, we can see that both heaven and hell are best thought of not as a reward or punishment for the kind of life we have lived, but as the logical

outcome of our relationship with God in this life. Heaven is not a reward for loving God any more than marriage is a reward for being engaged. And hell is not a punishment for turning one's back on Christ and choosing the road to destruction. It is where the road goes.[3]

Jesus gently but firmly bids us enter into a relationship with him that leads to eternal life. He calls us to recognize our own sinfulness—our natural inclination to put other things in a higher priority than knowing and loving God. He brings us to a sense of our humanity—realizing that we are not ultimately in power and control. He then reveals to us that he has assumed full responsibility for our sin. When we respond in repentance, belief and obedience to him, he enters into our lives and begins a lifelong process of changing us to be like him. God does not force us into relationship with himself. Jesus did not run after the rich young man who approached him in Matthew 11:22. He let the man go away sorrowful when his possessions held higher value for him than eternal life. Jesus faithfully proclaimed the gospel, but there is no record of his using high-pressure tactics with anyone. His example suggests that we can relax in our approach to dying patients. If a person refuses to discuss spiritual things or actively denies God, we must respect that choice. If we have been faithful in ministering God's love through word and deed, we need not feel guilty about a person's eternal destiny.

Perhaps the most honest position to take on the fate of unbelievers is to admit that we cannot know for certain. The Bible does not tell us exactly what will happen to those who have never heard the gospel, or the mentally handicapped, or babies or young children. When a person's commitment to Christ seems questionable, we need not necessarily despair. Only God knows the true spiritual state of a person. All that we know for certain is that God gives us the opportunity to respond in faith now, and he invites us to join him in spreading the joyful news of his love and mercy. It is not our place to assign people to heaven or hell. Our job is to proclaim and be faithful (Jas 4:17). What we do know for certain is that God loves each person far more than we ever could, and that he is just. We can trust those in our care to him.

Yes, death for the Christian is still an enemy. It separates us from our loved ones, sometimes much earlier than we expect. In the case of a stillborn baby

---

[3]Stephen H. Travis, *Christian Hope and the Future* (Downers Grove, IL: InterVarsity Press, 1980), 121.

or repeated miscarriage, death robs parents of the much-anticipated role of parenting a child. Death disrupts normal family functioning. It can be exorbitantly expensive, especially when preceded by a long illness. The process of dying can be ugly and painful. Death is filled with unknowns. Death often leaves behind unanswered questions. The most common question is *why*. But for the Christian there is hope in death.

The hope of eternal life is the knowledge that our relationship with Jesus Christ will remain unbroken in death. We have sampled the goodness of God here on earth. We look forward to basking in the pure, full presence of God after death, no longer afflicted by physical suffering, emotional struggles, or broken relationships. All that is true, honorable, just, lovely, gracious, excellent, and praiseworthy (Phil 4:8) will surround us. We will know the love of God in ways in which human love has never reached us. We cannot even imagine the depths of its goodness.

Think about what it would be like to go to a party with all the people you ever wanted to see, and to be able to have a mutually caring relationship with each one. Imagine experiencing the pure love and joy of being with your parents and siblings without any of the old dysfunctional patterns. Consider the deep friendships that somehow dissolved in pain and misunderstanding suddenly being restored to their original luster. In heaven, no longer will we know loneliness, fear, anger or frustration. We will be able to love and be loved as God loves us. What a party!

PRACTICAL CONSIDERATIONS

In the meantime, the church has been commissioned to be a small taste of heaven. When the church functions as God intends, it offers mutual love and support throughout life, and especially in times of crisis. We uphold one another in prayer as well as providing practical assistance. When families are coping with life-threatening illness, and up to the time of death, practical assistance may include offering food, transportation, housing, money, and companionship for the family. The funeral service serves to reassure the bereaved of the hope of eternal life and provides concrete human comfort and support.

Dr. Paul Johnson, a physician who faced a life-threatening illness, suggests these additional guidelines for Christians when supporting a dying person:

- Always tell the truth.
- Never set times.
- Listen with sensitivity.
- Respond to needs.
- Never allow the person to feel abandoned.
- Make yourself available.
- Don't give medical advice.
- If necessary protect persons from themselves (especially if they are self-medicating or not following their prescribed medical regimen).
- Always hold out hope.
- Provide spiritual support.[4]

Johnson describes his own feelings as he battled cancer:

> Partly it was embarrassment. All of a sudden I was different: someone somehow inferior, abnormal. Then, too, just as suddenly, I was the focus of attention, but it was a strange kind of attention. Not really personal, but impersonal, as I was the object of tests and examinations and all sorts of sterile routines. All of this seemed aimed at making me pull back, within myself, away from relationships which were now impersonal and professional rather than personal and caring.[5]

In this time of extreme isolation and loneliness, Sister Rosemary Donley's three nursing approaches in suffering will provide comfort and hope.[6]

First, we can offer compassionate accompaniment. We can listen carefully to the sick or dying person's needs and concerns, pray with the person, and share appropriate Scripture passages. We can work to facilitate reconciliation in broken relationships. Sometimes we may need to merely stay with the person and say nothing.

Donley's Nursing Approaches

- Compassionate accompaniment
- Bringing meaning to the situation
- Excellent physical care

---

[4]Larry Richards and Paul Johnson, *Death and the Caring Community: Ministering to the Terminally Ill* (Portland, OR: Multnomah, 1980), 61-62.

[5]Richard and Johnson, *Death and the Caring Community*, 14.

[6]Rosemary Donley, SC, "Nursing's Mission: Spiritual Dimensions of Health Care," *Journal of Contemporary Health Law and Policy* 7, no. 1 (1991): 207-17.

Second, we can help to bring meaning into the situation and to the person's life. Encouraging reminiscence, family sharing, and worship will focus the person's attention on what is most important in their life. Recalling favorite hymns, Bible passages, and family stories help to put a person's life into a larger context. We can facilitate visits from clergy if desired. If given a choice, many terminally ill patients will prefer to die at home, surrounded by family, as opposed to dying in a hospital. For the dying patient, such wishes should be clarified and every effort put forth to honor the patient's choice. Hospice care can be provided in the home as well as in the hospital, or even at a hospice house.

Finally, Donley says we can provide excellent physical care. Pain control and other comfort measures, as well as a pleasant environment, make it easier for a dying person to relax and to relate to loved ones. Gentle, loving touch is particularly important at this point. A backrub, a hand on the shoulder, or holding a person's hand communicates human warmth and care. Not only should we consciously work toward caring touch in our own interactions with the dying person, but we may also need to encourage family members and friends to touch. They may hesitate to do so for fear of hurting the person, or they may feel intimidated by the hospital environment and medical equipment.

Importantly, nurses can facilitate the fulfillment of patient and family wishes at the end of life. Singing hymns, reading Scripture, and praying together as their loved one is dying is part of coping with death for the Christian family. Final moments are both precious and memorable. The nurse should provide privacy for the family to be at the bedside of their loved one. Many hospitals provide a hospitality cart with light snacks and beverages for families as they keep vigil. Taking time to patiently answer a family member's questions in the midst of a busy shift is vital. Remember that the family will remember the care you provided long after you have forgotten them. During such stressful times as end of life, Christian nurses can minister through kindness, compassion, and love.

Nurses in churches have a particularly important role in educating the Christian community in how to care for dying people and their families. Family members may feel trapped and isolated if they are caring for someone at home. They may also need help to know how to provide the physical care the dying person requires. Simple things like giving a bed-bath, making an occupied bed, lifting, transferring and assisting the person with eating and toileting will likely feel overwhelming to a family member who has never done them before. We can offer instruction and support to them, as well as arranging volunteer help when needed. A nurse's assessment skills can be invaluable for a church congregation in knowing how to handle such situations.

Hospice nurses often provide an outstanding service to dying patients and their families. They manage pain, facilitate communication with the family and health care personnel; provide emotional and spiritual support; arrange for practical concerns such as transportation, housekeeping, and meal preparation; and offer follow-up care for the family. When a person is dying at home, the hospice nurses remain on call to assist the family, preparing them to know what to do at the time of death and supporting them in the process.

In the case of a sudden death, family members will not have the benefit of hospice care or any preparation for the sudden onslaught of emotions and tasks to be done. Our role, unless we are working within a congregational setting, will be brief and limited. The most important intervention we can make at this point is to connect the family with their faith community by calling their pastor or the hospital chaplain. Nurses in churches will be especially important in helping these families deal with grief and face the complex decisions they will have to make in the coming months.

Support for those facing a life-threatening illness can also be found through the delivery of palliative care services. Palliative care differs from hospice in that it is delivered alongside curative care. According to the Center to Advance Palliative Care (CAPC), the aim of palliative care is to help patients and families manage the stress of illness and provide relief from suffering through symptom management.[7] Palliative care is provided to respond to the patient's symptoms without regard for the prognosis. Well timed palliative care can reduce the symptoms of pain, shortness of breath, depression, fatigue, and anxiety that often accompany a life-threatening illness. Although experts advise that palliative care should begin at the time of a life-threatening or life-limiting diagnosis, many patients, and even health care providers, are reluctant to accept palliative care because they mistake it as being equivalent to hospice. Malloy, Ferrell, Virani, and Mazanec describe palliative care as

---

[7]"About Palliative Care," Center to Advance Palliative Care, accessed January 18, 2020, www.capc .org/about/palliative-care.

interprofessional specialty care that attends to and manages suffering.[8] The WHO defines palliative care as an approach that improves quality of life for patients and their families by providing physical, psychosocial, or spiritual care for those facing serious illness.[9]

In 2000, the End-of-Life Nursing Education Consortium (ELNEC) was launched with initial funding from the Robert Wood Johnson Foundation as a means to provide faculty and nursing students with evidence-based education related to palliative care.[10] In spite of efforts by advocates to improve the uptake of palliative care, there is still reluctance among some health care providers to order a palliative care consult. Thus, many patients still die without receiving the relief and comfort that palliative care provides. As patient advocates, nurses are uniquely positioned to champion palliative care for patients who are battling life-threatening illness and to help families understand that palliative care is supportive care for both the patient and the family.

Nurses in churches can also provide or arrange for instruction in the practical planning and decision making that need to take place surrounding death. Many congregations encourage their people to preplan funerals and keep their desires on file in the church office. Churches with senior citizen groups or faith community nurses may sponsor classes on how to handle Medicare, develop advanced directives and wills, or choose an extended-care facility. Many hospice organizations will send a speaker to church groups to explain their services. Churches may also sponsor grief support groups. If your own congregation does not offer these services, you can develop a list of community resources, including other churches, to which you can refer people.

The church and the individual members within it are in the business of life and living. For that reason, Christian fellowship is essential for the person who works with death and dying on a daily basis. Family caregivers need to

---

[8]Pam Malloy, Betty Ferrell, Rose Virani, and Polly Mazanec, "Promoting Palliative Care Internationally: Building Leaders to Promote Education, Practice, and Advocacy," *American Academy of Hospice and Palliative Medicine*, 2018, S141.

[9]"Palliative Care," World Health Organization, accessed September 25, 2020, www.who.int/health-topics/palliative-care.

[10]See "End-of-Life-Care (ELNEC)," American Association of Colleges and Nursing, www.aacnnursing.org/ELNEC.

attend worship and other church functions. Hospice volunteers or trained church members may be able to relieve them so they can get away. Nurses also need the support of the church. The constant exposure to death, which nurses in oncology, hospice and critical care face, can become overwhelmingly depressing. Bible study, prayer, worship, and mutual support and encouragement reaffirm the hope to which we are called—a hope that leads to life, not death.

Death is the last enemy. Even for Christians, death painfully interrupts and reorders our lives. However, though we grieve, it is not "as others do who have no hope" (1 Thess 4:13). We do not grieve alone. The Christian community surrounds and upholds us. We do not die alone. Jesus assured us, "Do not let your hearts be troubled. Believe in God, believe also in me. In my Father's house there are many dwelling places. If it were not so, would I have told you that I go to prepare a place for you? And if I go and prepare a place for you, I will come again and will take you to myself, so that where I am, there you may be also" (Jn 14:1-3).

In the face of death, Jesus offers us hope of eternal life. As Christian nurses, we offer that hope to those who walk through the valley of the shadow of death.

FOR FURTHER THINKING

1. Describe the first time you were present with someone who died. What were you thinking and feeling?

2. What do you fear most about your own death?

3. What do you hope heaven will be like?

THEOLOGICAL REFLECTION

1. Read Psalm 23, John 14:1-3, and Romans 8:31-39. These are the traditional Scripture readings at funerals and memorial services. What specific reasons for hope does each passage offer to believers?

2. Read 1 Corinthians 15:12-28. According to this passage, what difference did Christ's death and resurrection make for us?

3. Read 1 Corinthians 15:35-58. What does this passage say about what happens to the believer at death?

4. How is this Christian view of death and resurrection different from the idea of reincarnation? Why do you think the idea of reincarnation appeals to people today?

5. In the light of the passages above, what responsibility do you think Christian nurses should take in communicating the gospel to patients before they die?

Case Study: A Spirit Set Free

Karen, an experienced pediatric nurse, often struggled to answer grieving parents when they asked, "Why is my child suffering?" She often went home discouraged and angry at God. But David, age twelve, gave her a different perspective.

With a particularly unresponsive treatment type of leukemia, David endured rigorous treatments, nausea and vomiting, blood transfusions, painful bone marrow aspirations, and spinal taps. He spent a lot of time in the hospital alone. His parents were divorced. He lived with his mom and stepfather. Both parents worked and there were other children in the family. However, David also seemed to have an unusually hopeful spirit. Karen tried to spend extra time with David whenever possible, often on her own time.

Whenever David came for treatment, he brought along a large wooden cross that he would place near him for the duration of the treatment or hospitalization. He never talked about the cross; it was just always there. One night he was admitted to the hospital with a high fever. Karen noticed his name on the admission log when she arrived for work the next morning, so she visited him before starting her shift. He told her that the admission happened so quickly that he had forgotten to bring his cross with him. He asked her to get his wallet from his jeans' pocket in the closet, from which he pulled a card with a tiny metal cross on it. The card read, "This cross is to remind me that I must carry my own cross daily."

David's leukemia had relapsed and did not respond to any treatment. He was discharged with only palliative treatment to manage his discomfort. However, he was readmitted a few weeks later with uncontrolled bleeding. Transfusions were ordered, and he was to be discharged by noon the next day.

Karen visited him about midmorning. He told her how tired he was. They chatted for a few minutes and then Karen had to work, but she planned to return before he was discharged. As she started to leave, he asked if she could stay with him a little while longer.

David said he was cold and asked if Karen would hold him for a while. That seemed like an odd request for a twelve-year-old boy, but he seemed younger than his age. The cancer and the requisite treatment had left him thin, bald, and so pale that his skin looked transparent. There was a couch-bed in his room that parents used when they stayed overnight, so Karen sat on the couch with David on her lap.

They talked quietly for a few minutes, and then he was silent. Thinking that he had dozed off, Karen looked at him. She saw the expression on his face changing as she felt the weight of his body shifting. She knew that he hadn't fallen asleep. The essence that was David seemed to be escaping, like air out of a balloon.

David's death was a watershed moment in Karen's life as a Christian and a nurse. Witnessing David's spirit break free from human confinement and suffering felt like a gift. She knew he was going home to his heavenly Father.

Karen explained, "Over the years, I have continued to struggle spiritually and intellectually with the pain and torment children have to experience. As a Christian, I believe that human suffering, prayerfully turned over to God, releases an outpouring of grace that joins with the redemptive power of the Cross, to transform a broken world. But some days, it is incredibly difficult to remember the promises of the Father and trust Him. Each day I remember better, though, because a child named David changed my life."[11]

Discussion Questions

1. What makes caring for dying patients so difficult—especially when they are children?

2. What would you have said to David's parents and stepparents if they asked you, "Why does God allow David to suffer so much?"

3. Examine Karen's nursing care for David. In what ways does she demonstrate excellence?

---

[11] Adapted from Karen E. Wilson, "A Spirit Set Free: Learning About Death from David," *Journal of Christian Nursing* (2003): 18-19.

4. How would you have responded to David's cross? In what ways might Karen have encouraged him to talk about what it meant to him?

5. If David had been your patient, what further interventions might you have tried?

6. Why do you think this experience was so encouraging to Karen? What did David teach her about death?

PART FIVE

...

NURSING

PRACTICE OF CARE

13

NURSING AS
CHRISTIAN CARING

Purpose:	To identify the nature of Christian caring
Objectives:	After reading this chapter and completing the exercises, you should be able to:
	1. Define nursing according to the nursing literature
	2. Identify changes occurring in contemporary nursing
	3. Compare Christian nursing with secular nursing
	4. Explain the implications of Christian faith for nursing practice
Keywords:	nursing, caring, nuns, deaconesses, profession, ministry, compassionate care, character

THE FIRST TWELVE CHAPTERS OF THIS BOOK have examined the concepts in the nursing metaparadigm from a Christian perspective. Now the task remains to define nursing today. Who are we? What do we do? While the definition of nursing has gradually evolved over time, in recent years there has been a radical shift in perspective.

We have seen how nursing as a public role first developed in the Christian church but by the seventeenth century had degenerated into a sorry state. When Pennsylvania Hospital, the first hospital in America, opened in 1752, nursing care was provided by both male and female nurses who were expected to be "trustworthy and experienced" but had no formal training. Their duties, including preparing food and feeding patients, washing and ironing the linens, and keeping the rooms clean, were shared by the patients as they were able.[1] However, during this period, nursing occurred primarily within the

---

[1] Roberta Mayhew West, *History of Nursing in Pennsylvania* (Philadelphia: Pennsylvania State Nurses' Association, 1932), 6.

family as an extension of motherhood. Hospital nursing was not considered a respectable vocation for a young woman.

Emily Hitchens and Lilyan Snow contend that volunteer nurses during the American Civil War "invented nursing" out of necessity. They volunteered because they felt it was the right thing to do, because the wounds of battle required care. The care these nurses offered included "order, cleanliness, and food when it was possible, and simple being with at all times." Many of these nurses went on to establish schools of nursing after the war.[2]

As we have seen, the Crimean War forced Florence Nightingale to reinvent nursing. She defined nursing as having "charge of the personal health of somebody . . . [knowing] how to put the constitution in such a state as it will have no disease, or that it will recover from disease."[3] She believed that every woman was a nurse and wrote her little book *Notes on Nursing* to help them "think how to nurse."[4] The women she took with her to Scutari were not formally educated as nurses. Nightingale taught them after they arrived. Following the war she established the first secular school of nursing.

However, war alone did not define nursing. Catholic monastic orders maintained the role of nursing sisters throughout the history of the church. The nineteenth century brought a revival of nursing in the Protestant church, especially in northern Europe. The deaconess movement sprang up as a response to the gospel. These early deaconesses lived in community and cared for the sick and poor without charge. They established hospitals and schools of nursing, training many women (including Florence Nightingale).[5]

The nuns and deaconesses were never overly concerned about defining nursing; they just did it. When the nuns first arrived in America in the eighteenth century, they weren't trained as nurses but as teachers. But they found that the people they had come to teach needed health care, so they started a hospital and nursed. Others became social workers, but when health needs surfaced, they too became nurses.[6] The deaconesses demonstrated a

---

[2]Emily Hitchens and Lilyan Snow, "Caring: The Moral Response to Suffering," *Christian Scholar's Review*, 1994, 309.

[3]Florence Nightingale, *Notes on Nursing: What It Is and What It Is Not* (New York: D. Appleton, 1860), 3.

[4]Nightingale, *Notes on Nursing*, 3.

[5]Catherine Herzel, *On Call: Deaconesses Across the World* (New York: Holt, Rinehart & Winston, 1961).

[6]Suzy Farren, *A Call to Care: The Women Who Built Catholic Healthcare in America* (St. Louis: Catholic Health Association of the United States, 1996).

similar flexibility. Their primary commitment was not to a professional discipline, but to God and service.[7] This strength may have led to the eventual decline of Christian nursing. The pursuit of a "secular order" by Nightingale and the early public health nurses in America meant that nurses caught the optimistic spirit of the age more quickly than the call to Christian commitment.

In the early part of the twentieth century secular nursing was still not clearly defined, but to a large extent nurses became physicians' helpers, a role that still shapes the public image of nursing. In an attempt to provide nursing with a stronger identity, set standards for nursing education and an effort toward greater autonomy, nurses began to organize into state and national associations. A body of thoughtful literature developed as a growing number of professional nursing journals began publication. These associations and journals became a forum for discussing the nature of nursing. World War II set the stage for increasing activism and assertiveness among nurses, and by 1946 the American Nurses Association had a plan for the future that included improved working conditions, educational standards with federal subsidies, and increased professional organization.[8]

In 1955 the American Nurses Association approved a definition of nursing practice that was adopted by most state boards of nursing:

> The practice of professional nursing means the performance for compensation of any act in the observation, care, and counsel of the ill, injured, or infirm, or the maintenance of health or prevention of illness of others, or in the supervision and teaching of other personnel, or the administration of medications and treatment as prescribed by a licensed physician or dentist; requiring substantial specialized judgment and skill and based on knowledge and application of the principles of biological, physical, and social science. The foregoing shall not be deemed to include acts of diagnosis or prescription of therapeutic or corrective measures.[9]

This definition illustrated a clear break with the tradition of volunteer nursing and Christian communities providing care without charge. Professional

---

[7] C. Golder, *The History of the Deaconess Movement* (Cincinnati: Jennings and Pye, 1903).
[8] "Platform for the ANA," *American Journal of Nursing*, November 1946, 729.
[9] "ANA Board Approves a Definition of Nursing Practice," *American Journal of Nursing*, December 1955, 1474.

nursing required compensation. This focus on compensation would become a rising theme. Another significant contrast to the nursing of nuns and deaconesses also occurred. While the nurse's responsibilities of observing, caring, counseling, supervising and teaching seem to be a step toward autonomy, the definition engraved the physicians' helper role into nurse practice acts. Nurses were not allowed to diagnose or treat. Treatments and medications could be prescribed only by a physician.

While the ANA definition remained the legal definition of nursing, the 1950s and 1960s brought a ferment of thinking about the nature of nursing. New definitions began to emerge. They focused more on nursing's uniqueness and less on its subservience to medicine. Virginia Henderson's classic definition of nursing, discussed in chapter one, has been ingrained into nurses ever since it was adopted in 1960. Most nurses feel this definition in their gut. It identifies who we are, our concerns and our actions. It also allows for an increasing sense of autonomy.

All of these early definitions focus on maintaining and restoring health to the individual and assume a positive direction toward health (or peaceful death). But by 1980 new definitions began to proliferate. Some of them were based on radically different understandings of nursing concepts. The American Nurses Association's 1980 "Nursing: A Social Policy Statement" definition did not even articulate the promotion of human health as the goal of nursing care.[10] The statement defined nursing as the "diagnosis and treatment of human responses to actual and potential health problems."[11] It was an attempt to evade the prohibitions against diagnosing and treating disease in nurse practice acts.

In response to protests about the lack of focus in the 1980 definition, the 1995 revision of this statement maintains the original wording but adds that

---

[10]Rozella M. Schlotfeldt, "Defining Nursing: A Historic Controversy," *Nursing Research*, January–February 1987, 64-67.

[11]American Nurses Association, *Nursing: A Social Policy Statement* (Kansas City: American Nurses Association, 1980). According to Donna Diers's article "What Is Nursing?" in Joanne Comi McCloskey and Helen Kennedy Grace, eds., *Current Issues in Nursing* (St. Louis: Mosby, 1997), 6-7, this wording was first adopted by the New York State Nurses Association in 1976, on the recommendation of their counsel that "the diagnostic privilege was the *sine qua non* of independent practice." This statement set off the nursing diagnosis movement with its attempt to establish a unique taxonomy for nursing. The whole process was essentially a political movement to separate nursing from medicine.

more recent definitions "frequently acknowledge four essential features of contemporary nursing practice":

- attention to the full range of human experiences and responses to health and illness without restriction to a problem-focused orientation
- integration of objective data with knowledge gained from an understanding of the patient or group's subjective experience
- application of scientific knowledge to the processes of diagnosis and treatment
- provision of a caring relationship that facilitates health and healing[12]

This revision also states, "Nurses intervene to promote health, prevent illness, or assist with activities that contribute to recovery from illness or to achieving a peaceful death."[13] Although this definition seems more in line with Florence Nightingale's, nursing is no longer the calling of every woman. It is a "scientific discipline as well as a profession"[14] that requires education (with a baccalaureate degree recommended) and national examination for licensure. Furthermore, this definition takes a bolder step toward the issue of diagnosing and treating. However, its scope of practice remains fuzzy, with a "flexible boundary that is responsive to the changing needs of society and the expanding knowledge base of its theoretical and scientific domains."[15]

Nurse practice acts in most states now permit advanced practice nurses to make simple diagnoses and prescribe certain classes of drugs, further blurring the line between nursing and medicine.[16] Nurses can practice independently, own and manage extended-care facilities, establish their own companies to deliver care, and receive compensation from third-party payers. Insurance companies now hire nurses as case managers with the authority to grant or deny reimbursements for physician-ordered medications and treatments.

Nursing's frantic scramble to redefine itself in order to advance (or even survive), together with the current upheaval in health care delivery, presents

---

[12]American Nurses Association, *Nursing: A Social Policy Statement* (Kansas City: American Nurses Association, 1995), 6.

[13]American Nurses Association, *Nursing*, 13.

[14]American Nurses Association, *Nursing*, 7.

[15]American Nurses Association, *Nursing*, 12.

[16]"More Power to the Nurses," *Chicago Tribune*, April 14, 1997.

us with an opportunity to reassess where we have come in nursing and determine where we want to go. To do so, we need to back up and look at nursing through a Christian worldview. Reacting from the midst of the whirlwind and jumping on the current trends without thoughtful examination could prove disastrous for nursing. Many of today's trends are contradictory and lead to fragmentation of the profession. There is tremendous growth in the move toward more education (nursing master's degrees and doctorates), while in other sectors the trend is toward less education (institutional training and associate degrees). Nurses are gaining more autonomy (advanced practice, community health, entrepreneurship), but becoming more isolated and alienated from one another in the process. Faith-community nursing brings nursing back into the church, but it often finds funding to be minimal or nonexistent.

In the midst of all this defining and redefining, just what is Christian nursing? How do we gain the perspective needed to define it? Many contemporary nursing leaders (and theologians) are saying that we are defined by our stories. To some degree that definition works. Throughout nursing history we can catch a glimpse of what Patricia Donahue calls the nursing impulse, a uniting of "the head, the heart and the hands" to nurture health and overcome disease.[17] However, there are also low points and digressions in the story of nursing that we do not want to incorporate into our identity. Rather, we need to repent of our self-interest and neglect and turn again to Jesus Christ for our vision of nursing.

Instead of looking primarily to nursing history or even current practice to find our story, we must begin with God's story in the Scriptures, for that is where Christian nursing began. The term *nurse* in the Bible implied a woman who fed and cared for infants and young children, not today's professional role. However, health care figured prominently in the life and teachings of Jesus. He healed the sick, cared for the poor and oppressed, sought out those whom society rejected, and instructed his followers to go and do likewise. Health care—including the physical, psychosocial, and spiritual dimensions— soon became the concern of the whole church.

---

[17]M. Patricia Donahue, *Nursing: The Finest Art*, 2nd ed. (St. Louis: Mosby, 1996), 2-7.

> ### Christian Nursing Defined
>
> Christian nursing is a ministry of compassionate and restorative care for the whole person, in response to God's grace, which aims to foster optimum health (shalom) and bring comfort in suffering and death for anyone in need.

Several characteristics of Christian nursing stand out in the Scriptures. (1) Nursing is a response to God's grace that flows from a dynamic personal relationship with God. (2) It is a ministry of the church and functions in the context of the body of Christ. (3) It recognizes the role of sin in a world created good, and it seeks to restore justice and righteousness. (4) It views the person as created in the image of God. (5) It works toward the goal of shalom as ultimate health. (6) It is demonstrated in compassionate care that is characterized by the fruit of the Spirit. These characteristics, and the theological understanding of the concepts in the nursing paradigm presented in the first twelve chapters, will help us both to define nursing and to shape the future of nursing practice.

Based on these considerations, we will define Christian nursing as *a ministry of compassionate and restorative care for the whole person, in response to God's grace, which aims to promote and foster optimum health (shalom) and bring comfort in suffering and death for anyone in need.*

A Ministry

Ministry in the New Testament and the early church was understood to be the work of every Christian. The Greek term translated as ministry, *diakonia*, essentially means service. It incorporates everything from preaching the gospel to waiting on tables and delivering relief to the poor. Jesus demonstrated this spirit of service by washing his disciples' feet, then telling them to follow his example (Jn 13). In fact, the term *diakonos* (servant) is often used synonymously with *doulos* (slave). When Jesus' disciples began to seek power and privilege, he told them: "But it is not so among you; but whoever wishes to become great among you must be your servant, and whoever wishes to be first among you must be slave of all" (Mk 10:43-44).

The ministry of nursing is servant work. Sometimes it is dirty work like washing feet and emptying bedpans. It is the visiting nurse who returns on her day off to clean a patient's apartment, or buys dressings for a patient who can't afford them. It is the critical-care nurse who works double shifts to cover for a sick colleague. It is the nurse practitioner who gives up a lucrative position to work in an inner-city clinic that pays less than he made before his advanced practice certification. It is the nursing instructor who spends extra hours encouraging and counseling students. It is the nursing leader who pours tremendous time and energy into serving on a professional organization's task force to develop documents that will shape the future of nursing. It is the nurse who gets involved in the political system to work for justice in health care delivery.

To a large extent these servant-nurses remain unheralded and invisible.[18] But the key to servanthood comes in whom we are serving. Jesus said, "Truly I tell you, just as you did it to one of the least of these who are members of my family, you did it to me" (Mt 25:40). We are servants of the Lord Jesus Christ, who also said to us, "I do not call you servants any longer, because the servant does not know what the master is doing; but I have called you friends, because I have made known to you everything that I have heard from my Father" (Jn 15:15).

Within the body of Christ, each person is equipped with various gifts for ministry. Romans 12:6-8 lists ministry (*diakonia*) among other gifts: "We have gifts that differ according to the grace given to us: prophecy, in proportion to faith; ministry, in ministering; the teacher, in teaching; the exhorter, in exhortation; the giver, in generosity; the leader, in diligence; the compassionate, in cheerfulness." In this passage "ministering" more likely refers to nursing rather than to anything resembling ordained clergy (which did not exist in this period). The gifts are not mutually exclusive. Those who minister may also have gifts of prophecy, teaching, exhortation, generosity, leadership, or compassion. Paul simply instructs us to use the gifts God has given.

---

[18]Journalist Suzanne Gordon presents some interesting suggestions about this problem of invisibility in "What Nurses Stand For," *Atlantic Monthly*, February 1997, 88. "Because nurses observe and cushion what the physician and writer Oliver Sacks has called human beings' falling 'radically into sickness,' they are a reminder of the pain, fear, vulnerability, and loss of control that adults find difficult to tolerate and thus to discuss. . . . [Nurses] are our secret sharers. Even though they are our lifeline during illness, when control is restored the residue of our anxiety and mortality clings to them like dust, and we flee the memory."

First Corinthians 12:4-12 provides a more extensive explanation of spiritual gifts.

> Now there are varieties of gifts, but the same Spirit; and there are varieties of services, but the same Lord; and there are varieties of activities, but it is the same God who activates all of them in everyone. To each is given the manifestation of the Spirit for the common good. To one is given through the Spirit the utterance of wisdom, and to another the utterance of knowledge according to the same Spirit, to another faith by the same Spirit, to another gifts of healing by the one Spirit, to another the working of miracles, to another prophecy, to another the discernment of spirits, to another various kinds of tongues, to another the interpretation of tongues. All these are activated by one and the same Spirit, who allots to each one individually just as the Spirit chooses.
>
> For just as the body is one and has many members, and all the members of the body, though many, are one body, so it is with Christ.

Notice that the gifts are intended to fit together for the benefit of the whole body. Today when nurses are clamoring for autonomy, we have to recognize that Christian nursing is never an autonomous role. The Christian nurse functions as part of the body of Christ (and the health care team) and is always accountable to the church (even when in secular employment). Because health care is the concern of the whole church, the boundaries of nursing's ministry will always remain fuzzy.

The history of nursing and compassionate health care is intricately woven through church history—until fairly recently. It was when nursing moved away from its association with the church that it degenerated into an independent profit-making scheme practiced by the Sairey Gamps of Dickens's day. We are seeing a similar decline today as hospitals and health care agencies, which were once church-owned and operated, have become dependent on federal funds and then on conglomerate buyouts for survival. If nursing is a part of the body of Christ that has been particularly gifted with the ability and responsibility to care for the health needs of others, then one of our primary roles must be to awaken the church to its mission of healing. Jesus sent out his followers in Luke 10:8-9, saying, "Whenever you enter a town and its people welcome you . . . cure the sick who are there, and say to them, 'The kingdom of God has come near to you.'" Proclamation is only half of Jesus' commission. Demonstration of the gospel through compassionate health care is the other half.

COMPASSIONATE AND RESTORATIVE CARE

Jesus gave the most comprehensive description of compassionate and restorative care when he told the story of the good Samaritan in Luke 10:30-35:

> A man was going down from Jerusalem to Jericho, and fell into the hands of robbers, who stripped him, beat him, and went away, leaving him half dead. . . . But a Samaritan while traveling came near him; and when he saw him, he was moved with pity. He went to him and bandaged his wounds, having poured oil and wine on them. Then he put him on his own animal, brought him to an inn, and took care of him. The next day he took out two denarii, gave them to the innkeeper, and said, "Take care of him; and when I come back, I will repay you whatever more you spend."

The Samaritan in this story had no legal responsibility to stop and help. Two Jewish religious leaders had already passed by the wounded man without getting involved. The victim was presumably a Jewish man, and customarily Samaritans were considered enemies by the Jews. The man could have been a decoy set up by the robbers in order to claim another victim. Yet the Samaritan pitied the man and risked his own welfare to intervene, using his own limited supplies. Furthermore, he took his patient to an inn and stayed with him as long as he could, then provided for continuity of care after he left.

Although caring has always been central to nursing, there is little consensus about what caring means. One group of researchers identified twenty-three different definitions of caring in the nursing literature (and they missed a few). They divided these definitions into five major categories: caring as (1) a human trait, (2) a moral imperative, (3) an affect, (4) an interpersonal interaction, and (5) a therapeutic intervention.[19] Only the last one (under which only six definitions fit) involves any kind of physical care. How do these definitions compare with a Christian view of caring?

We do not need to look far to realize that caring for others is not intrinsic to human nature. Empirical evidence surrounds us attesting to the opposite; so does the biblical witness. Romans 3:23 tells us that "all have sinned and fall short of the glory of God." The good Samaritan was remarkable because his compassionate care stood in contrast to the normal human response

---

[19]Janice M. Morse, Joan Bottorff, Wendy Neander, and Shirley Solberg, "Comparative Analysis of Conceptualizations and Theories of Caring," *Image* (1991): 119-26.

(illustrated by the two religious leaders who did not stop to help). During a recent class for CPR recertification, the instructor told us, "Outside of a health care setting no one has to know that you are a nurse or that you are certified in CPR—the risks are just too great to get involved." Most of the class nodded in agreement. Caring for strangers is not intrinsic to human nature. Even within the health care setting, there seems to be a common human bent toward leaving the dirty work for the next shift.

On the other hand, the second category of definitions—caring as a moral imperative—may well develop in a culture shaped by strong moral virtues. Such was the case of the "nursing inventors" in the nineteenth century, who were influenced by the philosophy of Immanuel Kant. They sought to retain Christianity's values without the religious commitment, making it into a practical morality. However, caring as a moral imperative does not develop in a vacuum (or in a pluralistic society). It is not a general principle that seems obvious to every reasonable person. It develops in the context of a living relationship with Jesus Christ within the body of Christ, which informs the standards for the virtue of love (which in turn results in caring). Once the spiritual foundations fade from memory, the virtues begin to crumble. While the good Samaritan demonstrated caring, it was not out of any categorical imperative. He was simply "moved with pity."

Whose values set the moral standards for caring in today's nursing? In Eastern philosophy, caring happens primarily in the mind, through seeking enlightenment. For the naturalist, caring usually means doing what is "best" for society rather than the individual. To many postmodernists, morality is simply what seems good to an individual at the time. Without a common religious foundation, we lose our categories for categorical imperatives. When a person can pick and choose the basis for caring by personal preference, supporters tout previously unethical behavior such as partial-birth abortions and physician-assisted (and nurse-assisted) suicide as caring practices, or health maintenance organizations can justify huge profits at the expense of adequate coverage.

The third category, caring as an affect or emotion, is not very helpful in the real world of nursing. We are all faced with patients we just don't like. In fact, our first response to some patients may well be revulsion—but we still must care for them. When the good Samaritan cared for the wounded man beside the road, although he was moved with pity, he probably felt no great love for him. In fact, this patient was so repulsive that others crossed to the other side of the road instead of caring for him. The Samaritan's compassion was demonstrated instead by concrete physical acts of mercy—by touching the patient, cleaning his wounds, and staying with him while he recovered.

The fourth category, caring as an interpersonal interaction, depends on meaningful, respectful communication between the nurse and the patient. That works only if the patient is alert and cooperative. The wounded man in the good Samaritan story was left "half dead." I doubt that any meaningful interaction occurred. He was probably unconscious. We need to care for people even when they are unable to articulate their needs or care for us in return. Most nursing care is a one-way deal. We can delight in those rare encounters when we feel cared for in return by a patient, but we can't base our model of caring on reciprocal need-meeting.

Nursing theorists using a New Paradigm worldview often assume that caring comes naturally to nurses and that it occurs as a metaphysical event. It usually means just "being with" a person. Compassionate accompaniment is an important element in our nursing care—but we cannot stop there. Psychiatric nurse Verna Carson expresses concern about this view because "defining our caring role as 'being with' . . . seems to exclude the very important aspects of 'doing for' and 'doing with.'"[20] Dunlop also notes that the emerging concept of caring in nursing seems to "ignore the body and its associated physical care."[21] But this is not the understanding of caring we see in the Scriptures. What would have happened if the Samaritan had simply sat down at the side of the road with the wounded man without making any active interventions? Robbers or wild animals would probably have killed them both.

CARING IN THE BIBLE

The Bible gives us a very clear picture of what caring means, and it is essentially a therapeutic intervention. We learn about caring by looking at God. "Cast all your anxiety on him [God], because he cares for you" (1 Pet 5:7). How does God care for us? A brief biblical overview paints a vivid and comforting picture.

---

[20]Verna Carson, "Caring: The Rediscovery of Our Nursing Roots," *Perspectives in Psychiatric Care*, April–June 1994, 4-6.

[21]M. J. Dunlop, "Is a Science of Caring Possible?" *Journal of Advanced Nursing* 11 (1986): 661-70.

We begin in Genesis 1 where God creates a man and a woman, declares them *good* and enters into relationship with them. By Genesis 3, the man and woman have tested the limits and disobeyed God, bringing upon themselves all the ugly effects of sin—pain, suffering, and death. But already at this awful moment we begin to see God's care demonstrated. He makes clothes for them (Gen 3:21). Then the long history of God gently meeting his people's needs unfolds.

God's involvement in the lives of his people is practical and physical. In Hosea 11, we see God's care expressed in his calling Israel, teaching her to walk, holding her in his arms, healing her, easing her workload, and bending down to feed her. Jeremiah tells us that God restores health and heals wounds (Jer 30:17). Zechariah says that God cares for his flock by changing unjust systems (Zech 10:3). These themes are repeated in Matthew 6:25-31, where Jesus tells us that our lives and bodies are important to God and that he will provide food, clothing, and shelter to sustain us.

We see an interesting twist to the "just being with" understanding of care in Isaiah 43:1-3. Here God says that he created and formed us, called us by name, claims us as his own, then walks with us *to protect us* when we go through the tough experiences of life. This is no mere presence—it is a sacrificial involvement in our lives. That sacrifice culminates in God's being willing to give his Son to die for us in the crucifixion of Jesus.

Christian caring is not just an emotional tug, an intellectual concept, or a metaphysical event. It is hands-on, patient-centered, physical, psychosocial, and spiritual intervention to meet the needs of a patient regardless of how the nurse feels. In the process of nursing we may eventually develop a caring affect, but our ability to feel caring will continue to be challenged by the system and by obnoxious patients.

> *Christian caring is hands-on, patient-centered, physical, psychosocial, and spiritual intervention to meet the needs of a patient regardless of how the nurse feels.*

Our skill in caring develops as we receive care from others and ultimately as we grow in our understanding and acceptance of God's care for us. Caring is an act of faith, for it involves the risk of opening ourselves to another who may not want to care or be cared for. But unless we take that risk, we cannot claim to be truly nursing.

Nursing doesn't hold an exclusive claim on caring. Lots of people care—parents, friends, social workers, pastors, teachers. Paul told the Thessalonians, "We were gentle among you, like a nurse tenderly caring for her own children" (1 Thess 2:7). But nursing means providing compassionate and restorative care for the whole person in response to God's grace, which aims to foster optimum health and bring comfort in suffering for anyone in need. It means getting our hands (and often our clothing) dirty and putting ourselves at risk for the welfare of our patients. A body of knowledge, an attitude of service, and a vital relationship with God are required to make that caring truly Christian nursing.

FOR THE WHOLE PERSON

Christian nursing is holistic, caring for the person physically, emotionally, psychosocially, and spiritually. In fact, we know that ultimate healing cannot occur unless our patients are placed in the hands of Jesus, the great physician (Is 53:5). However, a nurse's background in the physical and social sciences, as well as the nursing arts, provides unique qualifications to care for the physical needs of others and to understand human responses to illness. Nursing, because of its concern for the whole person, is also uniquely positioned to coordinate communications among members of an interdisciplinary health care team.

A pastor recently told us about a pastoral call he made accompanied by Sue, a nurse from his congregation. He expressed amazement over how much more information Sue uncovered in one visit than he had gained in over a year. By simply observing the woman and her surroundings and initiating a brief conversation, Sue assessed that she had some potentially serious health problems and that she needed help with her diet, transportation, laundry, and housekeeping. Sue was then able to help her receive the services she needed from community agencies and volunteers in the church.

This pastor's story is one we have heard over and over. Nurses just have a different way of seeing, hearing, smelling, feeling, and perceiving—a skill that develops over years of experience. Perhaps that is one of our primary spiritual gifts. A comment made by a nurse visiting an extended-care facility illustrates this kind of perception. She stopped, looked around, and remarked, "This is a good nursing home. It smells good, and there is a light in the residents' eyes."

Two very simple observations, but they indicated that residents were receiving good physical care and also respect and loving attention.

We examined in chapter seven what it means to be human, but let's summarize the main points again. First, all people are created by God in his image (Gen 1:26) to live in loving relationship with God, self, and others (Deut 6:4-6; Mt 22:37-39) and as responsible stewards of the environment (Gen 1:26). Second, every person is separated from God by sin, but that relationship is restored by grace through faith in Jesus Christ, in whom we are redeemed and made holy by the Holy Spirit (Rom 3:22-28; 1 Cor 6:11). Third, the person is a physically, psychosocially, and spiritually integrated being with intrinsic value and significance (Ps 8:4-8; 1 Thess 5:23; Heb 2:11-17). Fourth, each person is responsible to live a healthful lifestyle (1 Cor 3:16-17; Eph 5:29) and to promote health (Ex 15:26; 3 Jn 2), but also to find meaning in suffering and death (Rom 5:3-5; 1 Cor 15:54; 1 Thess 4:13-14).

What It Means to Be Human

- Created by God in his image
- Separated from God by sin, but redeemed in Christ
- Physically, psychosocially, and spiritually integrated being with intrinsic value
- Responsible to live a healthful lifestyle
- Able to find meaning in suffering and death

Nurses care for all dimensions of the person as they relate to health and healing. If any of these aspects of the person is ignored, healing will usually be impeded. Therefore, nursing assessment must include not only biological functioning but social, emotional, and spiritual factors as well.

A RESPONSE TO GOD'S GRACE

The motivation for Christian nursing comes primarily from a sense of gratitude to God, not merely a reaction to human need or a sense of duty (although they too flow naturally from a grateful heart). We can say with the apostle John, "We love because he [God] first loved us" (1 Jn 4:19). The contrast between gratitude and duty results primarily in a difference in attitude and approach. When I care out of a sense of gratitude for what God has done for me, I can view the patient as a person of great value, worthy of my respect, interest, and attention. When I care out of a sense of duty, the patient becomes an object. I do what I have to do and get out. The spirit of that fine line is expressed in a letter written by a nurse in an extended-care facility—written to one of the patients, after he died.

> Your reputation preceded my meeting you, Robert. My coworkers called you "Starman"—they said they believed you were communicating with the stars. I found out what they meant. When I worked third shift and checked on you throughout the night, your eyes were always open, as though gazing into lost galaxies of time.
>
> Frankly, sometimes we felt repulsed by your twisted figure. Forgive our shallow thinking. Anyhow, thanks for allowing me to bathe you, to feed you and care for you.
>
> I cannot imagine having to be cared for through so many years, dependent on someone for all your life-sustaining needs. I pray that every hand that touched you touched with compassion, and every word spoken was with loving kindness. But I know as I write this, that was not the case. God forgive us.[22]

Even as we care out of a sense of gratitude, there is always a sense that God is still working on us, making us more like Christ (2 Cor 3:18). We don't always care in the way we would like to care. Sometimes only a sense of duty enables us to press on. We humbly struggle with our own sinfulness, our inability to truly care and to draw our strength from him (Phil 4:13).

When you care from a sense of gratitude for what God has done for you, you see patients with great value, dignity, and worth. "We love because he [God] first loved us" (1 Jn 4:19).

AIMS TO FOSTER OPTIMUM HEALTH

Health is being able to live as God created us to live—as an integrated whole, living in loving relationship with God, self, and others (Ps 16). Health cannot be separated into isolated compartments, and neither can nursing care. We deceive ourselves when we think that we can care only for physical needs while ignoring the emotional, spiritual, and

---

[22]Joy A. Bickle, "Starman," *Journal of Christian Nursing* (1995): 6.

social needs of our patients. If we are concerned only for the mechanical functioning of the body, we would do better as pure scientists or car mechanics. On the other hand, we cannot fully meet the health needs of anyone while ignoring physical needs. Pastors and counselors focus on the spiritual and emotional components of health, but only nurses incorporate all dimensions. We need not duplicate the services of other members of the health care team, but we often function as coordinators of care, making referrals, communicating across the disciplines, and keeping the whole person in view.

The presence of sin in the world and the predilection of each person to sin take a toll on health spiritually, physically, and psychosocially (Ex 20:5; Ps 32:3-4; Lk 5:17-25). Physical or psychosocial dysfunction can cause spiritual distress (Job 16:7-9; Ps 13–22). Nurses stand in a unique position to assess the interrelationship between these dimensions.

The intimacy required in caring for the body often leads patients to be more open in sharing emotional and spiritual concerns. For example, a woman who feels guilt over a past abortion may feel freer to confess her sense of guilt to the nurse, who already knows her medical history, than to a pastor whom she perceives as "too holy" to understand. A man with bleeding ulcers may be able to tell a nurse about his anger toward his son or his alcohol binges, but hesitates to seek professional counseling.

Nursing works toward the healing of the whole person in the context of communities. This broad understanding of health—shalom—is the goal of nursing. Furthermore, it is the goal of the entire Christian community and a sign of the kingdom of God (Rev 21:1-7). Within that broader view of health, nursing finds a unique place in keeping people healthy, holistically intervening to restore health, and enabling the body of Christ and the health care system to work together toward healing.

AND BRING COMFORT IN SUFFERING

Optimal health means enabling people to live as fully as possible while they are alive. However, despite increasing life spans in many countries, we are mortal beings. The human death rate is still 100 percent. We live in a world that has been corrupted by the effects of sin. Not all of our patients will get well. Some may live with severe physical and mental limitations due to brain damage, loss of limbs, suppressed immune systems, or other conditions.

Those with degenerative diseases may experience remissions, but the course of the illness causes their bodies and often their minds to deteriorate. If physical health is our only aim in nursing, we can feel only futility and despair in the face of these conditions.

Christian nursing also means providing comfort, hope, and compassionate presence for those who are suffering and will not recover. Two hospice nurses explain, "Caring requires a commitment . . . and a willingness to do the unlovely. Neither education nor experience quite prepare you for doing the unlovely. . . . Caring demands listening and observing with your whole person. . . . To care means to be trustworthy. . . . Caring is costly. It takes a great amount of physical, emotional, and spiritual energy."[23]

What *does* prepare us for doing the unlovely? How can we keep going when we cannot see physical improvement? Many in our society believe that the answer lies in ending the suffering by terminating life, but Christian nurses are not free to participate in active euthanasia. Only God has the authority to determine when a person should die. We can provide comfort to those who are suffering by keeping them clean, controlling their pain, turning and positioning them. We can advocate for discontinuing futile heroics and unnecessary painful treatments. We can stay with them, surround them with peace and beauty, facilitate relationships with their loved ones, encourage them spiritually, and walk with them through the valley of the shadow of death until we must entrust them into the hands of Jesus for the rest of the journey.

In order to provide that kind of care, we need to be walking moment by moment with Jesus ourselves. He is the only one who can prepare us and sustain us in the face of suffering and death. Otherwise they will overcome us. Death is an enemy with deceptive strategies. It tempts us either to seek it (through suicide or euthanasia) or to frantically hold it at bay (through futile heroics or placing hope in miracle cures). Only in Christ can we find realistic hope in the face of suffering and death—and the depth of character needed to provide compassionate accompaniment when hope for recovery is gone.

The Character of the Nurse

Based on the hope given in Christ Jesus and on the presence of the Holy Spirit, Christian nursing should be characterized by love, joy, peace, patience,

---

[23]Roberta Lyder Paige and Jane Finkbiner Looney, "Hospice Care for the Advanced Cancer Patient," *American Journal of Nursing* (1977): 1813-15.

kindness, goodness, faithfulness, gentleness, and self-control (Gal 5:22). This "fruit of the Spirit" results from a dynamic, personal relationship with God through Jesus Christ. We can't work it up on our own. The fruit develops as we put our faith into practice. When we don't feel loving, we act lovingly anyhow. Eventually our feelings may catch up with our actions. Joy and peace don't come naturally, especially in a chaotic working environment where staff do not trust or respect each other. But by focusing on Jesus we can begin to see God at work in difficult situations. Joy and peace grow in the light of eternity. Patience, kindness, goodness, faithfulness, gentleness, and self-control sound like characteristics of the ideal nurse. They too come with practice, refined in the furnace of difficult patients, substance-abusing nurse managers, surly nursing assistants, arrogant physicians, and diet kitchens who can't seem to get their orders straight.

Think about the way fruit develops on a tree. It begins as a lovely flower, characteristic of the tree producing it. Soon the blossoms fade, replaced by tiny fruit, which slowly grows larger and sweeter as the tree is nourished by the sun, the rain, and the soil. If it is picked prematurely, the fruit will be hard and sour and will not continue to grow. Left to ripen and protected from pests and injury, it will grow until it becomes soft, sweet, and nutritious.

Character develops in a similar way. God's Spirit causes "fruit" to blossom and grow in our lives. It is nurtured through prayer, Bible study, worship, and Christian fellowship, as well as through practicing being what God intended us to be. At times negative influences in the environment can damage or stunt the growth of the fruit; however, even then there is hope. Some of the best applesauce and apple pies have come from the less-than-perfect apples that dropped from the trees—and next year there will be a new crop. With a little pruning, spraying, fertilizing, and watering, the fruit will improve as the trees mature. Eventually we become "like trees planted by streams of water, which yield their fruit in its season" (Ps 1:3).

The common theme in all these aspects of Christian nursing is the glory of God. Nurses, committed to Jesus Christ and holistically caring for the sick, the poor, and the needy, demonstrate the character of God to the world. They bring the light of Christ into dark situations with humility, love, passion, and power.

FOR FURTHER THINKING

1. From your experience, how is "Christian nursing" different from any other nursing?

2. Describe someone you know who exemplifies Christian nursing.

3. How does your personal relationship with Jesus Christ affect:

    a. Your nursing care?

    b. Your ethical decisions?

    c. Your relationship with colleagues?

    d. Your personal and professional goals?

THEOLOGICAL REFLECTION

Read Matthew 9:12-13, Luke 4:18-19, Luke 10:8-9, and John 10:10.

1. What goals for ministry does Jesus give in these passages?

2. How could you apply each of these goals to your own nursing practice?

NURSING SATISFACTION

Are Christian nurses satisfied with nursing? According to a 2001 *Journal of Christian Nursing* website Nursing Satisfaction Survey (NSS), the answer is overwhelmingly yes. The results are surprising, especially when compared to surveys on the general nursing population.

In 2017, researchers surveyed almost 7,000 nurses, all members of the American Nurses Association, to investigate the association of burnout and career choice regret. Results revealed that 15 percent of respondents (one in seven) expressed regret at becoming a nurse, and 38.4 percent of the nurses reported at least one symptom of burnout.[24]

In contrast, respondents to the *JCN* survey report that 79 percent look forward to going to work each day. Overall, 86 percent find their work satisfying. Surprisingly, work setting made little difference in nursing satisfaction. However, spirituality had a strong bearing on nursing satisfaction. A desire to help others (92 percent), compassion for the sick (74 percent), and the opportunity to serve

---

[24]Liselotte Dyrbye et al., "An Investigation of Career Choice Regret Among American Nurses," *American Journal of Nursing* (2020): 24-33.

God (72 percent) were their top three reasons for choosing nursing as a career. Opportunities to meet spiritual needs of patients brought great satisfaction.[25] Interestingly, satisfaction with nursing increased with age.

The reasons *why* came out in the stories that some respondents attached to their surveys. Cheryl Munns, a faith community nurse in Wisconsin, gives a glimpse into how longevity contributes to nursing satisfaction.

> One night about fourteen years ago, while working in the ICU of a large hospital, a patient in his early fifties was admitted post cardiac arrest. He had been resuscitated by his daughter in their living room and was alert, with a stable cardiac rhythm, on admission. It was a slow night. He was my only patient for the night shift. His wife met him at the hospital, and I talked with her for a while. Since everything looked okay at that time, she decided to go home and get some sleep. I told her I would call if his condition changed.
>
> Shortly after she left, Jim's condition did change. He began having runs of ventricular tachycardia (v-tach), so the ICU resident and I were in his room constantly. We tried many different medications, but the runs of v-tach continued. During these episodes, Carl would become unresponsive after five to seven beats. However, if I saw a short run of v-tach beginning and told him to cough, he could convert his rhythm. So each time I saw v-tach on the monitor, I would say to him, "Carl, cough!"
>
> Finally, he asked me to stay with him. I sat next to his bedside, listening as he talked about his life, his wife and three children, and his fears about his heart condition. I asked him if he wanted his wife to come. He said, "no," that it would be best for her to get a good night's sleep.
>
> Again, he became unstable so we called the cardiologist. At that point, about 3:00 a.m., I called his wife and told her that she might want to come to the hospital. She said she would be there shortly. When I went back to his room, Carl asked if I would call his wife because he was afraid. I told him I already had. Carl made it through the night and, after a cardiac catheterization and other tests, he went home.
>
> About two months later, right before Christmas, Carl was brought in by ambulance on the day shift, after having another cardiac episode. Again, he was alert. I was assigned to Carl. He had an implantable defibrillator inserted, recovered nicely, and was home for Christmas.

---

[25]Judith Allen Shelly, "Measuring the Spirit of Nursing," *Journal of Christian Nursing* (2003): 14-17.

Carl and I have stayed in touch over the years. Eventually, I left the hospital and worked in a clinic. When Carl came for his cardiology visits twice a year, he would find where I was working, and we would talk.

A few years later, I was volunteering as a patroller at a local ski slope when we got a call about a skier with a severe leg injury. At the scene we discovered an eighteen-year-old boy in severe pain with a spiral tibia/fibula fracture. We called for an ambulance to meet us in the patrol room. As we worked on the boy, I talked with him. When he told me his name and where he was from, I asked if his dad was Carl. He said, "Yeah, do you know him?" When I told him who I was, he said, "You are the nurse who saved my dad's life."

Again, this young man was afraid. He asked me if I would ride in the ambulance with him, as he was there with friends and no family. We don't usually ride to the hospital with the patients, but I agreed. When I talked with Carl on the phone, he was surprised and relieved to hear my voice. He knew, then, that his son would be okay. The boy had surgery and made a complete recovery.

I think we all have times when our nursing career takes on a deeper meaning. The hospital experience with Carl was a spiritual nursing experience, one of the times in my twenty years of nursing that reinforces what I do as truly valuable, for me and for those in my care. I recently began working as a faith community nurse. It already has given me many wonderful opportunities to share both my faith and my nursing, and I know many more opportunities lie ahead.

Tamara Damron, an RN in West Virginia, also tells a story of how she grew into a more comfortable relationship with her profession.

I guess every nursing student has a vision of what their daily life will be like as a nurse. I'm old enough to have visions of white, with a sense of religious service. As an eighteen-year-old, I could see myself tending to those in a leper colony, a missionary to the sick and ailing. Upon graduation, though, I found myself feeling stupid and incompetent.

About six months later, I no longer felt as incompetent, but then my ideal met reality. I faced inadequate staffing, uncooperative coworkers and too many demands. With complaints from patients and families, I found myself to be more aligned with the staff, who seemed to feel "We're in the trenches together," rather than with the patients I wanted to serve. After six years in nursing, I was ready to throw my hands up and say, "No more."

I began to reevaluate. I reaffirmed my motivation and began to ask, "What is nursing?" I returned to school and began to study nursing theory. Orlando's

Nursing Process Theory helped substantially, enabling me to focus my energies in a cogent way. I also began to review my personal life and realized that I needed to grow spiritually. Spirituality used to be a way of life for me. However, once in nursing school, church attendance, prayer, and church activities gave way to studying for exams, and clinical and class time. I had little time left for my family or church.

Not much changed after graduation or for the next six years, as I worked night shifts and every other weekend. A book by Brother Lawrence, *The Practice of the Presence of God*, helped me to realize that it's not the situation that you find yourself in (positive or negative) but the awareness of your place in Christ and with Christ that brings peace. Now, I am trying to rely on God's power and grace.

Many years have passed since I graduated from nursing school. I have now regained my *vision* of nursing. The reality shock of nursing has given way to the beauty of what a nursing ministry can be. It is even better than the dreams of an eighteen-year-old who knew nothing of the world, other than that she wanted to be a nurse.

New graduates find themselves facing overwork, understaffing, unsympathetic colleagues, and lack of confidence in their clinical skills. Amazingly, though, 60 percent of them look forward to going to work each day, and 83 percent feel satisfied with their work in nursing. Staying in nursing over the long haul gives most nurses confidence in their abilities and a strong sense that they are helping others and serving God.

Interpersonal relationships contribute to both nursing satisfaction and dissatisfaction. Eighty-three percent say that their coworkers enjoy each other; however, about half sense a great deal of interpersonal conflict among staff. Most respondents do not feel that their colleagues share their satisfaction with nursing.

Sixty-nine percent feel that most of their colleagues are dissatisfied and that only about half of their coworkers are optimistic about nursing. Seventy-five percent find their supervisors helpful and supportive, but only 58 percent trust the administrators where they work. Over half (51 percent) feel their employers take advantage of them and that certain employees receive preferential treatment. This sense of injustice was felt most strongly by the twenty-three- to twenty-nine-year-olds (87 percent) and least by the forty- to forty-nine-year-olds (57 percent).

Surprisingly, work setting made little difference in nursing satisfaction, although optimism was slightly lower among hospital nurses. Faith community nurses showed no significant difference from nurses in hospitals, the community, extended care, clinics, or universities.[26]

DISCUSSION QUESTIONS

1. How does your experience in nursing compare with the survey results?

2. What are some concrete ways that you could encourage and support new graduates in your workplace?

3. How free do you feel to provide spiritual care? What causes you to hold back?

4. When you find yourself in the middle of a gripe session, how could you turn the tone around?

5. How could you apply the principles in Hebrews 10:24-25 in your nursing situation?

---

[26]Case study adapted from Shelly, "Measuring the Spirit of Nursing."

14

SPIRITUAL CARE

Purpose: To describe Christian spiritual care

Objectives: After reading this chapter and completing the exercises, you should be able to:
1. Describe a spiritual need
2. Define spiritual care
3. Identify six principles for spiritual intervention
4. Describe the ultimate aim of spiritual care

Keywords: spiritual care, compassionate presence, active listening, witness, prayer, Bible, body of Christ

IT WAS THE FIRST SUNDAY OF THE MONTH, and the volunteer faith community nurses were taking blood pressures at church after the worship service. Donna lingered in the hall until most of the other people left. Finally she peeked into the room where I (Judy) was putting away my equipment. "I guess I'd better have my blood pressure checked too," she said hesitantly.

Donna, age forty-three, had been coming every month, and I was worried about her. Although she was under medical care and on high doses of medication, her blood pressure stubbornly stayed around 230/120. Married and the mother of four children ranging in age from eighteen to ten, Donna was grossly overweight and had a different physical ailment every time I saw her.

Accident-prone and highly anxious, she began to tell me that she was sure she would die soon. Her mother had recently been hospitalized with a stroke, and her ninety-three-year-old grandmother had just died of breast cancer. We talked about her fears and then discussed some strategies for reducing her risk of stroke and cancer. But she did not think she could improve her diet or increase her level of activity. She was "too scared" to do breast self-examination or go for a mammogram. She blamed her hypertension and anxiety on her children. Her husband, though faithful, was unsupportive and passive.

Donna teaches kindergarten Sunday school and does an excellent job. She is sensitive to the children, showing particular skill with one child with autism. She vividly conveys God's love to the children but fears that God is angry with her. Her life feels like it's falling apart. When Donna comes to have her blood pressure checked, she is really seeking spiritual care.

On the other hand, Carol always felt she had her life under control. Bright, capable, and on a tenure track at a prestigious university at age twenty-six, she was popular with students and heavily involved with the student Christian fellowship on campus. When she began experiencing severe kidney infections, she followed her medical regimen precisely and fully expected to recover quickly.

Instead, her kidneys shut down permanently, requiring a transplant. All went well for about a year; then her body rejected the kidney. After a second transplant she returned to teaching and working toward her doctorate.

Although Carol lived for another fifteen years, she became acutely aware that her entire body was gradually failing. Finally she admitted that no amount of positive thinking would turn the process around. She called me from her hospital bed, saying, "You know that spiritual care you're always talking about? Well, please come—I need it right now." She died about six months later.

What can nurses offer in the way of spiritual care? In what way can nursing be a Christian ministry?

WHAT IS SPIRITUAL CARE?

Probably more than any other profession, nursing deals with giving hope to the hopeless. Although other professionals, such as physicians and clergy, also offer hope, it is the nurse who stands with the sick person for extended periods of time offering care and support when medical science can no longer offer a cure.

Spiritual care must be an integral component of caring for the whole person, and assessing spiritual needs should be included in the total nursing assessment. It is not a nice extra to tack on when we have time, nor should it have to be private and unrecorded. Let's look again at Jesus' approach to the paralytic brought to him by friends:

And just then some people were carrying a paralyzed man lying on a bed. When Jesus saw their faith, he said to the paralytic, "Take heart, son; your sins are forgiven." Then some of the scribes said to themselves, "This man is blaspheming." But Jesus, perceiving their thoughts, said, "Why do you think evil in your hearts? For which is easier, to say, 'Your sins are forgiven,' or to say, 'Stand up and walk'? But so that you may know that the Son of Man has authority on earth to forgive sins"—he then said to the paralytic—"Stand up, take your bed and go to your home." And he stood up and went to his home. When the crowds saw it, they were filled with awe, and they glorified God, who had given such authority to human beings. (Mt 9:2-8)

Jesus assessed that although the presenting problem appeared to be physical, the man's primary need at this point was spiritual—forgiveness of sins. Notice that his diagnosis and treatment did not meet with the approval of the community leaders, but he still had the confidence and courage to act on his convictions. Also notice the results. Not only was the man healed, both physically and spiritually, but the crowds glorified God. Good spiritual care should bring glory to God, and not mere comfort to the patient or acceptance with the health care community.

Sometimes spiritual care means simply being present, praying, sharing from Scripture, offering a word of witness and encouragement, or participating in a healing service. At other times it may include arranging referrals, planning creative strategies for follow-up care in the home, or helping a person become connected to a Christian community.

Myrtle, an eighty-five-year-old in excellent health, never missed a Sunday at church. She sang in the choir, attended a weekly Bible study, and served in various volunteer roles with enthusiasm. Then she fell on the ice and broke her arm. Suddenly she became a recluse. Stating that she knew the day would eventually come when she could no longer function and the Lord would take her home, she assumed that that time had now arrived.

When Jean, a nurse from her congregation, visited, she assessed Myrtle's physical needs. More important, she realized that Myrtle had a spiritual need: to know that God still had work for her to do. After listening to Myrtle and praying with her about her concerns, Jean was able to convince Myrtle that a broken arm was hardly life-threatening, and she would be able to get out and participate in her activities again. Before long, Myrtle was back at her seat in the choir.

What are spiritual needs? In *Spiritual Care: The Nurse's Role*, Shelly and Fish define a spiritual need as "the lack of any factor or factors necessary to establish and/or maintain a dynamic, personal relationship with God."[1] Although spiritual needs have a horizontal dimension (in relationship to other people), they are primarily vertical (in relationship to God). These include the need for faith, hope, and love (1 Cor 13:13), for confession and forgiveness (Jas 5:13-16), and for meaning and purpose (Rom 8:18; Eph 2:10; 3:18-19; Phil 2:13). God meets spiritual needs; we don't. But God works through people, including nurses, to communicate his grace to others. How can nurses provide spiritual care?

Christian spiritual care means facilitating a person's relationship with God through Jesus Christ. That will not always be a "comfort measure." In fact, it may well cause some temporary discomfort as a person becomes aware of sin before a holy God. In our highly secularized postmodern culture, the idea of proclaiming the gospel in a health care setting might seem inappropriate or even impossible; yet, if we truly believe what we claim to believe, salvation through Jesus Christ is the only cure for spiritual sickness.

Consider how inappropriate it would be to treat a festering abscess with palliative measures alone. You could give morphine to mask the pain, and the patient would feel much better, but the infection would probably keep spreading, causing serious complications and even death. In the same way, offering palliative spiritual interventions without addressing a person's relationship to Jesus Christ will provide only false comfort.

Spiritual care means putting people in touch with God through compassionate presence, active listening, witness, prayer, Bible reading, and partnering with the body of Christ (the church community and the clergy). It is never coercive or rude.

Spiritual care can be appropriate in both secular and Christian settings, and for both Christians and non-Christians. In practical terms, spiritual care is usually well received when it is offered in a spirit of gentleness and humility. Christian nurses have often provided spiritual care in secular settings without encountering any resistance from either patients or hospital administration. Sometimes, though, there is opposition.

---

[1]Judith Allen Shelly and Sharon Fish, *Spiritual Care: The Nurse's Role* (Downers Grove, IL: InterVarsity Press, 1988), 39.

When patients or family members come from other religious traditions, or no religion, they may refuse any offer of spiritual intervention. Some may request spiritual care from a representative of their own belief system. In such cases we must respect their preferences.

Sometimes that opposition comes when spiritual care is inappropriately offered. I (Judy) once had to report a nurse who, in addition to providing unsafe physical care, witnessed crassly and manipulatively to her patients. For example, she would ask preoperative patients, "If you die on the operating table, where will you spend eternity?" Most patients heard nothing beyond the first three words. They refused to sign the operative permits. To this day, I am sure she thinks she was terminated for her faithful Christian witness.

Other nurses have been censured for providing good spiritual care. Margie is one example. She was called into the hospital administrator's office and reprimanded for praying with a patient. The administrator learned of this through a glowing letter of appreciation from the patient, who wrote, "The nurses were so caring, especially Margie Johnson, who prayed with me before surgery." He instructed Margie to never pray with a patient again.

Margie belonged to a nurses' fellowship group, and she shared her story with them. The group began to pray for the hospital administration. Margie continued to pray with patients when she felt it was appropriate. Within six months the hospital chaplain approached the administrator with a plan for a continuing education class on spiritual care. He asked Margie to serve on a panel of responders. The administrator attended the event—and was persuaded to change his policy. He began encouraging nurses to provide spiritual care.

> *Spiritual care means putting people in touch with God through compassionate presence, active listening, witness, prayer, Bible reading, and partnering with the body of Christ.*

Not every story has such a happy ending. Some Christian nurses have continued to work under spiritually oppressive conditions. Others have chosen to change jobs to work in a more open environment. Our commitment to Christ demands that we remain faithful to him. At times we will need to keep our witness quiet, but we cannot with integrity deny our patients the hope of Jesus Christ because of human rules (Acts 4:19-20; 5:29).

Compassionate Presence

When the prophet Elijah ran from those who were persecuting him, he became exhausted, depressed, and a bit paranoid. God sent an angel, who "touched him" and then told him to "get up and eat" the food prepared for him (1 Kings 19:5). The angel persisted, coming repeatedly, constantly assessing and meeting Elijah's physical, emotional, and spiritual needs. The ultimate effect of this angel's intervention was to put Elijah in a position where he could hear personally from God.

In many ways our nursing care is similar to that angel's intervention. We meet patients where they are, provide the assistance needed at the moment, and constantly nudge them toward the goals God intends for them. Compassion means to *feel with* another person. Notice, though, that the angel did not stop there. Elijah wanted to die. He felt no hope. The angel did not offer assistance in dying! He came alongside Elijah, touched him, allowed him to rest, provided food and water, and sent him on his way when he was sufficiently recovered.

Darryl, thirty-two and dying of a drug-resistant infection, turned his head toward the window as his evening nurse, Sarah, entered the room. Most of the personnel he had encountered so far seemed distant and subtly contemptuous toward him. The nurse who cared for him on the day shift made such a production of her universal precautions that he knew she was afraid of catching the infection from him. But Sarah seemed different. She laid her hand on his shoulder, saying, "Darryl, you seem tense—would you like a backrub at bedtime?" He relaxed and turned toward her, gratefully accepting the offer.

In a similar way Sarah can offer Darryl her compassionate presence: giving him a backrub, feeding him when he is too weak to eat, and treating him as the valuable human being that God created him to be. If Darryl receives that kind of humane care, he will be much more open to consider the hope that God has for him in Christ Jesus, and much less compelled to seek assisted suicide.

Active Listening

Nurses have a reputation for being "fixers." When someone suffers, we want to *do something* to ease the pain and provide comfort. Often that response comes in the form of providing answers and solutions, just as Job's friends did.

After their harangues, Job called them "miserable comforters" (Job 16:2). He pleaded with them, "Listen carefully to my words. . . . Bear with me, and I will speak" (21:2-3). The monologue that followed was not easy to hear. Job complained against God. He spoke in utter despair. But through it all, God was doing an important work in Job's heart, while his friends sat silently, allowing him to speak. In the end he could affirm, "I had heard of you by the hearing of the ear, but now my eye sees you; therefore I despise myself, and repent in dust and ashes" (42:5-6). Following that confession, Job's life turned around. He regained health, possessions, and relationships.

Active listening includes hearing what a person is not saying as well as the actual thoughts and feelings articulated. An active listener expresses empathy, humility, and commitment to the other, even while sometimes challenging the ideas expressed, but the first and most important step is to keep your mouth shut. Compassionate listening often requires a personal vulnerability that leaves the listener open to rejection or ridicule. We are not talking here about reflective listening, where the nurse stands back and objectively facilitates a verbal catharsis. Instead we are suggesting an involved dialogue where the nurse enters into the patient's suffering and points the way to hope.

> *Active listening includes hearing what a person is not saying as well as the actual thoughts and feelings articulated.*

WITNESS

After careful, active listening, there are times when a word of witness is appropriate and helpful. Ruth Farr used such an approach with a suicidal patient. After carefully assessing the patient through reading her chart, listening and observing, Ruth related,

> In terms of therapeutic communication, I had no idea how to connect with this patient. Nevertheless, the Lord knew how. So it was up to him to provide an opening. If there was something he wanted me to say, I would need his help in knowing the right words to use. In a few minutes he answered my prayer. Her statement "I have to kill myself" was the cue.
> "What makes you think you have to kill yourself?" I asked.
> "Because I've done so many bad things," she answered.

"But you don't have to die for bad things you've done."

"Yes, I do. I have to be punished. God could never forgive me . . . I'll just have to die."

"But that's why Jesus died for you, so you won't have to die. All you need to do is ask him to forgive you."[2]

Most Christian nurses would not be so bold. Many psychiatric nurses would say that Ruth took a terrible risk by interjecting religious ideation (even though the patient initiated it) and that her solution was too simplistic. But Ruth was apparently listening to the prompting of the Holy Spirit. She clearly documented her intervention. The patient came to a major turning point in her illness, and subsequent nurses notes on the chart by Ruth's colleagues documented the patient's marked improvement.

Sometimes a word of witness can come in the form of a story. The prophet Nathan used that approach with King David after he arranged to have Uriah, the husband of Bathsheba, killed in battle. David had accidentally observed Bathsheba while she was bathing, and he wanted her. Being a man of action, David got what he wanted, and soon Bathsheba gave birth to David's son.

> And the LORD sent Nathan to David. He came to him, and said to him, "There were two men in a certain city, the one rich and the other poor. The rich man had very many flocks and herds; but the poor man had nothing but one little ewe lamb, which he had bought. He brought it up, and it grew up with him and with his children; it used to eat of his meager fare, and drink from his cup, and lie in his bosom, and it was like a daughter to him. Now there came a traveler to the rich man, and he was loath to take one of his own flock or herd to prepare for the wayfarer who had come to him, but he took the poor man's lamb, and prepared that for the guest who had come to him." Then David's anger was greatly kindled against the man. He said to Nathan, "As the LORD lives, the man who has done this deserves to die; he shall restore the lamb fourfold, because he did this thing, and because he had no pity."
>
> Nathan said to David, "You are the man!" (2 Sam 12:1-7)

In this case, David recognized his own sin and responded by immediately confessing and repenting, but he still had to pay the consequences for his behavior. Nathan went on to tell him that the baby would die. When the baby

---

[2]Ruth E. Farr, "I'll Just Have to Die," *Journal of Christian Nursing* (1994): 5-6.

became ill, David fasted and prayed, then fell into a deep depression. It was not until after the baby died that David recovered. If anyone on the scene had been doing research on whether prayer "worked" or measuring the effectiveness of witness as a nursing intervention by whether it produced peace, this case would not be regarded as a success. However, it became a turning point in his relationship with God.

A word of witness can also be telling our own stories of how God has met us in difficult times. For example, Cynthia, a nurse who has recovered from breast cancer, visits patients who have been newly diagnosed and leads post-mastectomy support groups. She always tells her own story, including how God has helped her through her struggles.

Deirdre is another example. Sexually molested by a male missionary colleague, she has begun to tell her story so that other abused women will find help and hope. Many women who are abused by Christian leaders become disillusioned with the church and may turn away from God and the Christian community. Deirdre's witness affirms God's love in the midst of a horrible experience.

Our witness should not be self-righteous or manipulative, but it can be bold. It includes who God is and what he has done for us in Jesus Christ. More personally, it expresses what God has done in our own lives. It can be very appropriate to humbly share with a patient how God has met us in times of suffering and need. At times when saying "I know what you are going through" does not connect, telling your story can knit a powerful bond and provide hope. It forms a fellowship of suffering that provides strength and encouragement to others who struggle to trust God in hard times. However, whenever we offer a word of witness, we must be sure that it is just that, for when it becomes preachy it loses its effectiveness.

Prayer—of Many Kinds

Prayer is making big press today. It shows up even in *Time* and *Newsweek*. Nurses, physicians, psychologists, and other health care professionals are conducting studies to show that prayer is "good for you" and that prayer "works."[3]

---

[3]*Newsweek*, January 6, 1992, 39-44; *Time*, June 24, 1996, 56-68; *Christianity Today*, January 6, 1997, 20-29. For abstracts on many of the research studies on prayer, see Dale A. Matthews, David B. Larson, and Constance P. Barry, *The Faith Factor: An Annotated Bibliography of Clinical Research on Spiritual Subjects* (Arlington, VA: National Institute for Healthcare Research, 1993).

Yet on closer observation the prayer being studied scientifically and advocated by everyone from physicians to talk-show hosts looks a lot different from Christian prayer.

Physician and prayer researcher Larry Dossey claims that it really doesn't matter where or to whom we direct our prayers.[4] He prefers to see God as impersonal and refers to God as *the Absolute*, saying, "The Absolute is radically beyond any description whatsoever, including gender. . . . The reader may insert . . . his or her preferred name for the Absolute—whether *Goddess, God, Allah, Krishna, Brahman, the Tao, the Universal Mind, the Almighty, Alpha and Omega, the One.*"[5]

Dossey contends that we should pray because it *works*, not because it maintains our relationship with a loving God. Since research seems to document that prayer is equally effective regardless of to whom it is addressed, he assumes that it really goes nowhere.[6] However, he recognizes a phenomenon of "negative prayer,"[7] while dismissing the reality of the spiritual world.

A quick check of internet resources on prayer shows 33,400,000 websites. Limiting the search to healing prayer reduces the number to 28,800,000. Exploring the websites uncovers things you never learned in Sunday school— everything from "Angel Answers to Spiritual Questions" (sample answer, "No, Jesus is not part of the Trinity"), "Funky Angel Healing Chakra Doll Prints" (only $2.50 each, in your choice of colors), "HALO Healing Light Order Online Prayer & Healing Ministry," to the more hopeful "Healing Prayer for the Community" (which turned out to be subtitled "Learn Wicca" and included a prayer addressed to the goddess Diana).

What is prayer? Why is it so popular? According to the Bible, prayer is communication with God. Interestingly, there are only 105 references to prayer in the whole Bible (122 to the word *pray*). Jesus taught us how to pray in Matthew 6 by giving the disciples this prayer:

> Our Father in heaven, hallowed be your name. Your kingdom come. Your will be done, on earth as in heaven. Give us today our daily bread. Forgive us our sins, as we forgive those who sin against us. Save us from the time of trial, and

---

[4]Larry Dossey, *Prayer Is Good Medicine* (San Francisco: HarperSanFrancisco, 1996), xiv.
[5]Dossey, *Prayer Is Good Medicine*, xiv.
[6]Dossey, *Prayer Is Good Medicine*, 31.
[7]Dossey, *Prayer Is Good Medicine*, 180-87.

deliver us from evil. For the kingdom, the power and the glory are yours, now and forever. Amen.[8]

While this prayer asks God for specific things, such as food, forgiveness, and protection, its primary focus is on a participation in God's kingdom that requires commitment and action on our part as well.

The Bible *does* tell us that God answers prayer. For example, Matthew 21:22 claims, "Whatever you ask for in prayer with faith, you will receive."

But prayer is not just asking God for things. It also involves praise, adoration, thanksgiving, confession, and meditation on God's Word. It is the language of relationship, not magic or manipulation.

The first time I (Judy) prayed out loud with a patient was unplanned. In fact, I was fearful of doing the wrong thing. I was a junior nursing student assigned to a seventy-year-old woman who was scheduled for surgery the next day. As I finished her morning care, she rather gruffly asked, "Are you a Christian?"

Self-consciously I admitted that I was. We had been sternly warned by our instructors that students were not to discuss religion with patients, and this conversation felt like I might be getting myself into trouble. Then the woman demanded, "Well then, you pray for me!"

I mumbled that I would pray for her when I returned to the dorm that evening.

"No," she responded, "You pray *now*, *here*!"

I hesitated, pulled the curtain and prayed.

Afterward she was a different person. The once fearful, demanding patient was now hopeful and at peace. When I told my clinical instructor, who was a Christian, about what happened, she personally affirmed me—but reminded me that such behavior was unprofessional.

Is it really appropriate to pray with patients? The obvious answer, if we truly believe that God is our loving Father, is—of course! We go to our loving heavenly Father with our concerns for those who are hurting. In so doing we admit our own limitations and acknowledge his love and control of the situation. In the Gospels we see a pattern of just such behavior. The centurion came to Jesus when his servant was sick (Mt 8:5-13); Jairus came on behalf of his daughter (Lk 8). Peter and the other disciples asked Jesus about Peter's mother-in-law's high fever (Lk 4:38). In Luke 9, a father appealed to Jesus for

---

[8] *The Book of Common Prayer* (New York: Oxford University Press, 1979), 364.

a second opinion after the disciples were unable to heal his son. In Mark 2, a group of friends actually tore the roof off a house in order to bring their paralytic friend to Jesus.

God has told us to come to him with our concerns for the sick and suffering. James writes,

> Are any among you suffering? They should pray. Are any cheerful? They should sing songs of praise. Are any among you sick? They should call for the elders of the church and have them pray over them, anointing them with oil in the name of the Lord. The prayer of faith will save the sick, and the Lord will raise them up; and anyone who has committed sins will be forgiven. Therefore confess your sins to one another, and pray for one another, so that you may be healed. The prayer of the righteous is powerful and effective. (Jas 5:13-16)

Notice here, though, that the One we address in prayer *does* matter. Prayer is more than a technique; it is a relationship with God that is enjoyed at good times as well as in periods of need. Furthermore, this conversation with God is not just a private conversation. It involves the Christian community and the confession of sin within that community. More than a physical cure, healing prayer results in forgiveness of sin and a restoration of relationship with God and his people.

When we pray for our patients, we bring them to the One who created them and loves them, the only One who can truly make them well. Not to do so would be irresponsible. Sometimes we will pray out loud at the bedside, but we should always pray for every patient in our care, even if it is while we walk down the hall to answer a call light, adjust an IV, or bathe a comatose patient. Visiting nurses have a wonderful opportunity to pray as they drive. Faith community nurses may have the added advantage of a prayer team and healing services.

BIBLE READING

The Scriptures can be a deep source of comfort and strength to the believer. The psalmist declares, "Your decrees are my heritage forever; they are the joy of my heart" (Ps 119:111). It is through the Scriptures that we find guidance and direction. Shared appropriately with patients, the Word of God can facilitate powerful spiritual healing.

Some were sick through their sinful ways, and because of their iniquities endured affliction; they loathed any kind of food, and they drew near to the gates of death. Then they cried to the LORD in their trouble, and he saved them from their distress; he sent out his word and healed them, and delivered them from destruction. (Ps 107:17-20)

On the other hand, the Word of God does spiritual surgery:

Indeed, the word of God is living and active, sharper than any two-edged sword, piercing until it divides soul from spirit, joints from marrow; it is able to judge the thoughts and intentions of the heart. And before him no creature is hidden, but all are naked and laid bare to the eyes of the one to whom we must render an account. (Heb 4:12-13)

Surgery causes pain before it heals. Sometimes the Bible will confront people with the painful news of their sin before they can hear the good news of salvation. Although we should never use Scripture to blame or attack others, God may well use it to convict people when we read it to them. We cannot measure the effectiveness of our spiritual interventions merely by whether we make patients feel good.

Norma Singer relates an experience where she used the Bible in her nursing care. Alma, a fifty-six-year-old woman admitted to the unit where Norma worked, asked if Norma could stay and talk with her for a few minutes. She poured out her concerns about her complicated medical history and a long list of fears, doubts, and guilt. Finally she expressed a fear of dying, because "I don't know what will happen to me!" Norma offered to pray for her, but Alma hesitated, then said, "See, nurse, I had an abortion a long time ago. And I just feel so guilty about it. I guess that's why I don't believe in prayer. Because of what I did."

"Abortion is covered," said Norma.

Then she talked with the surprised woman about God's forgiveness and how even abortion was covered by what Christ did for us on the cross. When a colleague paged Norma, she offered Alma a Bible, pointing out some passages to read about forgiveness. Throughout the day, whenever Norma passed the room, she noted that Alma was still reading the Bible. At the end of the shift, Norma again offered to pray with Alma. This time Alma eagerly agreed and prayed herself, confessing her sin and accepting Christ as Savior.[9]

---

[9]Norma Singer, "When Things Go Bump in the Night: A Story of Forgiveness," *Journal of Christian Nursing* (1997): 24-25.

In this story we see a beautiful example of the Word of God being "living and active" (Heb 4:12). Norma did not have to use it to back up her arguments, convince, or coerce Alma. The Bible alone did the work after Norma's solid groundwork had been laid.

We can use the Bible inappropriately. For example, just quoting our favorite verses without stopping to listen to the patient's concerns will not usually communicate caring or understanding. Too many patients have merely had their suffering compounded by an insensitive Christian who flippantly quoted part of Romans 8:28, "We know that all things work together for good." Furthermore, using the Bible to judge and condemn someone tends to communicate self-righteousness, not hope.

Notice in Norma's story that Alma already felt guilty and assumed God hated her. She needed to hear the good news that God would forgive her, regardless of how bad her sin had been. Reading the Bible convinced her that her sin was indeed covered. Norma's approach took that sin very seriously, but she let God do the judging. The Bible, not Norma, set the standard of righteousness for Alma.

For patients who are already familiar with the Bible, we can often serve them by allowing them to minister to us. Marlene, a visiting nurse, recently related how much she enjoys visiting a particular patient on a weekly basis. Beulah is homebound, but she demonstrates a hopeful attitude and a strong faith. Whenever Marlene visits, Beulah hands her a slip of paper with a Bible verse written on it, saying, "This is your verse for today." Invariably, the verse applies directly to her needs that day.

We can use the same approach with those in our care. A handwritten verse or colorful Bible portion, chosen specifically for an individual patient, will often be carefully read, digested, and treasured for years to come. It communicates God's Word, and it also demonstrates our own care and personal interest in the person.

In order to effectively use Scripture in our spiritual care, we need to be familiar with appropriate passages, spend time in personal and group study, and live in daily obedience to what we are learning from the Scriptures. Setting aside a time for daily personal Bible reading and prayer is essential, even in a hectic schedule. Studying the Bible in a small group provides us with insights from other believers. It also gives us the opportunity to practice talking to others about how the Bible applies to daily life, increasing our confidence for sharing with patients. We also need to learn from the experts, including listening to sermons, reading commentaries and books that provide Bible background and application, and perhaps taking courses in Bible and theology.

CHRISTIAN COMMUNITY

Partnering with the body of Christ—the church community and the clergy—is another important aspect of spiritual care. Mary Jane, who had been in poor health and homebound for several years, missed her involvement in her church. When nurses from the congregation visited to encourage her and to assess her changing needs, Mary Jane expressed frustration that she could not get out to church activities.

So the nurses brought the church to Mary Jane. She became the official volunteer coordinator, each week calling every person who had a part in the upcoming Sunday services, from children's choir members to ushers. She also initiated the congregation's prayer chain, cataloged books for the church library, and made crafts for special occasions. Mary Jane probably knew more about what was happening in the church than any of those who attended regularly. Her involvement with the church met a spiritual need for Christian community.

We are created in God's image, which means we are designed to live in relationship with God and with one another. We need the body of Christ, the church, in order to live healthy lives. When a person becomes institutionalized or homebound, the isolation from the church compounds the sense of brokenness. An important aspect of spiritual care is connecting our patients to the Christian community.

While visiting Korea we were amazed at how seriously the Korean churches take this responsibility. One Christian hospital in particular is surrounded by dozens of churches started for the express purpose of incorporating all the new Christians who came to know the Lord through the ministry of that hospital. Nurses can provide only a small, though significant, part of the whole spectrum of spiritual care. For the most part, that care will come through the church.

We can begin to connect patients with the church by asking whether they are associated with a church and whether their pastor knows about their present condition. Has their pastor, deacon, faith community nurse, or other member of their congregation visited recently? If not, would they appreciate it if a family member or the nurse notified the pastor about any important changes in their health status?

Recently Martha, an active member of my (Judy's) congregation who lived alone, became seriously ill. She panicked and called an ambulance but did not tell anyone in the church, because she was too weak to make any more phone calls and too embarrassed to bother anyone. The effective grapevine of a small community, along with the prompting of the Holy Spirit, finally got the word to the pastor and to me. A neighbor saw the ambulance and called a church member the next day. That woman tried calling Martha at home. When she got no answer, she began calling local hospitals until she located Martha, and then called the pastor to report. The pastor and I visited Martha in the hospital, and she deeply appreciated the time of fellowship and prayer and felt relieved that we could notify her friends and extended family.

Our visit also drew in Martha's hospital roommate, Eunice, who was also a Christian. We ended up all joining hands and praying together. Up to that point Martha and Eunice had not talked about their faith with one another. Following the visit, they began praying together.

Intentionally including the pastor and the church community in the health care team may facilitate the healing process. Nursing literature recognizes the importance of the church community in health care.[10] In many cases, the church is merely viewed as another community-based location for primary health care. However, even when the spiritual dimension of care is limited, patients may perceive the care they receive as more caring and holistic. Frank is a good example.

Another longtime member of our church and an adult-onset diabetic, Frank at age eighty had little interest in following a diabetic diet. He would fast before going for his blood glucose tests, but he ate whatever he wanted in between. I had noticed that his general health seemed to be deteriorating. When the parish nurses at church sponsored a health fair in conjunction with

---

[10]See for example, Margaret B. Clark, and Joanee K. Olson, *Nursing Within a Faith Community* (Thousand Oaks, CA: Sage, 2000); Sybil D. Smith, *Parish Nursing: A Handbook for the New Millennium* (New York: Haworth Pastoral Press, 2003); *Parish Nursing: Healthcare Ministry Within the Church* (Sudbury, MA: Jones and Bartlett, 2003).

the annual bazaar, I convinced Frank to come in to get his blood sugar tested. It was 542 mg/dl. We called his physician, who met him at the hospital emergency room. By the time Frank arrived at the hospital, his blood sugar was well over 600 mg/dl. His wife called me when they got home and reported that Frank had finally decided to take his diet seriously. "He wouldn't listen to me, but he is listening to you now," she remarked. Frank continues to check in periodically to tell me how his blood sugar is doing and assure me that he is sticking to his diet. In Frank's case there was little overt spiritual care offered. However, because we worship together and have a long-term friendship, Frank trusts me with his physical health.

Another way the church meets our patients' spiritual needs is through the sacraments. The Eucharist/Lord's Supper was intended to be a healing event, a celebration of Christian unity and the salvation provided in the death and resurrection of Jesus Christ. As such, we can call on the clergy to bring the sacrament of Communion to those in our care. However, Holy Communion is not magic and should never be offered lightly.

The sacraments, according to *The Book of Common Prayer*, are "outward and visible signs of inward and spiritual grace given by Christ as sure and certain means by which we receive that grace."[11] Augustine of Hippo defined them as "a visible sign of an invisible reality."[12]

Augustine categorized around thirty liturgical ceremonies as sacraments.[13] By the Middle Ages the church had distinguished seven: baptism, confirmation, Communion, marriage, penance, extreme unction, and ordination. Catholic churches still recognize all seven. Most Protestant churches recognize two sacraments: baptism and Communion (or the Eucharist or Lord's Supper). Except for baptism in the case of imminent death, most churches require ordained clergy to preside over the sacraments. However, nurses can be alert for appropriate opportunities to facilitate bringing clergy into the health care team so that the sacraments can be offered.

---

[11]*Book of Common Prayer*, 857.

[12]Irving Hexham, *Concise Dictionary of Religion* (Downers Grove, IL: InterVarsity Press, 1993), 193.

[13]C. O. Buchanan, "Sacrament," in *New Dictionary of Theology*, ed. Sinclair B. Ferguson and David F. Wright (Downers Grove, IL: InterVarsity Press, 1988), 607.

Spiritual Interventions

- Compassionate presence
- Active listening
- Witness

- Prayer
- Scripture
- Christian community

A Way of Life

We cannot underestimate the power of supportive presence in spiritual care—what Luther called the "mutual consolation of the saints."[14] This involves active listening, encouragement, expressing faith and hope, and compassionate physical care. Anticipating a person's physical needs, being willing to cheerfully handle foul-smelling excrement and bodily discharges, offering a gentle touch or a helping hand all communicate personal dignity and worth. They are just as much spiritual care as prayer and Bible reading. Perhaps one of the strongest drawing points of many alternative therapies is that practitioners spend extended time with the patient, paying particular attention to the body. However, only in the biblical worldview is the physical body viewed as reflecting the image of God and thereby worthy of respect and care.

Spiritual care is not a set of techniques, although we have many resources at our disposal. Spiritual care is a way of life that involves walking together with the Lord. Sometimes it is merely a listening ear or a gentle touch. At other times it requires more direct witness. The basic resources we have to offer are prayer, the Word of God, and the Christian community; however, the most important resource is God himself. The ultimate aim of our spiritual care is to bring people into a dynamic personal relationship with Jesus Christ and the fellowship of his people.

For Further Thinking

1. How would you describe the components of Christian spiritual care? How does this differ from *generic* spiritual care?

2. To whom are you accountable for the spiritual care you provide?

---

[14]Martin Luther, *Luther's Works*, vol. 2, *Lectures on Genesis: Chapters 6-14*, ed. Jaroslav Jan Pelikan, Hilton C. Oswald, and Helmut T. Lehmann (St. Louis: Concordia Publishing House, 1999), 335.

3. How do you measure spiritual outcomes?

4. Read the Joint Commission Standards for Spiritual Assessment online, available at: www.drdlevy.com/joint-commission-website-spiritual-assessment/. How could you incorporate these questions in your assessment of a patient in your care?

THEOLOGICAL REFLECTION

Read Matthew 9:2-8, Luke 4:18-19 (Isaiah 61:1-3), John 3:1-17, and Romans 8:5-6.

1. According to these passages, what is the significance of the spiritual dimension of a person?

2. Based on these Scripture passages, how would you define *spiritual care*?

3. Why should spiritual care be an integral aspect of nursing care?

   a. From God's perspective

   b. From a human perspective

4. How is spiritual care related to physical and psychosocial care?

Case Study: A Psalmist's View of His Spiritual Needs (Psalm 38)

O LORD, do not rebuke me in your anger,
  or discipline me in your wrath.
For your arrows have sunk into me,
  and your hand has come down on me.

There is no soundness in my flesh
  because of your indignation;
there is no health in my bones
  because of my sin.
For my iniquities have gone over my head;
  they weigh like a burden too heavy for me.

My wounds grow foul and fester
  because of my foolishness;
I am utterly bowed down and prostrate;
  all day long I go around mourning.
For my loins are filled with burning,
  and there is no soundness in my flesh.

I am utterly spent and crushed;
>   I groan because of the tumult of my heart.

O LORD, all my longing is known to you;
>   my sighing is not hidden from you.
My heart throbs, my strength fails me;
>   as for the light of my eyes—it also has gone from me.
My friends and companions stand aloof from my affliction,
>   and my neighbors stand far off.

Those who seek my life lay their snares;
>   those who seek to hurt me speak of ruin,
>   and meditate treachery all day long.

But I am like the deaf, I do not hear;
>   like the mute, who cannot speak.
Truly, I am like one who does not hear,
>   and in whose mouth is no retort.

But it is for you, O LORD, that I wait;
>   it is you, O LORD my God, who will answer.
For I pray, "Only do not let them rejoice over me,
>   those who boast against me when my foot slips."

For I am ready to fall,
>   and my pain is ever with me.
I confess my iniquity;
>   I am sorry for my sin.
Those who are my foes without cause are mighty,
>   and many are those who hate me wrongfully.
Those who render me evil for good
>   are my adversaries because I follow after good.

Do not forsake me, O LORD;
>   O my God, do not be far from me;
make haste to help me,
>   O LORD, my salvation.

DISCUSSION QUESTIONS

1. How does this psalmist-patient describe the reason for his suffering? How does he view his sin?

2. What physical symptoms does he exhibit?

3. What emotional responses accompany his illness? How has his illness affected his self-concept?

4. How does he perceive his friends and family? His enemies? God? Why do you think he felt as he did?

5. List all of the patient's expressed needs and develop a nursing care plan based on that self-assessment.

   a. What nursing diagnoses would you make?

   b. What interventions would be appropriate?

   c. What outcomes of care would you expect?

6. If this patient had expressed only the physical and emotional complaints, what questions would you ask him to determine if there were any underlying spiritual needs?

15

LOOKING TO THE FUTURE

Purpose: To envision a hopeful future for Christian nursing

Objectives: After reading this chapter and completing the exercises, you should be able to:
1. Identify three characteristics that contribute to high morale in nursing
2. Describe the factors influencing nursing education
3. Identify the problems inherent in scientific research in faith and health
4. Describe a practical theology of nursing

Keywords: future, context, integrity, nursing practice, nursing education, nursing metaparadigm, research, practical theology

STANDING IN LINE WHILE WAITING TO ENTER A THEATER, I (Judy) heard a voice calling, "Nurse! Nurse!" and saw a woman I did not recognize rushing toward me with a man in tow. When they arrived at my side, she said to the man, "This is my nurse." Then she turned to me and explained apologetically, "I wanted my husband to meet you." She then continued to her husband, "She is a good nurse; she brought me warm milk when I couldn't sleep, and then she prayed with me." At that point I remembered her. I had cared for her postoperatively over a year before.

Actually, this woman had been a rather difficult patient, not only due to her anxiety and insomnia, but because her condition initially required a great deal of complicated care. She had tested my nursing skills to the maximum. The warm milk and bedtime prayer offered the night before her discharge seemed insignificant to me compared with managing all the treatments, medications, tubes, and wires earlier in her hospitalization. Why did she view them as the mark of a good nurse?

What makes a *good nurse*? Is knowledge and skill enough? Where do the characteristics of care and compassion fit in? Who defines what constitutes a *good nurse*? In a time of rapidly changing roles and expectations, is there anything that remains constant in the definition of a good nurse?

Characteristics Nurses Need Most

- Compassion
- Competence
- Faith commitment
- Integrity
- Responsibility

How do nurses define a "good nurse"? In a survey of Christian nurses, we asked, what characteristics do nurses need most? Compassion rated highest (listed by 80 percent of participants), followed by competence (52 percent), faith commitment (26 percent), integrity (25 percent), and responsibility (10 percent).[1]

As we face the challenges of the chaotic health care environment, many nurses feel that we are losing something extremely important in the profession. The core of our identity seems to be eroding at the expense of cost-effectiveness and the constant pressure to do more with less. As the demands of the nursing role have escalated, and work environments have become increasingly stressful, research describing the effects of compassion fatigue, burnout, and secondary traumatic stress in nurses has surged. Compassion fatigue has been described by Beth Hudnall Stamm as encompassing two aspects: burnout (emotional exhaustion, detachment, hopelessness, and cynicism) and secondary traumatic stress (work-related trauma due to continued exposure to extremely stressful events).[2] The opposite of compassion fatigue has been labeled compassion satisfaction, described by Stamm as pleasure that is derived from doing work well. And yet, Kelly reminds us that "as nurses, simply being in the profession, places one at risk for compassion fatigue."[3]

What then, is the Christian nurse's response to the risk of compassion fatigue? Jesus set the moral standard for nursing by telling the story of the Good

---

[1]Judith Allen Shelly, "Health Ministries: A Dual Degree Program for Graduate Nursing Education," DMin diss., Lutheran Theological Seminary at Philadelphia, 1997.

[2]Beth Hudnall Stamm, *The Concise ProQOL Manual*, 2nd ed. (Pocatello, ID: ProQOL.org, 2010), 13.

[3]Lesly Kelly, "Burnout, Compassion Fatigue, and Secondary Trauma in Nurses: Recognizing the Occupational Phenomenon and Personal Consequences of Caregiving," *Critical Care Nursing Quarterly* 43, no. 1 (2020): 74.

Samaritan. That standard is no less than compassion—a compassion that demands competent care provided with commitment to the patient, integrity, and a deep sense of responsibility. We assert that as Christian nurses, our strength and resilience to combat the threat of compassion fatigue has its roots in faith. Repeatedly, God calls us to a life that is characterized by joy (Gal 5:22; Jn 15:11; 1 Pet 1:8) and compassion (Col 3:12). God has called us to care, and he will equip us to be compassionate. And although the work of nursing may be difficult, we can find joy in doing our work in the name of the Lord Jesus, giving thanks to God the Father through him (Col 3:17).

Nurses around the world celebrated 2020 as the International Year of the Nurse and the Midwife as proclaimed by the World Health Organization in recognition of the 200th birthday of Florence Nightingale.[4] Nightingale's legacy is worthy of recognition for her contribution to the profession of nursing. But as we reflect on the past, we cannot help but consider, What will nursing look like a hundred years from now? Or even fifty years from now? Economics will most certainly continue to shape health care delivery and access to health care. We will face alternating nursing shortages and job scarcity. As the population ages and chronic disease increases, specific nursing tasks will change. Technological developments will continue to escalate, and nurses will need to keep pace with all things digital. Artificial intelligence will do the work once done by humans. Virtual communication will replace face-to-face encounters as the use of telehealth increases. The milieu may be radically different. Christian nursing, however, will forever be a ministry of compassionate health care to anyone in need. We must not lose that! The mark of a good nurse will always be compassion—offering that cup of cold water (or warm milk) in the name of the Lord.

NURSING'S EXPANDING CONTEXT IN A COMPLEX WORLD

We have demonstrated throughout this book that nursing must view the person as holistic—a biopsychosocial and spiritual unity. That concept is not unique to Christian nursing. Have you ever met a nurse who saw only the physical aspect of care as that which defines nursing? We all know that when a person is hurting emotionally, all sorts of physical ailments crop up.

---

[4]"Year of the Nurse and the Midwife 2020," World Health Organization, accessed February 8, 2020, who.int/news-room/campaigns/year-of-the-nurse-and-the-midwife-2020.

On the other hand, physical conditions can affect the mind and the spirit. It's hard to concentrate or pray when you are hurting. Alzheimer's destroys the body and the mind. A serious diagnosis may cause a person to give up hope and die.

We have also examined the biblical understanding of shalom as it relates to health. Individuals, created by God with unique value and worth, find fulfillment in relationship with a human community. Most nurses today also acknowledge that we care for individuals in the context of families and communities. However, few have stopped to consider the full implications of that understanding. Of course, we support the family members who are present with our patients, we tap into community resources, and perhaps we even include their clergy in our care plans, but there is a larger perspective. Human connections—like families, communities, schools, and churches—function together to facilitate health. Nursing practice in the future must expand to include a broader participation in these extended relationships.

Health care delivery continues to evolve. As hospital stays become shorter, nurses are increasingly delivering primary health care to the places where people live, work, and worship. This focus on community health will empower people to accept more responsibility for their own health. There will be opportunities for faith community nursing to expand to facilitate a more comprehensive involvement of the church in health care—not only for congregational members but also for the poor and underserved in their communities and beyond.

First Corinthians 12:12-31 provides us with a glimpse of how God uses these interconnections. We are to be the body of Christ. Each organ functions uniquely, and they all need each other. Hearts can't do much good without lungs. Our bodies need nutrients digested and waste products excreted to sustain life. In a similar way, God puts individuals into relationships. For Christians, a primary connection is the church. Within the church, we support and care for one another. We can't just amputate a body part when it gives us trouble without affecting the whole body. When one part hurts, we all suffer. When one part receives honor, we all share in the glory.

The context of the church as a center for health care will continue to expand as economically driven health systems leave people confused and underserved. Even now, nurses are involved through counseling, leading support groups, teaching wellness, training lay caregivers, establishing and running centers for primary health care, referring people to appropriate resources, and advocating for them in the health care system. Nurses work in community-based health clinics and church-based health centers where the uninsured can come to receive free care and health screenings. These centers often provide more than health care. Nurses will continue to be the steady presence in the community to address the complex issues of poverty, decreased health literacy, food insecurity, substance abuse, and mental health issues.

Nurses will also always be involved in supporting families. None of these families is perfect. The first dysfunctional family appeared soon after creation and passed on their destructive family processes to all the generations that followed. Read the book of Genesis if you want to see the problem dramatically illustrated. However, the family is still the best place to find the love and nurture we need to prepare us for life. We then move out of our families of origin into new families, churches, and communities, only to reenact the same old patterns—both positive and negative.

As nurses we have the advantage of recognizing some of the dynamics involved in human relationships. To some degree we can be objective observers of the interrelationships between those processes. The skills we have learned in assessment, diagnosis, planning, intervention, and evaluation serve us well as we move into a new era of health care with shifting values, goals, and areas of practice. We are living in a time of increasingly broken relationships. The pain experienced in unstable families spills over into the church, the workplace, and the community at large. As nurses, we have some important contributions to make toward health and healing in each of these systems. For example, we can use our nursing skills to change unhealthy patterns in family dynamics through providing education and support for single parents and those affected by substance abuse, chronic illness, or grief.

As we move into the ever-expanding contexts of nursing—often not by our own choosing—we need to remember the biblical injunction, "Since we are surrounded by so great a cloud of witnesses, let us also lay aside every weight and the sin that clings so closely, and let us run with perseverance the race that is set before us, looking to Jesus the pioneer and perfecter of our faith" (Heb 12:1-2). The race is not easy. Many nurses are discouraged.

Maintaining Hope and Integrity in Nursing Practice

When we examine the state of health care, especially in the United States, it is easy to become discouraged and lose hope. In spite of the progress that has been made to care for the uninsured over the past two decades, there are still an estimated 30.7 million uninsured Americans.[5] The overall health of people is not improving even though health care spending is high. According to CMS.gov, in 2018 the United States spent just over $11,000 per person on health care, a number that represents approximately 17.7 percent of the nation's Gross Domestic Product.[6] Nonetheless, the United States experiences higher mortality rates and disease burden when compared to other large, wealthy countries.[7] Nurses are caring for patients with multiple comorbidities within the constraints of a complex health care system. The sources of stress are many. Among these are the burden of electronic documentation, insufficient staffing, the constant pressure to stay abreast of technology innovations, and the presence of unhealthy work environments. The phenomena of incivility and workplace bullying are rampant in institutions where healing and caring should be the first priority. It is not uncommon for new nurses to leave nursing as a result of their experience during their first year of transition to RN practice. In hopes to reduce RN turnover rates, nurse residency programs have sprung up in hospitals in an effort to mentor new nurses through what is often a stressful and difficult first year of transition to practice. A 2017 study of 1,464 newly licensed registered nurses revealed that only 83 percent of new nurses were retained in the first year of practice.[8]

---

[5]Micah Hartman, Anne B. Martin, Joseph Benson, and Aaron Catlin, "National Health Care Spending in 2018: Growth Driven by Accelerations in Medicare and Private Insurance Spending," *Health Affairs* 39, no. 1 (2020): 8-17.

[6]"National Health Expenditure Data: Historical," Centers for Medicare & Medicaid Services, December 17, 2019, www.cms.gov/Research-Statistics-Data-and-Systems/Statistics-Trends-and-Reports/NationalHealthExpendData/NationalHealthAccountsHistorical.

[7]Nisha Kurani, Daniel McDermott, and Nicolas Shanosky, "How Does the Quality of the U.S. Healthcare System Compare to Other Countries?," Peterson-KFF Health System Tracker, accessed February 8, 2020, www.healthsystemtracker.org/chart-collection/quality-u-s-healthcare-system-compare-countries/#item-start.

[8]Mary A. Blegin et al., "Newly Licensed RN Retention: Hospital and Nurse Characteristics," *The Journal of Nursing Administration* 47, no. 10 (2017): 508-14.

THREE COMMON THEMES

In the midst of this general sense of discouragement in nursing, some bright glimmers of hope continue to appear. When the *Journal of Christian Nursing* put out a call for brief articles on "Why I Love Nursing," the response was enthusiastic. What made these nurses different from their dispirited colleagues? Three common themes seemed to ring out from each of these authors: a sense of serving God by what they were doing, joy in their interpersonal relationships, and an ability to see the big picture.

The sense of serving God gave these nurses a vision of a greater mission and a willingness to suffer for it. This theme is perhaps most strongly voiced by those serving through their churches as faith community nurses. Over and over these nurses exclaim, "This is what I came into nursing to do!" Many of them have quit high-paying jobs in secular nursing to work for little or no pay. What are they doing? Their jobs include health assessments, screening, teaching, counseling, praying—and encouraging people to see the connection between faith and health.

Why Nurses Stay in Nursing

- Sense of serving God
- Interpersonal relationships
- Ability to see the big picture

On the other hand, many nurses are sensing God's call within their secular jobs. An oncology nurse recently told me (Kim), "I just have a passion for this. I have a peace that this is where I'm supposed to be. My faith is an important part of who I am, and so it has a huge impact on my career. It's my purpose to be a nurse." This nurse has sensed God's calling on her life and she is living out her purpose. Even on the most difficult days, as she cares for patients who are suffering, she feels joy in being able to do the "little things," like offering a sip of water, or turning a patient to keep him comfortable.

In a culture raised on a false gospel of "health and wealth," most of us have difficulty seeing God's hand in situations that involve pain, suffering, and deprivation. Some would go so far as to say that God is not blessing us if we must suffer loss or even discomfort. Nursing students frequently struggle with how to deal with the suffering and pain they see in their patients. I (Kim) encourage them to remember that as they care for patients, they are bringing comfort to ease the suffering during a time of vulnerability and fear. The apostle Paul encourages us further with his perspective reminding us to be light in a dark world. In writing to the Corinthian church he explained:

> For it is the God who said, "Let light shine out of darkness," who has shone in our hearts to give the light of the knowledge of the glory of God in the face of Jesus Christ. But we have this treasure in clay jars, so that it may be made clear that this extraordinary power belongs to God and does not come from us. We are afflicted in every way, but not crushed; perplexed, but not driven to despair; persecuted, but not forsaken; struck down, but not destroyed; always carrying in the body the death of Jesus, so that the life of Jesus may also be made visible in our bodies. For while we live, we are always being given up to death for Jesus' sake, so that the life of Jesus may be made visible in our mortal flesh. (2 Cor 4:6-11)

Although nursing in recent years has been viewed as a fairly well-paying, secure job, we have seen in earlier chapters that it did not begin this way. Throughout history, nurses have viewed their work as a calling from God and entered into the suffering of others to make a difference. To do that means challenging the forces of sin and evil in the world in the name of Jesus. Of course there will be opposition! Of course we will grow weary! The way will not be easy. But we will find a keen sense of mission and direction from God that gives us the hope to keep going when we feel afflicted, perplexed, persecuted, and struck down.

A second common thread in the testimonies of nurses who love nursing is *a delight in interpersonal relationships with patients and colleagues*. There is a deep sense of compassion for those who are suffering, an entrance into their lives to comfort and to care. These nurses tell stories of patients who were healed against all odds, and others who died in peace because of the nursing care they received. They relate incidents where they were able to help a colleague out of a tough situation or enable a health care team to work together in harmony. They also tell about how patients and coworkers encouraged them. That sense of mutuality makes them want to go to work each day, even in the midst of organizational change and personal injustices.

This same sense of joy inspired Paul in tough times. Consider 1 Thessalonians 2:19, "For what is our hope or joy or crown of boasting before our Lord Jesus at his coming? Is it not you?" The work he invested in the Thessalonians was rewarded by seeing their spiritual growth.

In the same way, we find joy and worth in our work by seeing patients get well, or die peacefully, and by working with a team that supports and respects one another. Paul continues in 1 Thessalonians 3:9, "How can we thank God enough for you in return for all the joy that we feel before our God because of you?" Seeing the fruit of our labors gives us the encouragement to keep going when the way becomes difficult.

The third common thread among nurses who love nursing is *an ability to see the big picture*. When crisis hits, they do not focus on what they are losing—they consider the needs and opportunities that arise out of the situation. They are willing to change and to take risks. Sometimes this means going back to school, moving to another area of nursing (or another location), or even breaking out into a completely new venture. These nurses have started nurse-managed clinics, extended-care facilities, and consultant services. Some have gone overseas as missionaries. Others have created new roles such as "spiritual care specialist" or "faith community nurse coordinator" within their present institutions.

Even in their retirement years, many nurses are making a difference by using their knowledge and skills to continue to serve others. It is often said, "Once a nurse, always a nurse"! We know of two nurses who had productive careers as nursing professors in a Christian college. They felt the call of God to start an inner-city clinic to serve the uninsured. This work is certainly not easy, but they rely on God to provide the resources and funding they need to keep their doors open.

A hospital staff nurse in Ohio writes, "I have chosen my goal—to serve Christ as a nurse. This has become my way of life, my ideal. I have a vision of the kind of nurse I want to be and I have the motivation I need—Christ. I am learning to trust him to help me achieve." She became a nurse after twenty years as a respiratory therapist. She knew that she might not find a job in nursing when she graduated, but she persevered because she knew God was calling her.

A home-health nurse in California saw people in her community falling through the cracks of the health care system, while at the same time several Christian nurses in her congregation lost their jobs to downsizing. She worked with them to set up a Christian home care agency that provides care at affordable rates.

It is encouraging to hear the testimonials of nurses who choose to see nursing as a calling and find joy in their vocation. In the face of challenge, it is time to reclaim our profession as a calling and to keep our vision for caring always before us. In the book *Guide to Nursing's Social Policy Statement*, Marsha Fowler describes the state of broken professions and eloquently calls for a restoration of "vocation as calling." She writes,

> Here, vocation as calling must be distinguished from *vocationalism*, a skills-based technicalism, with no roots in calling. In reclaiming the concept of vocation, the profession becomes part of the person's identity, the work meaningful, as "love of craft," and the occupation, more than just a job. . . . This is the nurse who loves nursing and who finds satisfaction, if not joy in service. Vocation is not only essential to civic professionalism, it also removes the possibility of runaway self-interest on the part of the professional.[9]

As Christian nurses, we recognize that our calling comes from God. Again, we turn to the apostle Paul, who writes,

> Not that I have already obtained this or have already reached the goal; but I press on to make it my own, because Christ Jesus has made me his own. Beloved, I do not consider that I have made it my own; but this one thing I do: forgetting what lies behind and straining forward to what lies ahead, I press on toward the goal for the prize of the heavenly call of God in Christ Jesus. (Phil 3:12-14)

The goal of nursing is not personal satisfaction; it is not maintaining the health care system as we have known it in the past few decades. Christian nursing has always been about pressing on toward the heavenly call of God in Christ Jesus—working toward shalom, announcing the in-breaking kingdom of God and demonstrating its presence through acts of justice and mercy. When we keep this goal in mind, we can look ahead with expectancy, knowing that when God calls us, he will lead us. He will equip us and ultimately work things together for good (Rom 8:28).

THE CHANGING FACE OF NURSING EDUCATION

As nursing practice changes, so must nursing education. Central to the task of nursing education is the need to clearly envision the knowledge, skills, and

---

[9]Marsha D. M. Fowler, *Guide to Nursing's Social Policy Statement: Understanding the Profession from a Social Contract to Social Covenant* (Silver Spring, MD: American Nurses Association, 2015), 65-66.

attitudes that will equip today's students to be tomorrow's practitioners. However, rather than looking at fads and trends, we might do well to re-examine the nursing metaparadigm from an eternal perspective—to develop a theology of nursing. In doing so, we gain insight into the trends and discernment over the fads.

It is God who calls us into nursing in the first place and gives us the wisdom and strength to endure when the going gets tough. Nursing education that neglects teaching this perspective leaves students without a moral foundation or clear motivation for nursing.

Nursing theory development is essentially a theological as well as philosophical process. So is curriculum development. Without a solid understanding of who God is and what he intends for us to be, we cannot develop appropriate nursing curricula or design the courses to prepare future nurses.

> *Without a solid understanding of who God is and what he intends for us to be, we cannot develop appropriate nursing curricula or design the courses to prepare future nurses.*

Part of the root cause of nursing's present confusion, and to a large degree, disintegration, comes from the absence of a guiding common theology. Some are trying to superimpose three opposing paradigms and come up with an "inclusive" whole. Others pick and choose eclectically, supposing that we can merely take what seems best from each. That simply won't work.

As we have seen, many of the current health care fads draw nurses toward spiritism and New Age thinking. Shifting moral values and ethical approaches, alternative therapies, new paradigms, and expanded roles lure nurses into seemingly attractive directions. Only a clear understanding of Christian theology, along with a vital faith relationship with God, will give us the discernment to choose wisely and faithfully from the increasing array of options available.

For nurse educators, especially those who teach in faith-based colleges and universities, opportunities abound to model Christian faith in the classroom, in the clinical area, and even one on one with students who may be struggling. Nurse educators can come alongside students to help them grow in their faith by sharing Scripture and offering to pray with them. One of the purposes of this book is to help students consider the concepts of person, health, environment, and nursing from a Christian lens. Nursing students must grapple with the difficult questions before they begin clinical practice so that they are well grounded in truth. Furthermore, students need to gain competence in practical theology—knowing how to share their faith, how to pray with patients and read Scripture appropriately, how to listen to the Spirit as well as the patient, and how to participate as colleagues in ministry along with the clergy and the body of Christ. Even students with strong personal faith need to learn how to practice Christian ministry in a health care setting.

The need for a theological foundation for nursing becomes especially evident in faith community nursing. Those who teach faith community nurses must be well grounded in theology as well as nursing. A nurse educator who happens to be a Christian is no more prepared to teach faith community nursing than a theologian who makes occasional hospital visits. We need a growing number of nurse-theologians who can view nursing through the eyes of faith, not only to teach faith community nurses, but also to shape the future of nursing and nursing education.

REVISITING THE NURSING METAPARADIGM

Once we have established a theological focus, nursing education needs to take seriously the biblical view of the environment, the person, and health. Several themes require special consideration: the goodness of creation, the effects of sin, the seen and the unseen aspects of the environment, the mandate God has given us as caretakers of creation, and the understanding of the person as an integrated whole, created to live in shalom with God, the human community, and the environment.

Mary Oesterle and Darlene O'Callaghan outlined some of the big questions in nursing education two decades ago:

1. In a health care system that is increasingly defining roles and responsibilities of assistive personnel, are basic skills such as bed-bath and bed-making principles essential content to a baccalaureate curriculum?

2. Why are we preparing students with an emphasis on practice in acute-care hospitals when the futurists identify them as becoming a collection of intensive care units, employing a limited number of our graduates?

3. Is nursing education congruent with the needs of the emerging health care environment?

4. Can we afford to structure our curriculum around specific content when knowledge changes so rapidly?

5. Why do we continue this focus on skills when assessment knowledge, critical thinking, decision making, and collaboration are essential processes of the future?[10]

It is in response to these questions that a Christian view of the nursing metaparadigm gives profound insight. Let's look at the first question. Yes, the reality for nursing today is that assistive personnel perform much of the physical care in the community, as well as acute-care settings. Many skills may become obsolete. Who needs mitered corners when we have fitted sheets? On the other hand, how many nursing students today have ever learned to make a bed properly? Can they teach the assistive personnel? Can they look at a patient and figure out that the decubitus on his sacrum may have something to do with lumps in the linens and improper positioning? Will they even see the skin breakdown if they do not spend time assessing the patient's skin while performing a bath?

Consider the perspective given by nurse educator Carol Bence as she addresses her graduating class:

> When we bathe another person we cross the intimacy barrier; something is shared. We get up close and personal with another human being. We enter his or her world. It is a humbling act for both the washer and the washee. It is an act of compassion. Too often, perhaps, we want to hurry through the bath so we can get on with the more important aspects of nursing. But perhaps it is in the simple ritual of the bath that we discover what it means to be a true nurse.[11]

As Christians we have a unique understanding of, and respect for, the human body. Our theology tells us that the body is important, warranting our nurture and care. In our rush to prepare managers and health promoters, we dare not neglect the seemingly mundane details of physical care.

In relating to other members of the health care team, Christian nurses have a model of servant leadership in Jesus Christ. Rather than seeking glory in the "more important roles" of the professional nurse, we have a responsibility to respect and support all members of the health care team. If we really care

---

[10]Mary Oesterle and Darlene O'Callaghan, "The Changing Health Care Environment: Impact on Curriculum and Faculty," *N&HC: Perspectives on Community* 12 (1996): 79-80.

[11]Carol Bence, "The Towel, the Bath," *Journal of Christian Nursing* (1997): 24.

for patients, then we must also care for all who are providing patient care. We also need to give them a good reason to respect us by demonstrating competency, confidence, and compassion.

To answer Oesterle and O'Callaghan's second question, we must be careful not to assume that students will be able to gain confidence in nursing skills and see the whole picture of health care without experience in a hospital setting. Many of the skills now required in home care and extended-care facilities were formerly practiced only in hospitals. With the high acuity of hospitalized patients and shorter hospital stays, nurses need more than skill. They need sound clinical judgment within the interprofessional health care team to deliver safe, quality care. Nurses must understand the complexities of systems and organizations, and become expert communicators and effective collaborators. Many nursing programs now use simulation to augment clinical time in the community and hospital. Advances in simulation technology make it possible for students to practice skills on a mannequin programmed to respond to student interventions. Thus, students can experience hands-on learning without fear of making a high-stakes error.

Nursing education will continually change to meet the needs of the emerging health care environment, including the growing field of informatics and health care technology. Students will also learn from a creative community experience, gaining expertise in assessment, critical thinking, decision making, and collaboration. Yet there must always be a body of knowledge and skill that makes a nurse a nurse. Of course skills will change! But the principles involved will easily transfer to new technologies and new contexts of care.

Nursing education also changes in response to research findings and standards set by our professional organizations. A body of evidence indicates that patients have lower mortality and fewer complications when cared for by a baccalaureate-prepared nurse. Thus, many hospitals now require a Bachelor of Science in Nursing degree as a condition of employment.

In the landmark report *The Future of Nursing: Leading Change, Advancing Health*, experts outlined several recommendations for the nursing profession to consider in order to effectively meet the health care needs of the nation.[12]

---

[12]Institute of Medicine, *The Future of Nursing: Leading Change, Advancing Health* (Washington, DC: The National Academies Press, 2011).

Among these recommendations was to double the number of nurses with a doctoral degree by 2020. Since the American Association of the Colleges of Nursing (AACN) endorsed the Doctor of Nursing Practice (DNP) degree as the clinical doctorate for nursing in 2006, the number of DNP programs has risen to nearly 350 nationwide.[13] What does this mean for the profession? Just as other professions have embraced doctoral-level education as entry for practice (pharmacists, physical therapists), advanced practice nurses must be educated at the doctoral level as well.

Another change on the horizon for nursing is a move toward competency-based education. The current "Essentials" documents that have guided nursing curricula for accredited programs are undergoing significant revision in an effort to more adequately prepare the nursing workforce across all levels of education.[14] Increasingly, accredited institutions offer nursing education programs, especially graduate education and degree completion programs, online. This trend will no doubt continue as nurses look for convenience and efficiency to earn advanced degrees.

As we consider the legitimate questions about how students will prepare for nursing in the next decade, we continue to focus our attention on what makes nursing, nursing. Obviously, it is not specific skills, nor a particular context, or even an immutable body of knowledge. We define Christian nursing as a ministry of compassionate care for the whole person in response to God's grace, which aims to foster optimum health (shalom) and bring comfort in suffering and death for anyone in need. The way we prepare nursing students must include the best of science, technology, the arts, and practical skills, which are consistent with a Christian worldview in order to nurture people toward health.

In the process we must not lose sight of the whole person or any dimensions of that wholeness. We must not neglect the care of the body or the care of the soul. We must also be careful to maintain shalom, for those in our care and all those within the nursing community. We must guard against preparing nurses to be lone practitioners without the support and accountability of a professional community as well as a Christian community.

---

[13]"DNP Fact Sheet," American Association of Colleges of Nursing, March 2019, www.aacnnursing.org/News-Information/Fact-Sheets/DNP-Fact-Sheet.

[14]"AACN Essentials," American Association of Colleges of Nursing, accessed February 15, 2020, www.aacnnursing.org/Education-Resources/AACN-Essentials.

Finally, we must consider the character of the nurse—those qualities that make a nurse. While critical thinking, decision making, and leadership skills are extremely important, our research shows that practicing nurses believe that the characteristics nurses need most are compassion, competence, faith, integrity, and responsibility. It is understandable that compassion ranks quite high as a desirable characteristic. What the public may not realize is that in many colleges and universities, the admission criteria for the nursing program is on par with the engineering department. Nursing education is gaining parity with the disciplines of science, technology, engineering, and math, commonly known today as STEM. Nursing programs are held to very high standards by state boards of nursing and accrediting bodies for "first time pass rates" on the National Council Licensing Examination (NCLEX), which is the exam that yields the RN credential. Such a high standard is actually a good thing. Nurses need to be knowledgeable and skilled in order to be competent safe clinicians.

The values of faith, integrity, and responsibility are consistent with what Jesus requires of us. In Matthew 22:37-39 Jesus tells us, "'You shall love the Lord your God with all your heart, and with all your soul, and with all your mind.' This is the greatest and first commandment. And a second is like it: 'You shall love your neighbor as yourself.'"

One of the greatest challenges for nursing education in the coming years will be shaping the character of students who have grown up in a culture that handicaps them in four ways:

- They have been given no standard of absolute truth.
- They have few models of love and faithfulness.
- They have absorbed a sense of personal entitlement that views selfless care for others as dysfunctional behavior.
- They have unprecedented levels of anxiety.

Nursing must return to its theological roots to maintain its heart and soul.

EXPLORING THE CHALLENGE BEFORE US: NURSING RESEARCH

Ever since nursing education entered the university through the door of science, nursing educators have been working to establish a body of knowledge unique to nursing through research. As we saw in chapter two, this orientation became the impetus for developing nursing theories. Most of the earlier nursing theories reflect the influence of naturalistic science. Because such theories could not adequately account for the human experience of health and illness, nurses broadened the scope of nursing theory. Qualitative research has gained credibility as an approach to describe the complex phenomena that are part of the human experience: hope, resilience, suffering, and grief as examples.

No matter the approach, nurse researchers need to be clear about the philosophical and theological underpinnings of the theories and research designs they use. Under pressure to complete theses and dissertations, Christian nurses may select research instruments without a clear understanding of their underlying philosophies. Research instruments are not neutral. The questions, and the things they are designed to measure, contain worldview and, possibly, religious assumptions that need to be discerned and explicitly described.

Investigators who use qualitative approaches such as phenomenology need to approach the research situation without being influenced by their own preconceived opinions and beliefs (i.e., bracketing). However, it is a challenge for researchers to free themselves of their own values and assumptions. In grounded theory methods however, there is the expectation that the researcher will show theoretical sensitivity, that is, to interpret the data from the lens of personal experience and knowledge about the topic being researched. It is essential for researchers to identify their worldview through a personal philosophy statement. It is through the dialogue between our experience and our prior understandings that we build our knowledge base. What keeps this dialogue from merely going in circles, for Christians, is that we can test our conclusions by God's revelation to us in Scripture. This is particularly important in studies involving psychosocial and spiritual concepts. Nurse researchers need to recognize, and acknowledge, their own presuppositions to be fair to those who read and use their work.

Good research will help nurses improve patient care as evidence informs clinical practice. All aspects of the person are legitimate areas for research—physical, psychological, social, and spiritual. The increasing interest in spirituality and health carries both positive and negative connotations, however. Christian spirituality pertains to the relationship of people with God. Expecting God to grant our requests with predetermined measurable results borders on idolatry. For example, measuring improved hemoglobin levels to determine whether God answers prayer would be inappropriate. However, research studies designed to show the correlation between health and religious practices, like prayer and church attendance, are legitimate, so long as they are presented only as descriptions of what people do and how they respond, not what God does. Positive correlations may indicate the general outcomes for people who love and obey God.

Studies about prayer can only be viewed from the human side. God, by his very nature, cannot be locked into a cause-and-effect study. Further, most studies purporting to show the value of prayer do not make any claims about the kind of god being addressed. Most of them simply account for any benefits on the basis of psychological effect of ritual. Some researchers, however, consider prayer as a means of linking into the universal consciousness. Christians who want to study any relationship between prayer and health should differentiate between a biblical understanding of prayer and the use of prayer as a manipulative technique (see the previous discussion on prayer in chapter fourteen).

Research studies on spiritual needs of patients abound. Usually patients are asked what they see as their spiritual needs. In other instances, nurse researchers use questionnaires with built-in assumptions about the nature of spiritual needs. In both approaches the identified spiritual needs may not be the real needs of patients. For example, the Bible has much to say about godly sorrow and repentance from sin. Repentance and sin are not usually the focus of nursing studies. In fact, most studies of spiritual needs focus on patients' psychological needs rather than a relationship between God and the person. Christians need to come to their research with a biblical understanding of the spiritual.

Finally, Christian nurses must be humble about their findings. We know that the full meaning of being human cannot be captured in research. The person, the environment, health, and nursing can only be fully understood in relationship with God. Discovering the fullness and implications of that relationship is a lifelong process. In fact, it cannot fully be accomplished in this life. In the meantime, we walk in faith.

EVIDENCE-BASED PRACTICE

What is our responsibility for evidence-based practice? As Christian nurses, we strive for excellence in all that we do, whether we are giving medications at the bedside, leading a unit-based committee, or teaching a patient's family how to change a dressing. Part of being excellent is taking responsibility to stay abreast of the best evidence for practice. Nurses must be committed to lifelong learning. We need to be open to learning new ways of doing things, even to the point of taking the initiative to do the hard work of appraising research evidence for practice. Most nurses frown at the suggestion that they should read research articles to determine best practice. Even though research and evidence-based practice methods are included in most nursing curricula, many practicing nurses do not feel adequately prepared to search the literature, critique the articles, and synthesize the evidence to determine best practice. The future of nursing depends on nurses who are clinician-scholars. We must take ownership of our practice, and that includes honing our skills in evidence-based practice.

As we have seen, nursing grew out of the life and teachings of Jesus Christ. If this is so, then we need to look at the ministry goals and outcomes of Jesus. According to the Scriptures, Jesus expressed a threefold mission of[15]

- healing the sick,
- restoring the relationship between God and his people, and
- restoring people to the human community.

In today's nursing, we'd call that whole-person care—attending to the physical, spiritual, and psychosocial needs of those in our care. In surveying the healing accounts listed from the Gospels and Acts in table 10.1, it appears that Jesus and the apostles would have no trouble being accredited as effective health care providers. They met physical needs 100 percent of the time. Everyone who sought healing was physically cured. In 97 percent of the situations, the biblical accounts indicate that the healed persons were restored to their communities as functioning members. Lepers came out of their legally imposed isolation. Blind beggars went back to their families. The disabled got up and walked home. The other 3 percent may have also been restored, but it was not documented.

Interestingly, only 82 percent of cases in the New Testament recorded that spiritual needs were met. Sometimes the issue just didn't come up, such as when Jesus healed Peter's mother-in-law of a high fever (Mt 8:14-15), or when he restored a Roman soldier's severed ear (Lk 22:47-51). However, when Jesus

---

[15]For Jesus' ministry goals see Mt 9:12-13; Lk 4:18-19; Jn 10:10.

healed the ten lepers, although all ten were cured of leprosy, only one came back to thank him. To that man Jesus replied, "Get up and go on your way; your faith has made you well" (Lk 17:11-19). There was fuller dimension to his healing that the other nine did not experience.

So what does this mean for Christian nursing? We, too, have a threefold ministry. Excellence in physical care ranks high in the mix, but it is incomplete without good psychosocial support and spiritual care. We won't cure every client physically (even The Joint Commission doesn't hold us to that standard). Our evidence may be even less apparent when it comes to patching up families and communities. We may feel pretty discouraged about the evidence for spiritual outcomes, but once in a while God uses us in amazing ways. When that happens, we are usually caught off-guard and taken by surprise.

> *We have a threefold ministry—excellence in physical care ranks high in the mix, but it is incomplete without good psychosocial support and spiritual care.*

The ultimate outcome of good spiritual care is always restoration of a person's relationship with God. That may include better physical and emotional health, but we may not see those results. Being restored to God usually does include reconciliation in human relationships, the ability to forgive others and accept forgiveness, to love and be loved. It brings fresh meaning and purpose to life and a sense of hope.

A PRACTICAL THEOLOGY

Asked to summarize his theology, the eminent theologian Karl Barth once replied, "Jesus loves me—this I know for the Bible tells me so."[16] In the face of a complicated technological society and an uncertain future, we might do well to stick with such a basic assertion. God's love, demonstrated for us in the person of Jesus Christ and recorded in the Bible, provides the core of our theological stance.

Because God's love is active and empowering, our theology must also be practical and dynamic. In nursing, knowing God's love impels us to care for

---

[16]See Roger E. Olson, "Did Karl Barth Really Say 'Jesus Loves Me, This I Know . . .'?," *Patheos*, January 24, 2013, www.patheos.com/blogs/rogereolson/2013/01/did-karl-barth-really-say-jesus -loves-me-this-i-know.

anyone in need, as it has inspired nurses for the past two thousand years. That includes seeking out and caring for the poor, the weak and the disenfranchised of society. It may involve joining the political process to advocate for those who cannot defend their own rights.

Nursing demonstrates God's love in a ministry of compassionate care for the whole person—physical, psychosocial, and spiritual. It aims to foster optimum health and bring comfort in suffering and death. The health toward which we strive is part of the greater work of God to bring completeness, soundness and well-being (shalom) to the total person—in relationship to God, self, others, and the environment. Nursing is a work of God's grace. We are privileged to share in that work.

For Further Thinking

1. What is your vision for the future of nursing? Write your vision and share it with others.

2. How does knowing Jesus Christ shape your vision?

Theological Reflection

Read Jeremiah 29:1-14.

1. According to Jeremiah, God *sent* his people into exile. What difference would it make to you to know that God had actually put you into a difficult situation?

2. How did God instruct the Jewish exiles to live while in exile (verses 4-9)? Consider the significance of each command—both to the exiles and to their Babylonian neighbors.

3. Apply these same instructions to your work situation. What difference would it make if you followed the same principles there?

4. What hope is offered in verses 10-14? What promises does God make to his people?

5. As you consider your own future as a nurse, what are your greatest hopes?

6. According to verses 12-14, what responsibilities do you have in reaching that hope?

7. What is God's part?

8. How can you share that hope with others?

CASE STUDY: NURSING'S FUTURE—SEVEN CHRISTIAN NURSING LEADERS SHARE THEIR VISION

A healing resource for the world. My vision for nursing is that we are a healing resource for the world. Nurses provide more than 80 percent of all direct care worldwide, yet frequently when world health is discussed, nurses are not involved. At times the emphasis on what we do leaves no room in the public's perception for what we know and our ability to maximize the knowing and doing of others. However, our in-depth client relationships enable us to be effective health care leaders with individuals, communities, and nations. In my vision, there is no service without effective decision making in which nurses are key players.

With a vision of nursing shaping and leading in health care, public health could lead the world health agenda. I see nurses as designers, monitors, and caregivers in this health care system.

To accomplish this, Christian nurses should daily demonstrate the power of Jesus Christ. This includes four types of power. *Informational power* includes the message of hope, salvation, and eternal peace that is skillfully communicated through words and behaviors with mutual respect across race, age, gender, faith, and other areas of diversity. *Legitimate power* comes through our license to practice, but more so through the blood of Christ and the empowerment of the Holy Spirit. *Charismatic power* enables us to show the joy we have in serving Christ through delivering quality care to patients with smile power and pure enjoyment in healing. *Extended power* is inviting others to join God's family. It is not enough that we are heirs to the incredible power of a living Savior; we must share it, pointing the way to salvation and praising the Son of God, Jesus Christ.

Beverly Malone, PhD, RN, FAAN, Chief Executive Officer for the National League of Nursing, formerly General Secretary of the Royal College of Nursing, United Kingdom, past president of the American Nurses Association and former Deputy Assistant Secretary for Health, U.S. Department of Health and Human Services.

• • •

An instrument of God. My vision for nursing is that every nurse should experience Jesus Christ as his or her personal Savior and Lord and, in turn, be an instrument of God. I envision nursing as a life-receiving, life-promoting, and life-accomplishing practice, where every nurse cares as Jesus cares for each of us—with compassionate heart, competent faith, conscientious deeds, and a committed call to care. The client we serve is the center and core object of nursing, and may be overwhelmed by illness and death or in a confused, forgotten state. That's why the scope of nursing is wide and deep—not limited to curing and treating—extending to caring and to healing.

Susie Kim, DNSc, RN, FAAN, formerly professor, chairperson of Psychiatric-Mental Health Nursing Division, Ewha Womans University, Seoul, Korea. She was editor of Korean Journal of Nursing Science and Gidok Kanho (Christian Nursing), past president of the Korean Academy of Nursing, and the 2001 recipient of the International Council of Nurses Nightingale International Achievement Award. Dr. Kim lived her vision. She developed an outstanding example of community health care for long-term psychiatric patients. With funding from the United Nations Development Program (UNDP), she set up four community-based mental health centers. Psychiatric nurses run the adult daycare centers and follow up with home visits. On Sundays one of these centers also serves as a church for long-term psychiatric patients and their families. The pastor felt called to this ministry after his young-adult son developed chronic schizophrenia. These community centers help patients learn to function so they can get back into society. Christian psychiatric nurses encourage them as they gradually get back into normal life. After retirement Dr. Kim founded a school of nursing in Malawi.

● ● ●

A clay jar. My vision for nursing comes from Paul's biblical teaching that those who know Jesus possess a great treasure. Paul reminds us, however, that it is a treasure held in "clay jars," so that it may be clear that the extraordinary power belongs to God and does not come from us (2 Cor 4:7). This message gives us the mandate to let the light of Christ, which has shone in our hearts, be reflected in all activities of our nursing ministry. These activities may be the academic work of teaching and writing, the leadership roles of administration and management or the treasured ministry of direct, hands-on care.

By attempting to live out scriptural teachings to the best of our abilities, Christian nurses can profoundly influence the profession for Jesus Christ. In this era of complex health care systems fraught with political, financial, and ethical dilemmas, the practice of Christian nursing must stand out as a shining beacon of selfless commitment to the needs of others as mandated by Jesus. Christian nurses must be leaders in the art and science of loving care and compassion in whatever area of practice they find themselves.

At times, this may take a toll on the Christian nurse—both physically and emotionally. But the gospel teaches that although suffering may result from Christian ministry, the rewards are great.

Sr. Mary Elizabeth O'Brien, PhD, RN, FAAN, AHN, professor emeritus, The Catholic University of America School of Nursing, Washington, DC. She is the author of Spirituality in Nursing: Standing on Holy Ground *and numerous other publications on spirituality and nursing. Sr. Mary Elizabeth is a compassionate nurse, as well as a dedicated teacher, mentor, and writer.*

• • •

Encouraging others. My vision expanded remarkably when I allowed Christ into my life. Through Jesus' example, I understood holistic care in a new way and gained an appreciation for the profound interrelationship of body, mind, and spirit. I realized that using aseptic techniques to close a wound and administering a medication on schedule weren't enough. Time and effort had to be devoted to ministering to the suffering spirits.

Walking with Christ redefined my priorities. Being top in my field, holding a high-power, high-status position doesn't seem as important as serving. I take time to minister to nurses, nursing assistants, and others who provide care, to lighten their loads, offer a word of encouragement, and recognize the ways their daily contributions positively affect lives.

My hope is that nurses will recapture and reignite the vision of nursing as a healing art rather than allowing insurers, accountants, administrators, and planners to define care, quality, and our roles. Christian nurses have a special role in influencing the profession for Jesus Christ. We do this through proclaiming Jesus Christ as our Savior and by sharing stories in welcoming languages and styles. More important, we influence by practicing nursing the way Jesus would if he were in our shoes. This means answering a call light in a room to which we're not assigned, taking time to hold a hand and finding blessing in a situation instead of complaining. It also means taking care of ourselves and encouraging colleagues to do the same, sharing our time, talents, and money to aid those in need, starting each shift with prayer for staff and patients, and loving the unlovable. By living out our ordinary lives in extraordinary ways, we leave the sweet fragrance and everlasting light of Jesus Christ wherever we go and cast an enlightened vision for nursing.

Charlotte Eliopoulos, RNC, MPH, CDONA / LTC, past president, American Holistic Nurses' Association, author of Gerontological Nursing.

• • •

A special calling. My knowledge and relationship with Jesus Christ influences my life and all its activities. My religious insights have increased my compassion and patience, and my religious beliefs about justice and the rights of people have motivated me to work for a better health care system. Today I work to secure access to health care for the 43.6 million people in our country without health insurance.

I believe nursing is a vocation, a special calling to assist the sick and to work for a better and just society. As a nurse, I have been educated and socialized to prevent and to treat illness, to care for the sick and to manage their illness experience. Education and professional associations have expanded my opportunities to achieve these goals through practice, education, research, and policy development.

My vision of nursing as a calling, a profession, and a ministry urges me to be prepared and competent, to act in the best interest of patients and students, to collaborate with others to assure access and quality care for patients and their families, and to educate the next generation of nurses to practice in a more just health care system.

Sr. Rosemary Donley, PhD, APRN, FAAN, is professor and and holds the Jacques Laval Chair for Justice for Vulnerable Populations at Duquesne University School of Nursing and is past president of the National League for Nursing and Sigma International Honor Society of Nursing.

• • •

A Christ-centered ministry. I have a vision for nursing to be a Christ-centered ministry. Nursing is an avenue to be part of what God has been doing throughout history—caring for those who are suffering and ill. Through nursing care that represents Jesus, people can discover that God cares and is present with them. Nurses practicing Christ-centered nursing, in collaboration with other colleagues in health care, have the potential to make a profound difference in the moral and ethical issues we face. God can transform nursing and health care through nurses empowered by the Holy Spirit.

In the words of Matthew 5:13-15, we are to represent Jesus in the world (including nursing) by being *salt* and *light*. Salt preserves, brings out inherent flavor, and creates thirst. Our lives should demonstrate these same characteristics. Biblical values preserve our Christian heritage in nursing and bring vital direction to our profession. Christian attitudes and behavior infuse peace, joy, and hope in nursing environments and help nurses find fulfillment in their work. Light reveals, heals, and dispels darkness and fear. Our good deeds reveal God's character and standards for righteousness. Being light may include God using us to help heal broken lives and relationships. The light of God's wisdom reveals truth and gives discernment in difficult situations.

Based on Jeremiah 29:1-11, Christian nurses can influence the future of nursing in six ways:

- building healthy nursing environments, where we can practice nursing with integrity and faithfulness
- serving within the community of nursing by becoming involved in institutional committees and nursing organizations
- praying for our nursing colleagues and leaders
- developing a Christian worldview and living out our beliefs with grace and truth
- trusting that God has plans "to give you a future with hope" (Jer 29:11)
- seeking God's will and direction

God is gathering Christian nurses from all nations to worship and honor the Lord almighty. It is exciting to envision what will happen!

Mary Thompson, MSN, RN, former director, Nurses Christian Fellowship, USA, a ministry of InterVarsity Christian Fellowship/USA; former president, Nurses Christian Fellowship International.[17]

---

[17]Adapted from Kathy Schoonover-Shoffner, "Global Leaders Cast a Vision for Nursing," *Journal of Christian Nursing* (2004): 22-27.

• • •

Looking to the future: What's next in nursing? As long as I can remember, my mother always talked about how wonderful it would be to be a nurse. She always wanted to be a nurse but in the 1940s, the opportunities for Black women to go to college were few to none. My mother chose another vocation and became a cosmetologist. Her conviction and respect for nurses came in 1958 when her mother, Elcie, was diagnosed with diabetes. My mother had married and was living in Chicago. She returned to Arkansas to care for her mom and to seek proper medical care. At the time, few Blacks had health insurance or access to health care. Most relied on the local midwife and home remedies. When my mother arrived, she realized that her mother was desperately ill. She sought out another Black family who had access to services that were not available to those who lived in rural areas. With their assistance, she was able to get her mother transported two hours away to the state's medical center. Although, she was able to get treatment, the long untreated complications resulted in her death at age fifty-eight.

This experience created in my mom a deep respect for the nursing profession. As she watched the nurses care for her mother, she realized how a nurse could affect a person's life. A year later, I was born. From my earliest days, I recall my mother encouraging me to be a nurse. She would tell me how wonderful nurses were and how they helped people. She would say, "Nursing is the most noble profession." Although my mom never became a nurse, she nurtured a love and respect for nursing in me. And today I am still improving the lives of people as a Christian nurse, fostering healing, not only to the body but also the soul.

Understanding nursing concepts from a Christian worldview is critical in developing future nurse leaders. Nursing as a profession is at a crossroads; the ability to lead in an ever-changing environment will require a focus on care outcomes, increased diversity of the workforce, competency based-learning, digital fluency, and point of care.

The framework that God has given me to lead effectively is *WIT*. Equipping Christian nurses to lead in a world of constant change will require three key attributes: wisdom, integrity, and transparency, easily remembered as WIT. *Wisdom* is having experience, knowledge, and good judgment to make sound, effective, and right decisions. *Integrity* is a moral compass characterized by the use of ethical principles to exhibit honesty, trustworthiness, and impeccable character. Finally, *transparency* is operating in such a way that others can to see how and why decisions are made and pursue specific goals. Transparency involves being straightforward, unambiguous, open, plain-spoken, and forthright. WIT defines the reason for my mother's convictions about the nobleness of the nursing profession.

Honoring God by caring for people where they are and exercising WIT will set us apart as Christian nurses and ground us in difficult times. With this level of commitment and leadership proficiency, nurses will successfully navigate changes and uncertainties as we approach the next revolution in health care, education, and nursing.

My mother was right! The ability to touch people's lives at their most happy and most vulnerable moments allows nurses to care for people in whatever health environment they reside.

Lepaine Sharp-McHenry, *DNP, RN, is dean and professor at the Simmons University College of Natural, Behavioral, and Health Sciences.*

Discussion Questions

1. With which of these vision statements do you most identify? For what reasons?

2. Each of these leaders has chosen to accept positions of influence in secular nursing organizations. How have you been involved with nursing organizations? To what extent have you been able to speak within these organizations from a Christian perspective?

3. Nursing organizations often take positions on issues that individual members may not fully endorse. How would you respond if an organization in which you were a member endorsed an ethical position that you could not support?

4. Mary Thompson led a Christian professional nursing organization. What advantages and limitations do you see in a specifically Christian professional organization?

   a. For influencing nursing as a whole

   b. For supporting and encouraging members

5. In what ways do you think Christians can most effectively work toward a positive future for nursing?

   a. In nursing practice

   b. In nursing education

   c. Through research

   d. By contributing to the nursing literature

   e. Through nursing organizations

   f. By influencing health policy

Appendix

GUIDELINES FOR EVALUATING ALTERNATIVE THERAPIES

THE FOLLOWING QUESTIONS CAN BE GUIDELINES for evaluating holistic health modalities. They provide us with a systematic way to assess the potential religious philosophical problems hiding behind alternative therapies.[1]

MODALITY

1. What techniques are necessary to practice the modality (meditation, "mindfulness," mind control, and so on)? Meditating on a portion of Scripture, the character of God, or the "peace of Christ" may be helpful; emptying the mind or using more mystical techniques can be dangerous.

2. Are assumptions made regarding human nature or the nature of ultimate reality? If so, are they compatible with Scripture? Techniques that purport to manipulate energy often explain it as being the Holy Spirit. Remember, the Holy Spirit is God, and we cannot manipulate God; instead we submit, request, and obey.

3. Are these assumptions clearly evident to all observers, or must one be involved with the modality to determine what they are? Most alternative therapies are experientially based. Spiritual assumptions will not be evident until a person has practiced them for a while. However, nursing literature is expressing these assumptions more overtly as public acceptance increases.

4. Has the technique been subjected to peer-reviewed scientific research, and have results been confirmed by subsequent studies? Keep in mind that poor research can prove almost anything. Some (most) alternative therapies are based on anecdotal evidence.

---

[1] Adapted and expanded from Arlene Miller, "Evaluating Holistic Health Modalities," in Judith Allen Shelly and Sandra D. John, *Spiritual Dimensions of Mental Health* (Downers Grove, IL: InterVarsity Press, 1983), 51-52.

5. What is the level of intervention (e.g., etiology, symptom relief)? Does it merely serve to make the person feel good temporarily? Might it mask symptoms that need urgent medical attention?

PRACTITIONER

1. What is the practitioner's worldview? Does he or she try to persuade clients to accept this worldview? In 2 Corinthians 4:2 Paul says, "We have renounced the shameful things that one hides; we refuse to practice cunning or falsify God's word; but by the open statement of the truth we commend ourselves to the conscience of everyone in the sight of God." There is a big difference between surreptitious persuasion and true evangelism, which is essentially telling the good news about Jesus without manipulation or deceit.

2. Does the practitioner claim a particular source of power? If so, is it compatible with Christian belief? A colleague recently attended a continuing nursing education program, approved by the state nurses' association, where the instructor claimed that her content on "healing touch" had been channeled to her by a spirit guide. If supernatural powers are involved, are they from God or from the evil one?

3. Does the practitioner demonstrate an awareness of possible underlying religious or mystical assumptions and their implications? Or does the practitioner unlink the modality from these beliefs? For example, many meditative practices come from Hindu or Buddhist beliefs of union with universal or cosmic energy.

CLIENT

1. Does practicing the modality require a change in lifestyle? If so, does the change appear to be positive or negative? Is the change compatible with Christian beliefs? Changes might include modifying meditation techniques, arranging furniture to facilitate the proper flow of energy, adapting nutritional diets (e.g., eating a balance of "hot" and "cold" foods), withdrawing from personal relationships, joining a community and participating in its group rituals, or following a certain spiritual teacher.

2. Does health improve? Is suffering relieved? To what extent? For how long? Although effectiveness holds a powerful attraction, it should not be the only criterion. Many things that make us feel good are not good for us.

3. Are there any short- or long-term adverse side effects (physically, mentally, or spiritually)? Hillstrom throws some interesting light on the benefits of Eastern meditation. She describes research studies indicating that there is no difference between the brainwaves of people who are meditating and those who are merely resting or sleeping. She continues, "Significantly, there are also studies indicating that Eastern-style meditation can have adverse and long-lasting physical and psychological consequences." These effects include headaches, insomnia, gastrointestinal upsets, anxiety, depression, confusion, mental and physical tension, and inexplicable outbursts of anti-social behavior.[2] Numerous meditators have themselves told us that entering into meditation without a spiritual guide is dangerous because of the physical and psychological side effects. Christians who attempt these meditative techniques often report an inability to pray or comprehend the Bible.

RESULTS

1. What is the stated explanation for the results?

2. Is the explanation generally accepted by health professions, or is it subject to controversy?

3. Do the explanations for the results seem to contradict scriptural teaching in any way?

4. What are other possible explanations?

Note: We are not including prayer in this alternative therapy evaluation. As Christian nurses we believe that God hears and answers prayer, even from non-Christians whose hearts are searching and open to him. In his infinite wisdom and loving compassion, God answers these prayers for our good and his glory. Sometimes these answers seem miraculous, and we receive what we prayed for. At other times the prayer is not answered in the way we hoped. We may realize, often later, that it was for the best. However, we may never understand in this life. Yet we continue trusting and obeying him.

---

[2]Elizabeth Hillstorm, *Testing the Spirits* (Downers Grove, IL: InterVarsity Press, 1995), 116-20.

INDEX